GYNECOLOGIC CANCER

M. D. ANDERSON
CANCER CARE
SERIES

Series Editors

Aman U. Buzdar, MD   Ralph S. Freedman, MD, PhD

M. D. ANDERSON CANCER CARE SERIES

Series Editors: Aman U. Buzdar, MD, and
Ralph S. Freedman, MD, PhD

K.K. Hunt, G.L. Robb, E.A. Strom, and N.T. Ueno, Eds., *Breast Cancer*

F.V. Fossella, R. Komaki, and J.B. Putnam, Jr., Eds., *Lung Cancer*

J.A. Ajani, S.A. Curley, N.A. Janjan, and P.M. Lynch, Eds.,
Gastrointestinal Cancer

K.W. Chan and R.B. Raney, Jr., Eds., *Pediatric Oncology*

P.J. Eifel, D.M. Gershenson, J.J. Kavanagh, and E.G. Silva, Eds.,
Gynecologic Cancer

Patricia J. Eifel, MD,
David M. Gershenson, MD,
John J. Kavanagh, MD,
and Elvio G. Silva, MD
Editors

The University of Texas M. D. Anderson Cancer Center,
Houston, Texas

Gynecologic
Cancer

Foreword by Maurie Markman, MD

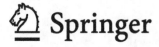 Springer

Patricia J. Eifel, MD
Department of Radiation Oncology
The University of Texas
M. D. Anderson Cancer Center
1515 Holcombe Blvd., Unit 1202
Houston, TX 77030-4009, USA

John J. Kavanagh, MD
Department of Gynecologic Medical
    Oncology
The University of Texas
M. D. Anderson Cancer Center
1515 Holcombe Blvd., Unit 1364
Houston, TX 77030-4009, USA

David M. Gershenson, MD
Department of Gynecologic Oncology
The University of Texas
M. D. Anderson Cancer Center
1515 Holcombe Blvd., Unit 1362
Houston, TX 77030-4009, USA

Elvio G. Silva, MD
Department of Pathology
The University of Texas
M. D. Anderson Cancer Center
1515 Holcombe Blvd., Unit 85
Houston, TX 77030-4009, USA

Series Editors:
Aman U. Buzdar, MD
Department of Breast Medical
    Oncology
The University of Texas
M. D. Anderson Cancer Center
Houston, TX 77030-4009, USA

Ralph S. Freedman, MD, PhD
Department of Gynecologic Oncology
The University of Texas
M. D. Anderson Cancer Center
Houston, TX 77030-4009, USA

Library of Congress Cataloging-in-Publication Data

A C.I.P. Catalogue record for this book is available from the Library of Congress.

Gynecologic Cancer

ISBN-10: 0-387-28794-9   e-ISBN-10: 0-387-28796-5
ISBN-13: 978-0387-28794-2   e-ISBN-13: 978-0387-28796-6

Printed on acid-free paper.

DEDICATION

This book is dedicated to the memories of Dr. Felix Rutledge and Dr. Gilbert Fletcher, who together farsightedly developed the model for the multidisciplinary approach to gynecologic cancers, which has benefited countless patients worldwide.

FOREWORD

There is perhaps no better model of the importance of multidisciplinary interactions in the care of cancer patients than that found in the management of gynecologic malignancies. From the critical importance of primary surgical cytoreduction of advanced ovarian cancer preceding the administration of cytotoxic chemotherapy to the now-standard use of cisplatin as a radiosensitizer delivered with external-beam radiation therapy in the treatment of locally advanced cervix cancer, oncologists involved in the care of gynecologic cancer patients must understand the optimal utilization of multiple treatment modalities.

For more than 5 decades, the gynecologic cancer program at M. D. Anderson Cancer Center has been an innovative leader in helping to establish the standards of care in this group of malignancies and in developing novel surgical, pharmacological, and radiotherapeutic approaches to improve both the survival and quality of life of women diagnosed with a gynecologic cancer.

This well-written and comprehensive text describes the current management of female pelvic tumors, with chapters authored by nationally and internationally recognized senior leaders in their fields, as well as by more junior M. D. Anderson faculty who will soon be responsible for the new advances that will, without question, characterize the future of clinical research in gynecologic malignancies.

Maurie Markman, MD
Vice President for Clinical Research
The University of Texas M. D. Anderson Cancer Center

PREFACE

The treatment of gynecologic cancers has improved owing to strong multidisciplinary efforts over the years. These efforts have resulted in a sharp reduction in both the incidence and mortality of invasive cervical cancer and marked improvements in early detection of the disease. Now, emphasis is being placed on fertility preservation, and options are being explored in cervical cancer as well as in other cancers where this may be possible.

The treatment of vulvar cancer, which can be quite debilitating in its advanced stages, has followed an approach similar to that of breast cancer, where radical surgery has given way to a multimodal approach that emphasizes quality of life as well as survival.

The introduction of paclitaxel was a major development in the primary treatment of ovarian cancer. This monograph also describes the appropriate use of other cytotoxic drugs for the treatment of recurrence or for palliation. As this book goes to press, there is more cogent evidence that intraperitoneal platinum-based therapy is likely to become a part of the standard treatment in this disease. In addition to therapy advances, there have been improvements in diagnostic tools and their application in ovarian cancer.

We would like to acknowledge Walter Pagel, director of the Department of Scientific Publications at M. D. Anderson Cancer Center, for his role in continuing to make the M. D. Anderson Cancer Care Series a success. We would also like to thank the volume editors, Drs. David M. Gershenson, Patricia J. Eifel, John J. Kavanagh, and Elvio G. Silva, and the authors of this first monograph on gynecologic cancer for their significant efforts to assemble what we believe will be a most useful and important resource for any physician who diagnoses and treats gynecologic cancer.

Aman U. Buzdar, MD
Ralph S. Freedman, MD, PhD

PREFACE

This book represents the culmination of a process that has evolved over almost 6 decades since Felix Rutledge and Gilbert Fletcher first stepped onto the scene at M. D. Anderson Cancer Center. Their shared vision of a multidisciplinary approach to caring for gynecologic cancer patients has not only persisted to the present but has, indeed, flourished.

Gynecologic Cancer is the most recent—but not the only—work to detail the practice of gynecologic cancer care at M. D. Anderson. Proceedings of M. D. Anderson's Clinical Conferences on Cancer focused on gynecologic cancer were published in 1962, 1969, and 1987. These books principally outlined the M. D. Anderson multidisciplinary approach to the clinical management of gynecologic malignancies. In addition, Dr. Fletcher's *Textbook of Radiotherapy*, published in 1980, and a 1976 textbook authored by Dr. Rutledge, J. Taylor Wharton, and Richard Boronow—*Gynecologic Oncology*—further described treatment techniques and recommendations.

Over the past several years, the face of M. D. Anderson's Gynecologic Oncology Multidisciplinary Program has changed markedly. The faculty is much larger in number and considerably more diverse. Although evidence-based medicine is the guiding principle in clinical decision making, a myriad of clinical scenarios exist for which there is no single therapeutic strategy. In such instances, differing viewpoints are healthy, and the wealth of experience gained from a large-volume practice is a tremendous asset. Also, the value of the peer-review process used in our Multidisciplinary Planning Conference and Clinic cannot be overestimated.

Of course, the treatment recommendations and practice guidelines included in this text are anchored on past clinical trial research and are continually updated as results of new trials become available. Although the clinical trial portfolio of our multidisciplinary group is ever changing and little discussed here, research-driven patient care is of critical importance in advancing our mission.

Also, we would like to acknowledge and thank Dawn Chalaire, ChaRhonda Chilton, Stephanie Deming, Kim M. Dupree, Manny Gonzales, Vickie J. Williams, and Chris Yeager of the Department of Scientific Publications for editing and compiling this volume.

On behalf of all the contributors to this book, it is a pleasure to present this new work that reflects M. D. Anderson practice early in this new millennium. And finally, we dedicate this book to all the women with gynecologic cancer who have undergone treatment at M. D. Anderson over the past 60-plus years.

David M. Gershenson, MD
Patricia J. Eifel, MD
John J. Kavanagh, MD
Elvio G. Silva, MD

CONTENTS

CONTRIBUTORS

Michael W. Bevers, MD, Associate Professor, Department of Gynecologic Oncology

Diane C. Bodurka, MD, Associate Professor, Department of Gynecologic Oncology

Russell Broaddus, MD, PhD, Assistant Professor, Department of Pathology

Jubilee Brown, MD, Assistant Professor, Department of Gynecologic Oncology

Eduardo Bruera, MD, Professor and Chair, Department of Palliative Care and Rehabilitation Medicine

Thomas W. Burke, MD, Professor, Department of Gynecologic Oncology

Michael T. Deavers, MD, Associate Professor, Department of Pathology

Michele L. Donato, MD, Associate Professor, Department of Blood and Marrow Transplantation

Patricia J. Eifel, MD, Professor, Department of Radiation Oncology

Michele Follen, MD, PhD, Professor, Department of Gynecologic Oncology

Ralph S. Freedman, MD, PhD, Professor, Department of Gynecologic Oncology

David M. Gershenson, MD, Chair and Professor, Department of Gynecologic Oncology

Revathy Iyer, MD, Associate Professor, Department of Diagnostic Radiology

Anuja Jhingran, MD, Associate Professor, Department of Radiation Oncology

John J. Kavanagh, MD, Chair Ad Interim and Professor, Department of Gynecologic Medical Oncology

Andrzej P. Kudelka, MD, Associate Professor, Department of Gynecologic Medical Oncology

Charles F. Levenback, MD, Professor, Department of Gynecologic Oncology

Karen H. Lu, MD, Associate Professor, Department of Gynecologic Oncology

Anais Malpica, MD, Associate Professor, Department of Pathology

Andrea Milbourne, MD, Assistant Professor, Department of Gynecologic Oncology

Pedro T. Ramirez, MD, Assistant Professor, Department of Gynecologic Oncology

Lois M. Ramondetta, MD, Associate Professor, Department of Gynecologic Oncology

Hui T. See, MD, Postdoctoral Fellow, Department of Gynecologic Medical Oncology

Elvio G. Silva, MD, Professor, Department of Pathology

Florian Strasser, MD, ABHPM, Clinical Fellow, Department of Palliative Care and Rehabilitation Medicine

Charlotte C. Sun, DrPH, Assistant Professor, Department of Gynecologic Oncology

Xipeng Wang, MD, Postdoctoral Fellow, Department of Gynecologic Medical Oncology

J. Taylor Wharton, MD, Professor, Department of Gynecologic Oncology

Judith K. Wolf, MD, Associate Professor, Department of Gynecologic Oncology

1 MULTIDISCIPLINARY CARE OF PATIENTS WITH GYNECOLOGIC CANCERS

David M. Gershenson, John J. Kavanagh,
Patricia J. Eifel, and Elvio G. Silva

CHAPTER OUTLINE

CHAPTER OVERVIEW

Almost from the establishment of M. D. Anderson Cancer Center, gynecologic cancer care has been characterized by a multidisciplinary approach. This chapter will briefly describe the current organization and infrastructure of patient care and clinical research within the Gynecologic Oncology Multidisciplinary Program.

INTRODUCTION

One of the first—if not the very first—multidisciplinary collaborations at M. D. Anderson Cancer Center began in 1948 when Dr. Felix Rutledge and Dr. Gilbert Fletcher, both legendary figures in their respective fields (gynecologic oncology and radiation oncology), started a "Disposition Clinic" in which patients with cervical and uterine cancers were seen and evaluated by them jointly and therapy decisions were formulated. This legacy of multidisciplinary care has permeated the fabric of gynecologic cancer care at M. D. Anderson ever since. For the first 40-plus years of its existence, this collaborative venture was in the form of a biweekly clinic in which new patients with cervical and uterine cancers were seen. Typically, patient summaries would be presented by the gynecologic oncology fellow outside the examination room, after which the patient would be examined by both the gynecologic oncologist and the radiation oncologist. Beginning in the 1990s, the clinic was expanded to include all patients with gynecologic cancer who required a treatment decision. In addition, a multidisciplinary conference attended by gynecologic oncologists, radiation oncologists, medical oncologists, and pathologists was added in the hour preceding the clinic. Presentation of cases, accompanied by pathology slide review, was shifted to the conference, thereby leaving more time during the clinic to counsel patients and their families.

This introductory chapter will briefly describe the current organization and infrastructure of the multidisciplinary care of women with gynecologic malignancies at M. D. Anderson. Because research is such an integral part of the patient care delivered at M. D. Anderson (so-called research-driven patient care), the gynecologic oncology multidisciplinary research infrastructure and process are also described. In addition, practice guidelines for the 3 major gynecologic cancers—endometrial, ovarian, and cervical—are presented.

ORGANIZATION OF MULTIDISCIPLINARY CLINICAL TRIAL RESEARCH

Clinical trial research is one of the highest priorities of the Gynecologic Oncology Multidisciplinary Program. Research-driven patient care requires an organization and infrastructure to support the myriad research activities and regulatory and oversight functions. The Gynecologic Oncology Multidisciplinary Program has several working groups that meet on a monthly basis to consider proposed protocols and to monitor ongoing studies. These working groups include the following: (1) Ovarian/ Peritoneal/Fallopian Tube, (2) Uterine/Gestational Trophoblastic Disease, (3) Cervix/Vulva/Vagina, (4) Health Services Research, (5) Surgery, (6) Radiation Oncology, and (7) Gynecologic Oncology Group Operations. Thus, we have both organ-site and modality groups that review and approve protocols. Once a protocol is approved by the appropriate working group, it is forwarded to the Program Steering Committee for review and approval. It then is forwarded to the institutional Clinical Research Committee for scientific review and, finally, on to the Institutional Review Board.

The role of the working groups is to develop a portfolio of studies that fit into the framework of the multidisciplinary program's strategic plan. The primary criteria used by each working group for setting the research agenda are scientific merit and advancing the field. Other important considerations include protocol prioritization (relative to competing studies) and the funding source. Research design and protocol prioritization are also reviewed critically by the Program Steering Committee.

GYNECOLOGIC ONCOLOGY MULTIDISCIPLINARY PLANNING CONFERENCE

Since the mid-1990s, new patients have registered for appointments in the Gynecologic Oncology Center through either self-referral or physician referral. Approximately 1,400 new patients are seen in the center annually. These include patients with newly diagnosed disease who are coming to M. D. Anderson for definitive treatment and patients with either newly diagnosed cancers or recurrent disease who are seeking a second opinion. Following a history and physical examination, patients undergo further evaluation and testing, and pertinent clinical material obtained elsewhere, including pathology slides and imaging studies, is reviewed. Patients subsequently return to the Gynecologic Oncology Center for discussion of treatment options and final disposition.

On Tuesday and Thursday afternoons, a Multidisciplinary Planning Conference is convened. This conference is attended by physicians from the relevant specialties—gynecologic oncology, medical oncology, radiation oncology, and pathology—as well as by research nurses, advanced practice nurses, nursing staff, pharmacists, health service research investigators, and trainees. Each patient's case is presented, pathology slides are reviewed, and treatment options are discussed. Emphasis is placed on potential eligibility for clinical trials. These case discussions and resultant recommendations form the foundation for the discussions with patients and family members in the clinic. The outcome of the case discussions may be a unanimous consensus, a consensus, or no consensus at all. The latter outcome occurs most commonly in cases of patients with unusual or rare tumors or with conditions for which there is no standard therapy.

GYNECOLOGIC ONCOLOGY MULTIDISCIPLINARY PLANNING CLINIC

Following the Multidisciplinary Planning Conference, patients are seen by the attending physician, accompanied by a fellow, resident, or advanced practice nurse, in the Multidisciplinary Planning Clinic. Patients who are potential candidates for radiation therapy or chemoradiation are generally seen and examined jointly by the attending physician and radiation oncologist. All patients and their families are seen for a final disposition and discussion of treatment recommendations. Patients who may be candidates for clinical trials also are provided by the appropriate research nurse with the information needed for them to give informed consent. Typical outcomes of the planning clinic include scheduling of primary or secondary surgery, enrollment on a clinical trial, initiation of a new systemic therapy, and initiation of chemoradiation. In addition, subsequent consultations may be sought with such services as pain management, nutrition, physical therapy, psychosocial services, and enterostomal therapy.

Gynecologic Cancer Practice Guidelines

Practice guidelines for the 3 major gynecologic malignancies—endometrial, ovarian, and cervical cancer—were first developed collaboratively several years ago by the Gynecologic Oncology Multidisciplinary Program. Subsequently, these guidelines have been reviewed and updated approximately annually by the respective organ-site working groups. These guidelines are outlined in the appendix and are meant to describe the M. D. Anderson approach to treatment of these 3 cancers within several different clinical settings. Of course, these guidelines do not cover every possible clinical scenario nor do they address the myriad types of less common or rare gynecologic cancers.

As with all M. D. Anderson treatment guidelines, the gynecologic cancer practice guidelines are based, whenever possible, on information from phase II and III clinical trials. Of course, in instances where no standard has emerged from clinical trial data, the guidelines are based on clinical experience only. As noted above, however, whenever possible, patients are encouraged to participate in clinical trials. A complete listing of current clinical trials of the Gynecologic Oncology Multidisciplinary Program can be found on M. D. Anderson's Web site: www.mdanderson.org.

APPENDIX: M. D. ANDERSON CANCER CENTER TREATMENT GUIDELINES FOR ENDOMETRIAL CANCER, EPITHELIAL OVARIAN CANCER, AND CERVICAL CANCER

These practice guidelines are based on majority expert opinion of the Gynecologic Oncology Center faculty at M. D. Anderson Cancer Center. The guidelines were developed using a multidisciplinary approach that included input from the following medical oncologists, radiation oncologists, and surgical oncologists:

Endometrial Cancer

Diane C. Bodurka, MD, Jubilee Brown, MD, Thomas W. Burke, MD, Patricia J. Eifel, MD, Anuja Jhingran, MD, Karen H. Lu, MD, Lois M. Ramondetta, MD, and Judith K. Wolf, MD

Epithelial Ovarian Cancer

Diane C. Bodurka, MD, Jubilee Brown, MD, David M. Gershenson, MD, John J. Kavanagh, MD, Karen H. Lu, MD, Anil K. Sood, MD, and Judith K. Wolf, MD

Cervical Cancer

Diane C. Bodurka, MD, Patricia J. Eifel, MD, Anuja Jhingran, MD, Charles F. Levenback, MD, Pedro T. Ramirez, MD, Lois M. Ramondetta, MD, and Judith K. Wolf, MD

Clinicians are expected to use independent medical judgment in the context of individual clinical circumstances to determine any patient's care.

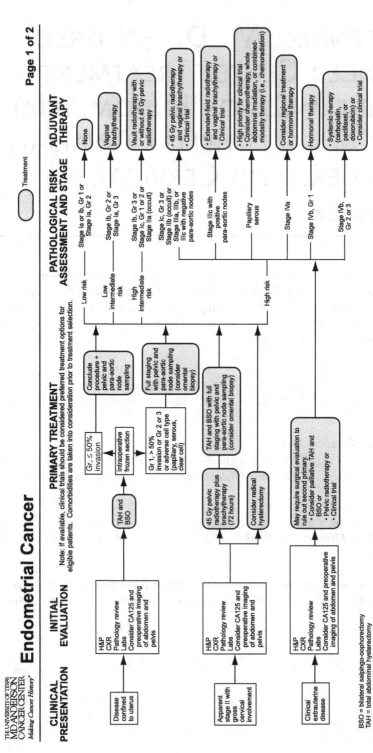

THE UNIVERSITY OF TEXAS
MD ANDERSON
CANCER CENTER
Making Cancer History

Endometrial Cancer

⬭ Treatment

PRIMARY TREATMENT

Note: If available, clinical trials should be considered preferred treatment options for eligible patients. Comorbidities are taken into consideration prior to treatment selection.

CLINICAL PRESENTATION — **INITIAL EVALUATION** — **PATHOLOGICAL RISK ASSESSMENT AND STAGE** — **ADJUVANT THERAPY**

Disease confined to uterus

H&P
CXR
Pathology review
Labs
Consider CA125 and preoperative imaging of abdomen and pelvis

TAH and BSO

Intraoperative frozen section

Gr, ≤ 50% invasion

Conclude procedure + pelvic and para-aortic node sampling

Gr 1, > 50% invasion or Gr 2 or 3 or adverse cell type (papillary, serous, clear cell)

Full staging with pelvic and para-aortic node sampling (consider omental biopsy)

Low risk
- Stage Ia or Ib, Gr 1 or 2: **None**
- Stage Ib, Gr 2 or Stage Ia, Gr 3: **Vaginal brachytherapy**

Low intermediate risk — Stage Ia, Gr 2 or Stage Ia, Gr 3

High intermediate risk
- Stage Ib, Gr 3 or Stage Ic, Gr 1 or 2 or Stage IIa (occult): **Vault radiotherapy with or without 45 Gy pelvic radiotherapy**
- Stage Ic, Gr 3 or Stage IIb (occult) or Stage IIIa, IIIb, or IIIc with negative para-aortic nodes: **45 Gy pelvic radiotherapy and vaginal brachytherapy or · Clinical trial**

Stage IIIc with positive para-aortic nodes: **Extended-field radiotherapy and vaginal brachytherapy or · Clinical trial**

Papillary serous: **High priority for clinical trial · Consider chemotherapy, whole abdominal irradiation, or combined-modality therapy (i.e., chemoradiation)**

Apparent stage II with gross cervical involvement

H&P
CXR
Pathology review
Labs
Consider CA125 and preoperative imaging of abdomen and pelvis

45 Gy pelvic radiotherapy plus brachytherapy (72 hours)

Consider radical hysterectomy

TAH and BSO with full staging with pelvic and para-aortic node sampling (consider omental biopsy)

High risk

Clinical extrauterine disease

H&P
CXR
Pathology review
Labs
Consider CA125 and preoperative imaging of abdomen and pelvis

May require surgical evaluation to rule out second primary
- Consider palliative TAH and BSO or
- Pelvic radiotherapy or
- Clinical trial

Stage IVa: **Consider regional treatment or hormonal therapy**

Stage IVb, Gr 1: **Hormonal therapy**

Stage IVb, Gr 2 or 3: **Systemic therapy (carboplatin, paclitaxel, or doxorubicin) or · Consider clinical trial**

BSO = bilateral salpingo-oophorectomy
TAH = total abdominal hysterectomy

Please refer to American College of Obstetricians and Gynecologists (ACOG) guidelines for patient referral.

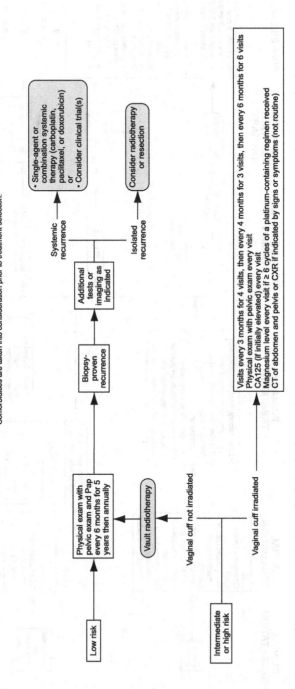

THE UNIVERSITY OF TEXAS
MD ANDERSON
CANCER CENTER
Making Cancer History

Endometrial Cancer

◯ Treatment

SURVEILLANCE

Note: If available, clinical trials are considered preferred treatment options for eligible patients.
Comorbidities are taken into consideration prior to treatment selection.

Low risk → Physical exam with pelvic exam and Pap every 6 months for 5 years then annually

Intermediate or high risk

Vaginal cuff not irradiated → Vault radiotherapy

Vaginal cuff irradiated → Visits every 3 months for 4 visits, then every 4 months for 3 visits, then every 6 months for 6 visits
Physical exam with pelvic exam every visit
CA125 (if initially elevated) every visit
Magnesium level every visit if ≥ 6 cycles of a platinum-containing regimen received
CT of abdomen and pelvis or CXR if indicated by signs or symptoms (not routine)

→ Biopsy-proven recurrence → Additional tests or imaging as indicated

Systemic recurrence → • Single-agent or combination systemic therapy (carboplatin, paclitaxel, or doxorubicin) or • Consider clinical trial(s)

Isolated recurrence → Consider radiotherapy or resection

Please refer to American College of Obstetricians and Gynecologists (ACOG) guidelines for patient referral.

Practice Outcomes   V6   08/18/2004

THE UNIVERSITY OF TEXAS
MD ANDERSON
CANCER CENTER
Making Cancer History®

Epithelial Ovarian Cancer

Note: Clinical trials are considered preferred treatment options for eligible patients.

◯ Treatment

CLINICAL PRESENTATION | **INITIAL EVALUATION** | **PRIMARY TREATMENT** | **PATHOLOGICAL STAGING** | **PRIMARY ADJUVANT THERAPY** | **SURVEILLANCE**

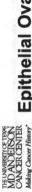

Pelvic mass

Diagnosis by previous surgery

INITIAL EVALUATION:
- CBC
- Chemistry profile
- CXR
- Verify most recent mammogram
- CA125
- Ultrasound or CT of abdomen and pelvis if suspicion of cancer
- Barium enema or colonoscopy if clinically indicated

- CXR
- CA125
- CT of abdomen and pelvis if clinically indicated

PRIMARY TREATMENT:
- Laparotomy, TAH, and BSO with comprehensive staging or
- If stage I and patient desires fertility, USO and staging biopsies or
- If stage II-IV and medically stable, cytoreductive surgery or
- If patient unable to tolerate surgery, consider chemotherapy

Previous surgery and staging appropriate

Previous surgery and/or staging incomplete:
1. Uterus not removed
2. Adnexa not removed
3. Omentum not removed
4. Documentation of staging inadequate
5. Other suboptimal effort

Options based on individual patient characteristics:
- Immediate chemotherapy or
- Chemotherapy followed by interval cytoreduction or
- Re-explore for cytoreduction

PATHOLOGICAL STAGING:
- Stage Ia or Ib
  - Grade 1 (Low grade) → No adjuvant therapy
  - Grade 2 or 3 (High grade) → Taxane and platinum agent for 6 cycles
- Stage Ic → Taxane and platinum agent for 6 cycles
- Stage II, III, or IV
  - Taxane and platinum agent for 6 cycles or
  - Clinical trial, if available

SURVEILLANCE:
- Visits every 3 months for 4 visits, then every 4 months for 3 visits, then every 6 months for 6 visits
- Physical exam with pelvic exam every visit
- CA125 (if initially elevated) every visit
- CBC annually
- Magnesium level if indicated
- CT of abdomen and pelvis or CXR, if indicated by signs or symptoms (not routine)

Stage II

Stage III or IV → Annual checkup. See Consolidation on page 2

BSO = bilateral salpingo-oophorectomy
TAH = total abdominal hysterectomy
USO = unilateral salpingo-oophorectomy

THE UNIVERSITY OF TEXAS
MD ANDERSON
CANCER CENTER
Making Cancer History®

Epithelial Ovarian Cancer

( ) Treatment

Note: Clinical trials are considered preferred treatment options for eligible patients.

CONSOLIDATION TREATMENT

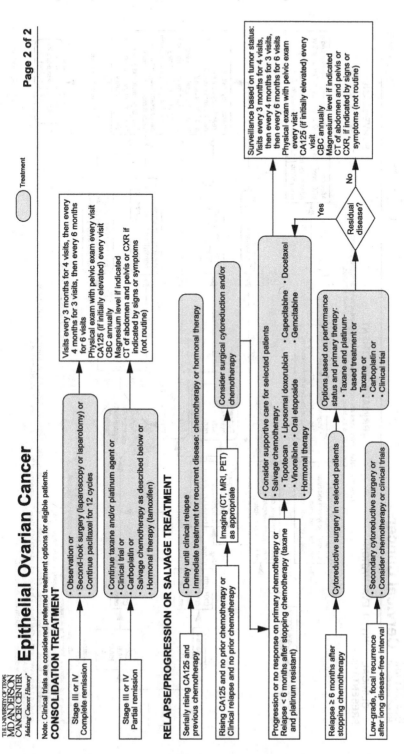

Stage III or IV
Complete remission
→
- Observation or
- Second-look surgery (laparoscopy or laparotomy) or
- Continue paclitaxel for 12 cycles
→
Visits every 3 months for 4 visits, then every 4 months for 3 visits, then every 6 months for 6 visits
Physical exam with pelvic exam every visit
CA125 (if initially elevated) every visit
CBC annually
Magnesium level if indicated
CT of abdomen and pelvis or CXR if indicated by signs or symptoms (not routine)

Stage III or IV
Partial remission
→
- Continue taxane and/or platinum agent or
- Clinical trial or
- Carboplatin or
- Salvage chemotherapy as described below or
- Hormonal therapy (tamoxifen)

RELAPSE/PROGRESSION OR SALVAGE TREATMENT

Serially rising CA125 and previous chemotherapy
→
- Delay until clinical relapse
- Immediate treatment for recurrent disease: chemotherapy or hormonal therapy

Rising CA125 and no prior chemotherapy or
Clinical relapse and no prior chemotherapy
→
Imaging (CT, MRI, PET) as appropriate
→
Consider surgical cytoreduction and/or chemotherapy

Progression or no response on primary chemotherapy or
Relapse < 6 months after stopping chemotherapy (taxane and platinum resistant)
→
- Consider supportive care for selected patients
- Salvage chemotherapy:
  - Topotecan
  - Vinorelbine
  - Hormonal therapy
  - Liposomal doxorubicin
  - Oral etoposide
  - Capecitabine
  - Gemcitabine
  - Docetaxel

Relapse ≥ 6 months after stopping chemotherapy
→
Cytoreductive surgery in selected patients
→
Options based on performance status and primary therapy:
- Taxane and platinum-based treatment or
- Taxane or
- Carboplatin or
- Clinical trial
→
Residual disease?
— Yes →
— No →

Low-grade, focal recurrence after long disease-free interval
→
- Secondary cytoreductive surgery or
- Consider chemotherapy or clinical trials

Surveillance based on tumor status:
Visits every 3 months for 4 visits, then every 4 months for 3 visits, then every 6 months for 6 visits
Physical exam with pelvic exam every visit
CA125 (if initially elevated) every visit
CBC annually
Magnesium level if indicated
CT of abdomen and pelvis or CXR, if indicated by signs or symptoms (not routine)

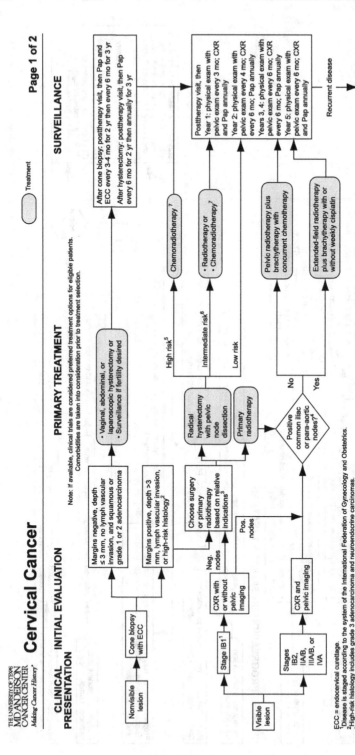

THE UNIVERSITY OF TEXAS
MD ANDERSON
CANCER CENTER
Making Cancer History

Cervical Cancer

Page 1 of 2

⬭ Treatment

CLINICAL PRESENTATION — **INITIAL EVALUATION** — **PRIMARY TREATMENT** — **SURVEILLANCE**

Note: If available, clinical trials are considered preferred treatment options for eligible patients. Comorbidities are taken into consideration prior to treatment selection.

Nonvisible lesion → Cone biopsy with ECC →

- Margins negative, depth ≤ 3 mm, no lymph vascular invasion, and squamous or grade 1 or 2 adenocarcinoma → • Vaginal, abdominal, or laparoscopic hysterectomy or • Surveillance if fertility desired → After cone biopsy: posttherapy visit, then Pap and ECC every 3-4 mo for 2 yr then every 6 mo for 3 yr; After hysterectomy: posttherapy visit, then Pap every 6 mo for 2 yr then annually for 3 yr

- Margins positive, depth >3 mm, lymph vascular invasion, or high-risk histology[2]

Visible lesion → Stage IB1[1] → CXR with or without pelvic imaging
- Neg. nodes → Choose surgery or primary radiotherapy based on relative indications[3]
  - Radical hysterectomy with pelvic node dissection
  - Primary radiotherapy
- Pos. nodes

Stages IB2, IIA/B, IIIA/B, or IVA → CXR and pelvic imaging → Positive common iliac or para-aortic nodes?[4]
- No
- Yes → Extended-field radiotherapy plus brachytherapy with or without weekly cisplatin

High risk[5] → Chemoradiotherapy[7]

Intermediate risk[6] → • Radiotherapy or • Chemoradiotherapy[7]

Low risk → (Pelvic radiotherapy plus brachytherapy with concurrent chemotherapy)

SURVEILLANCE:
Posttherapy visit, then
Year 1: physical exam with pelvic exam every 3 mo; CXR and Pap annually
Year 2: physical exam with pelvic exam every 4 mo; CXR every 6 mo; Pap annually
Years 3, 4: physical exam with pelvic exam every 6 mo; CXR every 6 mo; Pap annually
Year 5: physical exam with pelvic exam every 6 mo; CXR and Pap annually

Recurrent disease → Multidisciplinary planning (see page 2 of guideline)

Practice Outcomes   V6   05/11/2005

ECC = endocervical curettage.
[1] Disease is staged according to the system of the International Federation of Gynecology and Obstetrics.
[2] High-risk histology includes grade 3 adenocarcinoma and neuroendocrine carcinomas.
[3] Relative indications in favor of radiotherapy are adenocarcinoma grade 3, positive nodes, extensive lymph vascular invasion, and deep stromal invasion on MRI.
[4] Retroperitoneal para-aortic/pelvic lymphadenectomy in selected patients.
[5] High-risk factors are positive nodes, positive margins, and parametrial involvement.
[6] Intermediate-risk factors include lymphovascular invasion, increasing size, and stromal invasion. Reference: Sedlis A, et al. A randomized trial of pelvic radiation therapy versus no further therapy in selected patients with stage IB carcinoma of the cervix after radical hysterectomy and pelvic lymphadenectomy: A Gynecologic Oncology Group study. Gynecologic Oncology. 1999;73(2):177-183.
[7] Concurrent weekly cisplatin or cisplatin with fluorouracil.

THE UNIVERSITY OF TEXAS
MD ANDERSON
CANCER CENTER
Making Cancer History

Cervical Cancer

RECURRENT CANCER

SURVEILLANCE

Note: If available, clinical trials are considered preferred treatment options for eligible patients. Comorbidities are taken into consideration prior to treatment selection.

◯ Treatment

Pelvic recurrence

No prior radiotherapy

Prior radiotherapy

Radiotherapy with possible curative intent with consideration of chemoradiation

Recurrence in central pelvis
- Consider total pelvic exenteration or
- Clinical trial or
- Chemotherapy

Metastasis to other sites
- Clinical trial or
- Chemotherapy or
- Supportive care

Isolated extrapelvic recurrence
- Resection or
- Radiotherapy or
- Combined-modality therapy

Posttherapy visit, then
Year 1: physical exam with pelvic exam every 3 mo; CXR and Pap annually
Year 2: physical exam with pelvic exam every 4 mo; CXR every 6 mo; Pap annually
Years 3, 4: physical exam with pelvic exam every 6 mo; CXR every 6 mo; Pap annually
Year 5: physical exam with pelvic exam every 6 mo; CXR and Pap annually

Stage IVB
- Palliative pelvic radiotherapy or
- Palliative chemotherapy or
- Palliative chemoradiation

Multidisciplinary planning

2 PREVENTION AND EARLY DETECTION OF ENDOMETRIAL AND OVARIAN CANCERS

Karen H. Lu

CHAPTER OUTLINE

CHAPTER OVERVIEW

For both endometrial and ovarian cancer, diagnosis of disease at an earlier stage results in a higher cure rate. More than 70% of women with endometrial cancer are diagnosed with stage I disease because irregular vaginal bleeding is an early symptom. However, fewer than 25% of women with ovarian cancer are diagnosed with stage I disease. Strategies for the prevention and early detection of these cancers are different for women in the general population who are at average risk versus those known to be at increased risk of the disease, such as women with inherited cancer susceptibility syndromes. Women with Lynch syndrome have a 40% to 60% lifetime risk of endometrial cancer and a 10% to 12% lifetime risk of ovarian cancer. They are advised to participate in screening programs as well as to consider surgical prevention. Women with hereditary breast-ovarian cancer syndrome have a 15% to 40% lifetime risk of ovarian cancer and are also advised to consider intensive screening and surgical prevention options. For women at high risk as well as those at average risk of endometrial and ovarian cancer, oral contraceptives are an excellent chemopreventive agent.

INTRODUCTION

In 2005, an estimated 79,480 women will be diagnosed with a gynecologic malignancy in the United States, and 31,010 women will die of a gynecologic cancer (Jemal et al, 2005). This chapter focuses on the prevention and early detection of endometrial and ovarian cancers. Papanicolaou testing and identification of premalignant cervical lesions are discussed in chapter 3.

ENDOMETRIAL CANCER

Endometrial cancer is the most common gynecologic cancer. In 2005, an estimated 40,880 women will be diagnosed with uterine cancer, and 7,310 women are expected to die of the disease (Jemal et al, 2005). Women in the general population have an approximate 3% lifetime risk of developing endometrial cancer. Importantly, 70% of women with endometrial cancer are diagnosed with stage I disease. This is so primarily because post-menopausal or irregular vaginal bleeding is an early symptom of endometrial cancer. Currently, endometrial biopsy performed in the office setting is recommended for women who present with postmenopausal or irregular vaginal bleeding. Endometrial biopsy in the office setting, which consists of endometrial sampling using a Pipelle, has been shown to have sensitivity equivalent to that of dilatation and curettage (Dijkhuizen et al, 2000). If an endometrial biopsy in the office setting is not feasible or the amount of tissue obtained is inadequate, dilatation and curettage is recommended.

Prevention for Women at Average Risk

For women at average risk of endometrial cancer, 2 primary prevention strategies can be instituted. First, oral contraceptives have been shown to decrease the risk of endometrial cancer by 50%. Second, patients should be encouraged to maintain a normal weight, given that obesity is so strongly associated with an increased risk of endometrial cancer.

Prevention and Screening for Women with Lynch Syndrome

Certain individuals are at increased risk of endometrial cancer, and in these women, specific strategies for the early detection and primary prevention of endometrial cancer can be instituted. Hereditary nonpolyposis colorectal cancer syndrome, or Lynch syndrome, is an inherited autosomal dominant cancer susceptibility syndrome (Aarnio et al, 1999). Women with Lynch syndrome are at significantly increased risk of endometrial, colon, and ovarian cancers. Recent studies have shown that women with Lynch syndrome have a 40% to 60% lifetime risk of endometrial cancer, a 40% to 60% lifetime risk of colon cancer, and a 10% to 12% lifetime risk of ovarian cancer. Given this increased risk, the proper identification of these women is crucial. Indications that a family may be affected by Lynch syndrome include (1) multiple individuals in the same lineage with colon or endometrial cancer or one of the less common Lynch syndrome cancers (ovarian, stomach, or ureteral cancer), (2) an individual in the family who has had more than 1 Lynch syndrome cancer, e.g., a woman with a history of colon and endometrial cancer, or (3) an individual in the family diagnosed with a Lynch syndrome cancer before the age of 50 years.

Clinical genetic testing for *MLH1*, *MSH2*, and *MSH6*, the genes responsible for Lynch syndrome in the majority of families, is now available. For both men and women who carry a mutation in 1 of these genes, yearly colonoscopy has been shown to decrease the mortality rate from colon cancer. In women who are known carriers of a mutation in 1 of these genes, appropriate counseling regarding endometrial and ovarian cancer prevention and early detection should be given, although the efficacy of specific prevention or screening strategies for endometrial or ovarian cancer in women with Lynch syndrome has not been proven.

Consensus statements recommend that women with Lynch syndrome undergo annual transvaginal ultrasonography and endometrial biopsy beginning at age 25 to 35 years (Burke et al, 1997). For prevention, young women of childbearing age can consider taking an oral contraceptive. Although the effectiveness of oral contraceptives in decreasing the rate of endometrial or ovarian cancer in women with Lynch syndrome has not been proven, oral contraceptives have been shown to decrease both endometrial and ovarian cancer risk in the general population. When childbearing is complete, a total abdominal hysterectomy and bilateral salpingo-oophorectomy should be recommended for women with Lynch syndrome. In addition, in women undergoing colon cancer surgery who have completed childbearing, prophylactic total abdominal hysterectomy and bilateral salpingo-oophorectomy should also be considered. Most importantly, women with Lynch syndrome should be taught the symptoms of early endometrial cancer and counseled to understand the necessity of an endometrial biopsy should they develop postmenopausal or irregular vaginal bleeding.

Prevention and Screening for Women Taking Tamoxifen

Women who are taking tamoxifen are also at increased risk of endometrial cancer. Tamoxifen has been shown to significantly decrease the risk of breast cancer recurrence in women with a history of breast cancer. In addition, in the National Surgical Adjuvant Breast and Bowel Project P-1 trial, tamoxifen was shown to decrease primary breast cancer occurrence in women at increased risk (Fisher et al, 1998). While the benefits of taking tamoxifen to reduce the risk of primary breast cancer or breast cancer recurrence have been proven, women need to be counseled that tamoxifen increases the risk of endometrial cancer. Tamoxifen is a selective estrogen receptor modulator that has anti-estrogenic effects on the breast and pro-estrogenic effects on the uterus. The risk of endometrial cancer in women taking tamoxifen is approximately 2 to 3 times the risk in women not taking tamoxifen.

Currently, recommendations for women taking tamoxifen include a discussion of early symptoms associated with endometrial cancer, including postmenopausal, irregular, or heavy vaginal bleeding. Patients who present with these symptoms need to undergo an endometrial biopsy. A number of studies have looked at transvaginal ultrasonography for screening of asymptomatic women taking tamoxifen. Tamoxifen increases the thickness of the endometrial stripe; however, this increase is mostly associated with subendometrial cyst formation and has not been well correlated with endometrial cancer. Therefore, we do not recommend routine ultrasonographic screening for asymptomatic women taking tamoxifen.

Prevention and Screening for Obese Women

Obesity is strongly linked to an increased risk of endometrial cancer. Women who are 50 pounds over their ideal body weight are 10 times more likely to develop endometrial cancer than are women at their ideal body weight. In addition, obese women are more likely to have irregular periods and may not seek gynecologic care specifically for this symptom. Gynecologists who care for obese women should counsel them regarding their increased risk and the need to report any postmenopausal, irregular, or heavy bleeding. Also, an endometrial biopsy should be performed when symptoms of postmenopausal, irregular, or heavy bleeding are reported.

Ovarian Cancer

The incidence of ovarian cancer is low, with 1 case of epithelial ovarian cancer occurring for every 2,250 postmenopausal women in the United States annually. For each individual woman, the lifetime risk of ovarian cancer is approximately 1 in 70, or 1.4%. However, epithelial ovarian cancer is highly fatal. In 2005, an estimated 22,270 women will be diagnosed with ovarian cancer and approximately 16,210 women will die of the disease (Jemal et al, 2005). The high mortality rate from ovarian cancer is due to the fact that approximately 70% of women are diagnosed with stage III or stage IV disease, for which the chances of long-term cure are less than 20%. However, more than 90% of patients diagnosed with stage I ovarian cancer can be cured.

Screening for Women at Average Risk

Clearly, an effective strategy for the early detection of ovarian cancer would significantly decrease mortality from the disease. Currently, however, no screening strategies have been proven to decrease mortality from ovarian cancer. CA-125 serum assay is approved for monitoring recurrence in women with ovarian cancer, but it lacks sufficient sensitivity and specificity to be an effective screening tool. Half of the women with early-stage ovarian cancer will not have an elevated CA-125 level. In addition, several common gynecologic conditions, including uterine leiomyoma, endometriosis, and pelvic inflammatory disease, elevate the CA-125 level. Large population-based studies have assessed the use of transvaginal ultrasonography for ovarian cancer screening. These studies found that transvaginal ultrasonography has limited specificity for the detection of ovarian cancer. Therefore, at this time, women at average risk of ovarian cancer are not offered routine screening. Recently, there has been an emphasis on educating women to be aware of the symptoms of ovarian cancer, which include bloating, an increase in abdominal girth, a change in bowel or bladder habits, and abdominal or pelvic pain. A recent study by Goff et al (2004) demonstrated that women with ovarian cancer have an increase in the frequency and severity of these symptoms compared with the general population of women presenting to their primary care physicians.

Prevention and Screening for Women with Hereditary Breast-Ovarian Cancer Syndrome

While the lifetime risk of ovarian cancer for women in the general population is 1.4%, women with hereditary breast-ovarian cancer (HBOC) syndrome have an approximately 15% to 40% lifetime risk of ovarian cancer (Ford et al, 1998). Mutations in the BRCA1 and BRCA2 genes account for the majority of inherited ovarian cancers. Individuals with a BRCA1 gene mutation have a 20% to 40% lifetime risk of ovarian cancer, while individuals with a BRCA2 mutation have a 15% to 20% lifetime risk of ovarian cancer. It is crucial to identify individuals from families that may have an increased risk of breast and ovarian cancer. Red flags for HBOC syndrome include (1) multiple individuals in the same lineage with breast cancer or ovarian cancer, (2) individuals with peritoneal cancer or fallopian tube cancer at any age, (3) 1 individual in the family with both breast and ovarian cancer, and (4) premenopausal breast cancer or ovarian cancer in women of Ashkenazi Jewish heritage. Clinical genetic testing for BRCA1 and BRCA2 mutations is available. When possible, genetic testing should be performed on a family member with breast or ovarian cancer. If a mutation in BRCA1 or BRCA2 is identified in a family member with cancer, other family members who have not had an HBOC syndrome cancer can then undergo genetic testing to predict their risk of cancer.

Multiple studies in the past few years have focused on appropriate screening and prevention strategies for individuals at high risk of ovarian cancer.

Bilateral salpingo-oophorectomy has been shown in 2 studies to significantly decrease the risk of ovarian cancer (Kauff et al, 2002; Rebbeck et al, 2002). Women who have completed childbearing should be counseled to undergo prophylactic bilateral salpingo-oophorectomy. The surgical procedure should include removal of both ovaries and both fallopian tubes. Full visualization of the pelvis and the paracolic gutters is important. We recommend performing abdominal and pelvic washings. The decision to remove the uterus or not is controversial, and we discuss the pros and cons with each patient. Regardless of the specific procedure used, a pathologist should be notified when a prophylactic bilateral salpingo-oophorectomy is being performed. We ask that pathologists, rather than taking representative samples from the ovaries and fallopian tubes, fully section the entire ovary and fallopian tube for histologic review. Multiple authors have reported that the risk of an occult ovarian cancer in these high-risk specimens is approximately 5% to 10%.

Much effort has been focused on screening for ovarian cancer in women with HBOC syndrome. However, no screening program has been demonstrated to decrease mortality from ovarian cancer in women at high risk. An ongoing large screening study is investigating the use of a CA-125 algorithm in women at high risk. Rather than using a single cut-off value to indicate the need for further diagnostic testing, the CA-125 algorithm determines risk on the basis of the trend in CA-125 values over time.

Other strategies currently being assessed for screening for ovarian cancer in women at high risk include the use of multiple serologic markers, proteomic strategies, and the combination of CA-125 and ultrasonography. No definitive outcomes have been reported thus far. Finally, oral contraceptives are a reasonable chemoprevention strategy in women at high risk of ovarian cancer. Contraceptive pills have been shown to decrease the risk of ovarian cancer by 50% in women at high risk.

At M. D. Anderson Cancer Center, we have a weekly High-Risk Ovarian Cancer Screening Clinic where we stress a multidisciplinary approach to the care of patients at high risk of ovarian cancer. We work closely with genetic counselors, breast medical oncologists, and breast surgeons. Patients are referred by Clinical Cancer Genetics and the High-Risk Breast Cancer Clinic as well as by other clinicians at our institution. In addition, family members of our ovarian cancer patients participate in the program. The initial visit consists of 2 parts: risk assessment and discussion of management strategies. Risk assessment includes obtaining a thorough family history as well as reviewing other risk factors for ovarian cancer. Individuals whose family history is suggestive of HBOC syndrome are counseled about genetic testing. On the basis of the results of the patient's risk assessment, we discuss appropriate management strategies, including oral contraceptives and prophylactic surgery. We also discuss the current limitations of screening for ovarian cancer and review the symptoms of ovarian cancer. We emphasize the importance of participation in multi-institutional studies for patients at high risk of ovarian cancer. Patients at high risk come back to the clinic every 6 months for a CA-125 assay and transvaginal ultrasonography. They are also referred to the High-Risk Breast Cancer Clinic for breast cancer screening and prevention.

SUMMARY

Women in the general population have a 3% and 1.4% risk, respectively, for endometrial and ovarian cancer. Educational efforts should be focused on teaching women to seek medical attention for postmenopausal, irregular, or heavy vaginal bleeding as well as for persistent abdominal symptoms including bloating, increased girth, a change in bowel and bladder habits, or abdominal or pelvic pain. Women in specific high-risk groups, including women taking tamoxifen and obese women, should be counseled regarding their increased risk of endometrial cancer and the signs and symptoms of the disease. Finally, women whose risk of endometrial or ovarian cancer is extremely elevated owing to hereditary predisposition should be counseled about specific chemopreventive and surgical prevention options as well as participation in screening studies.

KEY PRACTICE POINTS

- Women with postmenopausal, irregular, or heavy vaginal bleeding should undergo an endometrial biopsy in the office setting to rule out endometrial cancer. If a biopsy is not feasible or an adequate tissue sample cannot be obtained, a formal dilatation and curettage should be performed.
- The lifetime risks of endometrial and ovarian cancer in women in the general population are 3% and 1.4%, respectively. Routine screening is not recommended for women at average risk.
- Women with Lynch syndrome have a 40% to 60% lifetime risk of endometrial cancer and a 10% to 12% lifetime risk of ovarian cancer. Annual endometrial biopsy and transvaginal ultrasonography should be performed in these women. When childbearing is complete, a hysterectomy and salpingo-oophorectomy should be considered.
- Women taking tamoxifen do not need to undergo routine screening but should have an endometrial biopsy if they have postmenopausal, irregular, or heavy vaginal bleeding.
- Women who are obese should be counseled to lose weight to decrease their risk of endometrial cancer.
- Oral contraceptives decrease the risk of ovarian and endometrial cancer by 50% in women in the general population and are a reasonable chemopreventive agent for women at increased risk as well.
- Women with HBOC syndrome should be advised to undergo prophylactic bilateral salpingo-oophorectomy when childbearing is complete. Pathologic review of the surgical specimens should be thorough, given the increased risk of occult ovarian and fallopian tube cancers in this population.

Suggested Readings

Aarnio M, Sankila R, Pukkala E, et al. Cancer risk in mutation carriers of DNA-mismatch-repair genes. *Int J Cancer* 1999;81:214–218.

Burke W, Petersen G, Lynch P, et al. Recommendations for follow-up care of individuals with an inherited predisposition to cancer: I. Hereditary nonpolyposis colon cancer. Cancer Genetics Studies Consortium. *JAMA* 1997;277:915–919.

Dijkhuizen FP, Mol BW, Brolmann HA, Heintz AP. The accuracy of endometrial sampling in the diagnosis of patients with endometrial carcinoma and hyperplasia: a meta-analysis. *Cancer* 2000;89:1765–1772.

Fisher B, Costantino JP, Wickerham DL, et al. Tamoxifen for prevention of breast cancer: report of the National Surgical Adjuvant Breast and Bowel Project P-1 Study. *J Natl Cancer Inst* 1998;90:1371–1388.

Ford D, Easton DF, Stratton M, et al. Genetic heterogeneity and penetrance analysis of the BRCA1 and BRCA2 genes in breast cancer families. The Breast Cancer Linkage Consortium. *Am J Hum Genet* 1998;62:676–689.

Goff BA, Mandel LS, Melancon CH, Muntz HG. Frequency of symptoms of ovarian cancer in women presenting to primary care clinics. *JAMA* 2004;291:2705–2712.

Jemal A, Murray T, Ward E, et al. Cancer statistics, 2005. *CA Cancer J Clin* 2005;55:10–30.

Kauff ND, Satagopan JM, Robson ME, et al. Risk-reducing salpingo-oophorectomy in women with a BRCA1 or BRCA2 mutation. *N Engl J Med* 2002;346:1609–1615.

Narod SA, Risch H, Moslehi R, et al. Oral contraceptives and the risk of hereditary ovarian cancer. Hereditary Ovarian Cancer Clinical Study Group. *N Engl J Med* 1998;339:424–428.

Rebbeck TR, Lynch HT, Neuhausen SL, et al. Prophylactic oophorectomy in carriers of BRCA1 or BRCA2 mutations. *N Engl J Med* 2002;346:1616–1622.

3 PREINVASIVE DISEASE OF THE LOWER GENITAL TRACT

Andrea Milbourne and Michele Follen

CHAPTER OUTLINE

CHAPTER OVERVIEW

The Papanicolaou test has become almost universally accepted as the best available screening tool for detecting and preventing cervical cancer. The evaluation of patients and interpretation of Pap test results have remained controversial, however. In this chapter, we will focus on the workup and follow-up of patients with an abnormal Pap test result and so-called "special cases." The workup of these patients usually involves a complete physical examination and a detailed medical history, which is updated at every visit. All patients undergo genital cultures and colposcopy of the cervix, upper vagina, and vulva with colposcopically directed biopsies. On the basis of these biopsies, we determine the course of treatment. Most patients with preinvasive disease are followed up for a total of 2 years after appropriate treatment. Most of the treatments that we perform are outpatient, in-clinic procedures.

INTRODUCTION

Preinvasive disease of the female lower genital tract includes cervical, vaginal, vulvar, and perianal dysplasia (squamous as well as glandular lesions). It is thought that the human papillomavirus (HPV) is a causative agent in most, if not all, cases of dysplasia. Although only a handful of HPV serotypes have been associated with the development of cervical cancer, any woman with dysplasia deserves a full colposcopic evaluation, since many patients are exposed to more than 1 strain of HPV and reflex HPV typing is not routinely performed in the case of abnormal Papanicolaou test results.

Since the adoption of the Pap test as a tool for cervical cancer screening, the incidence of cervical cancer has decreased. About 50 million women undergo cervical cancer screening with the Pap test annually in the United States, and the test has become almost universally accepted as the best available screening tool for detecting and preventing cervical cancer. The evaluation of patients and interpretation of Pap test results have remained controversial, however.

In most instances, colposcopy with colposcopically directed biopsies has been accepted as the "gold standard" of cervical evaluation. It is, however, a technique that requires practice and experience as well as the acceptance of certain standards. Therefore, considerable variation in the quality of the procedure, depending on the operator, remains the norm.

In our colposcopy clinic at M. D. Anderson Cancer Center, we see only referred patients; thus, this chapter does not include screening recommendations. Instead, we will focus on the workup and follow-up of patients with an abnormal Pap test result. Also, some time will be spent on the evaluation and follow-up of so-called "special cases."

EVALUATION OF PATIENTS WITH AN ABNORMAL PAP TEST RESULT

Every new patient who enters our clinic undergoes a complete history and physical examination. We make every attempt to address the patient's health concerns, as well as refer her for appropriate screening, such as mammography or colorectal screening. The complete history, physical examination, and review of systems are important for a number of reasons. For example, often a patient's immunodeficiency will become apparent during this patient-provider interaction. On average, our patients with preinvasive disease are followed up every 6 months for 2 years. It is important to have a clear follow-up protocol with the appropriate personnel in place to track the patients. Colposcopy patients, unfortunately, seem to have universally poor compliance and tend to miss many appointments. It therefore takes a considerable amount of time and effort to follow-up on these patients. If an infrastructure is not in place, many patients will "fall through the cracks" and be lost to follow-up. This can lead to potentially disastrous consequences for both the patient and the provider.

To ensure accuracy, we prefer that all cytologic and pathologic specimens obtained elsewhere be reevaluated by one of our gynecologic pathologists at M. D. Anderson. We are aware that many times this results in extra cost for the patient; however, we think that the added expertise of our specially trained gynecologic pathologists is worth the extra cost. We also perform HPV typing on all new patients, not as a guide to therapy but as part of our research studies.

High-Grade Squamous Intraepithelial Lesions

All patients referred to us for the evaluation of a high-grade squamous intraepithelial lesion identified on a Pap test undergo a complete history and physical examination, including repeat evaluation of the cytologic specimen, cervical cultures, colposcopy, vaginoscopy, vulvoscopy, biopsies of all abnormal areas, and an endocervical curettage (ECC). We also offer HIV testing to these patients. At the patient's first follow-up visit, we explain the findings to the patient as well as the necessary treatment.

If histologic evaluation reveals cervical intraepithelial neoplasia (CIN) II or higher with negative findings on ECC, we recommend a loop electrosurgical excision procedure (LEEP). If there is CIN II or higher with positive findings on ECC, we recommend a LEEP cone (LEEP with "top hat") treatment. Both LEEP procedures are performed in the office under local anesthesia (lidocaine with epinephrine), and the patient is examined for healing 1 month after treatment.

If the patient has positive ectocervical margins, we usually follow up with a Pap test and colposcopy every 6 months. We use cauterization to obtain hemostasis after the LEEP procedure, which causes considerable thermal injury to any neoplastic cells in the LEEP bed; thus, many times the patient will have normal findings at follow-up. If the patient has positive endocervical margins, we may offer retreatment or follow-up with a Pap test, colposcopy, and ECC at 6 months. The choice often depends on the patient's age. Younger patients have a much higher risk of cervical incompetence after retreatment, which increases the risks associated with pregnancy; thus, follow-up testing is often chosen for younger patients. If the patient is older, on the other hand, she has a much higher risk of persistent dysplasia; thus, retreatment is often preferable. It is important to remember, however, that an older patient has a much higher risk of developing cervical stenosis after multiple excision treatments.

Usually, we only recommend hysterectomy as treatment for high-grade dysplasia in older patients with persistent dysplasia. Thus, we rarely perform or recommend hysterectomy as primary treatment for young patients with high-grade squamous intraepithelial lesions because the lesions can recur at the vaginal cuff. We offer hysterectomy only after we have obtained negative margins or are unable to evaluate the endocervix owing to stenosis or lack of sufficient remaining cervical tissue.

Low-Grade Squamous Intraepithelial Lesions

Patients with low-grade squamous intraepithelial lesions (LGSIL) require a lot of reassurance. Often the patient arrives with a preconceived notion that it is only a matter of time before she will develop cervical cancer. Thus, in evaluating patients with LGSIL, it is most important to rule out an underlying higher-grade lesion and to reassure the patient that the detected cellular changes can be managed or treated, if necessary. Approximately 25% of patients with LGSIL on a Pap test will have a higher-grade lesion; we therefore perform an ECC on all new patients with LGSIL. This is in addition to any indicated biopsies and regardless of whether the colposcopy was satisfactory.

If the patient has a higher-grade lesion (CIN II or higher), we treat her according to the grade of that lesion (see "High-Grade Squamous Intraepithelial Lesions" above). If all results point to a CIN I or lower lesion, we usually recommend that the patient be followed up every 6 months for 2 years. In our experience, many patients with LGSIL have complete resolution of the dysplasia during the 2-year follow-up period, especially if the patient is young.

We rarely recommend treatment for LGSIL and only offer it to patients who have persistent dysplasia for more than 2 years.

Atypical Squamous Cells of Undetermined Significance

The newer recommendations for screening call for HPV typing only in patients over the age of 30 years who have a finding of atypical squamous cells of undetermined significance (ASC) on a Pap test. However, we still have many patients referred to us, either by themselves or by their primary physicians, because they are uncomfortable with any abnormal Pap test result. These patients, like all our new patients, undergo a complete history and physical examination, with cervical cultures, colposcopy, biopsies, and ECC. We perform an ECC on all our patients with an ASC Pap test result because there is a 10% to 15% chance of an underlying higher-grade lesion. After a thorough pathologic review of the referral Pap sample and our evaluation, we determine if further workup or treatment is necessary.

Atypical Cells of Undetermined Significance—Cannot Rule Out High-Grade Dysplasia

Patients with a Pap test result of atypical cells of undetermined significance in which high-grade dysplasia cannot be ruled out (ASC-H) undergo the same evaluation as patients with ASC and undergo an ECC. However, patients with ASC-H undergo immediate colposcopy, unlike patients with ASC, who can have either a repeat Pap test or HPV test-ing. Again, depending on the results, patients with ASC-H may receive treatment or undergo continued evaluation.

Atypical Glandular Cells of Undetermined Significance

All patients referred to us with the Pap finding of atypical glandular cells of undetermined significance (AGC) undergo a complete history and physical examination, colposcopy, appropriate biopsies, and ECC. If the patient is over age 35 years or she has irregular menses or is obese, she will also undergo an endometrial biopsy. The majority of patients with AGC have a squamous lesion; however, a small percentage of them have unde-tected endometrial hyperplasia or even endometrial cancer or an adeno-carcinoma of the cervix. If all of the biopsy results are negative, we perform a LEEP cone procedure and/or pelvic ultrasonography or follow up on the patient conservatively, depending on her risk factors, age, and reproduc-tive status. If no abnormality is found, patients with AGC are followed up every 6 months with a Pap test, colposcopy, and ECC for a total of 2 years.

If a patient is found to have adenocarcinoma in situ, she will have a cone biopsy. Many surgeons prefer a cold-knife cone biopsy to ensure pristine margins; however, with sufficient experience a LEEP cone proce-dure can be performed with satisfactory results. In the event that only glandular dysplasia is detected, we may offer the patient a hysterectomy, again depending on her age and reproductive status. In a small cohort of patients who for various reasons did not want a hysterectomy, we found no evidence of recurrence after a minimum follow-up of 1 year. These patients had clear margins on their cone biopsies, with the distance from dysplasia to margin greater than 10 mm.

EVALUATION OF SPECIAL CASES

Pregnant Patients with an Abnormal Pap Test Result

Pregnant patients with an abnormal Pap test result undergo the same eval-uation as nonpregnant patients, the only exception being that they do not undergo an ECC. This is avoided for 2 reasons: (1) in most pregnant patients, a satisfactory colposcopy is possible, since the transformation zone is everted during pregnancy; and (2) the risk of bleeding and contractions, and thus premature labor or spontaneous abortion, is significant for pregnant patients undergoing ECC. We perform a biopsy on most patients at their first visit to rule out invasive disease and to have a baseline cervical biopsy.

Our pregnant patients with CIN I are followed up every 3 months until delivery, patients with CIN II are followed up every 2 months until delivery, and patients with CIN III are followed up every month until delivery. Patients are reevaluated at 6 to 8 weeks after delivery. If treat-ment is indicated, they undergo the appropriate treatment at that time.

Very rarely, if there is a suspicion of invasive cancer and colposcopically directed biopsies could not rule it out, we will perform a LEEP or a cold-knife cone biopsy on a pregnant patient. These procedures are performed with the knowledge, input, and presence of the referring obstetrician or a maternal-fetal specialist.

Vaginal Dysplasia

In our clinic, we see many patients who for various reasons have had a hysterectomy and then develop vaginal intraepithelial neoplasia (VAIN). All referred patients undergo a complete history, physical examination, and colposcopy with colposcopically directed biopsies. On the basis of the histopathologic findings, the patients are then treated appropriately. For patients with VAIN I, we often prescribe estrogen vaginal cream and repeat evaluation every 6 months with a Pap test and colposcopy. Patients with VAIN are often older and either naturally or surgically postmenopausal. Although many of these patients are taking oral estrogen replacement therapy, they often still have an atrophic vaginal vault. The addition of vaginal estrogen will often "plump up" the vaginal mucosa sufficiently to resolve low-grade dysplasia.

Patients with higher-grade dysplasia are also treated with vaginal estrogen, as this allows us to perform excisional biopsies and upper vaginectomies much more safely. We usually perform excisions in patients with VAIN III, and often in those with VAIN II, in the operating room. If the patient is not a surgical candidate or has had surgery in the past for vaginal dysplasia, we often opt for treatment with 5-fluorouracil (5%) topical cream. This treatment, like laser ablation, is often not as successful as surgical excision but is a viable option for elderly or medically debilitated patients. We advise our patients to use the cream once weekly for 5 months and to return after 6 months for a reexamination and colposcopy. We find that this treatment regimen is better tolerated and less painful than daily or twice-weekly treatment. We have found that after the 5-month treatment interval, many patients still have some excoriation at the vaginal cuff that requires more vaginal estrogen treatment to heal.

Many patients with VAIN have persistent dysplasia despite treatment. It is important not to overtreat these women but rather to attempt to reassure them. As long as they are being followed up on a regular basis, any progression can be readily identified and addressed.

Vulvar Dysplasia

Vulvar dysplasia and vulvar cancer are often perceived to be diseases of elderly women. The demographics of the disease are changing, however, and more and more young women are being diagnosed with vulvar dysplasia. Additionally, vulvar dysplasia does not have a uniform appearance and therefore is often misdiagnosed as a benign condition. Furthermore, many women do not perform vulvar self-examinations and thus do not notice any skin changes until the disease has progressed. Often vulvar dysplasia will start with very innocuous symptoms, such as pruritus or burning, or be completely asymptomatic. Unfortunately, in too many cases women are falsely reassured by their primary provider that the lesions are normal and there is "nothing to worry about." It is important to understand that many young women may be immunocompromised for any number of reasons, such as pregnancy, steroid treatment for autoimmune diseases, connective tissue disorders, organ transplantation, Crohn's disease, or HIV/AIDS. All of these women are at increased risk for developing vulvar dysplasia.

The vulva and perineum should be examined at every annual Pap test, and patients should be encouraged to perform self-examinations on a bimonthly basis. If there is any question about a lesion, a vulvoscopy should be performed, including an examination of the rectum. Importantly, acetowhite changes take longer to become evident on the vulva and perineum; thus, acetic acid should be applied at least 5 minutes prior to a colposcopic examination. The colposcopic findings of vulvar dysplasia are very similar to those of cervical dysplasia. Acetowhite epithelium, mosaicism, and abnormal vessels can all be seen on the vulva as well as on the perineum.

Even more so than colposcopy, vulvoscopy requires that the provider have considerable experience to be able to recognize and differentiate between the different levels of dysplasia. Often, it is difficult to differentiate dysplasia from other, benign vulvar conditions such as lichen sclerosus, lichen simplex chronicus, or hyperkeratosis. If there is any question remaining after vulvoscopy, a biopsy of the lesion should be performed. A 3- to 6-mm dermatological punch biopsy can be easily accomplished after infiltrating the area with 1% lidocaine with epinephrine. Hemostasis can be maintained with silver nitrate and Gelfoam or a suture, if necessary.

Vulvar intraepithelial neoplasia (VIN) I lesions do not require any treatment, only observation, and often will resolve on their own. VIN II and VIN III lesions should be excised to be certain that there is no occult invasion. A wide local excision can be performed as an outpatient procedure using minimal anesthetic. So long as the lesion appears to be completely excised, negative margins are not necessary, since the inflammation resulting from healing will often clear up any positive margins. Additionally, any resection should preserve as much of the natural anatomy of the woman's genitals as possible. If necessary, a plastic surgeon experienced in vulvar reconstruction ought to be consulted.

If a large area of the vulva is involved, especially if the lesions are multiple and not confluent, laser ablation can be performed. This should only be done after confirmation that there is no invasion and should probably be reserved for younger patients, since vulvar cancer is more common in women over the age of 50 years. In patients with HIV/AIDS, who often have large areas of dysplasia, laser ablation is often less disfiguring and less traumatic than a wide local excision, and wound infections are very rare.

Postoperatively, patients—especially those who undergo laser ablation—should be instructed in proper hygiene and wound care. Follow-up for all patients treated for VIN will often be protracted, but they should undergo a colposcopy at least every 6 months and more frequently if the patient is immunocompromised. It is equally important to instruct patients to perform self-examinations, since they are often able to detect abnormalities.

Additionally, women with vulvar dysplasia should be reassured about their appearance, as women often feel that they look abnormal after a wide local excision. This, of course, is one more reason to attempt the best cosmetic result possible during surgery.

CONCLUSION

In conclusion, preinvasive disease of the lower genital tract is much more common than often assumed. It affects women of all socioeconomic levels and age groups. All women deserve to have regular genital screening. Although dysplasia is sexually transmitted, it need not and should not be a stigma, since between 50% and 85% of the sexually active population have at one point in their lives been exposed to HPV. It is important to remember that exposure does not mean disease and that dysplasia can regress. This is often true in immunocompromised patients, whose dysplasia will regress once their immune status improves.

KEY PRACTICE POINTS

- Patients with an abnormal Pap test result need and deserve a thorough evaluation by a skilled clinician and colposcopist.

- In most instances, colposcopy with directed biopsies has been accepted as the "gold standard" of cervical evaluation, but it requires practice and experience as well as the acceptance of certain standards.

- All patients referred to us for the evaluation of a high-grade squamous intraepithelial lesion identified on a Pap test undergo a complete history and physical examination, including repeat evaluation of the cytologic specimen, cervical cultures, colposcopy, vaginoscopy, vulvoscopy, biopsies of all abnormal areas, and ECC.

- When evaluating patients with LGSIL, it is most important to rule out an underlying higher-grade lesion and to reassure the patient that the detected cellular changes can be managed or treated, if necessary.

- We perform an ECC on all our patients with an ASC Pap test result because there is a 10% to 15% chance of an underlying higher-grade lesion.

- Pregnant patients with an abnormal Pap test result undergo the same evaluation as nonpregnant patients, the only exception being that they do not undergo an ECC.

- Patients with VAIN are treated with vaginal estrogen; patients with higher-grade dysplasia may also undergo excisional biopsy and upper vaginectomy.

- Young women who are immunocompromised are at increased risk for developing vulvar dysplasia.

SUGGESTED READINGS

American Cancer Society. *Cancer Facts and Figures*. Atlanta, GA; 1997.

Benedet JL, Miller DM, Nickerson KG, Anderson GH. The results of cryosurgical treatment of cervical intraepithelial neoplasia at one, five, and ten years. *Am J Obstet Gynecol* 1987;157:268–273.

Dunn JE Jr. The relationship between carcinoma in situ and invasive cervical carcinoma: a consideration of the contributions to the problem to be made from general population data. *Cancer* 1953;6:873–876.

Gad C. The management and natural history of severe dysplasia and carcinoma in situ of the uterine cervix. *Br J Obstet Gynaecol* 1976;83:554–559.

Gunasekera PC, Phipps JH, Lewis BV. Large loop excision of the transformation zone (LLETZ) compared to carbon dioxide laser in the treatment of CIN: a superior mode of treatment. *Br J Obstet Gynaecol* 1990;97:995–998.

Kashgarian M, Dunn JE, Jr. The duration of intraepithelial and preclinical squamous cell carcinoma of the uterine cervix. *Am J Epidemiol* 1970;92:211–222.

Kaufman RH, Adam E, Icenogle J, Reeves WC. Human papillomavirus testing as triage for atypical squamous cells of undetermined significance and low-grade squamous intraepithelial lesions: sensitivity, specificity, and cost-effectiveness. *Am J Obstet Gynecol* 1997;177:930–936.

Kinlen LJ, Spriggs AI. Women with positive cervical smears but without surgical intervention. A follow-up study. *Lancet* 1978;2:463–465.

Koss LG. Natural history of carcinoma in situ and related lesions of the cervix. In: Koss LG, ed. *Diagnostic Cytology and Its Histopathologic Bases.* 3rd ed. Philadelphia, Pa: JB Lippincott; 1979:305.

Koutsky LA, Holmes KK, Critchlow CW, et al. A cohort study of the risk for cervical intraepithelial neoplasia grade 2 or 3 in relation to papillomavirus infection. *N Engl J Med* 1992;327:1272–1278.

Kurman RJ, Henson DE, Herbst AL, et al. Interim guidelines for management of abnormal cervical cytology. The 1992 National Cancer Institute Workshop. *JAMA* 1994;271:1866–1869.

Lorincz AT, Reid R, Jenson AB, Greenberg MD, Lancaster W, Kurman RJ. Human papillomavirus infection of the cervix: relative risk associations of 15 common anogenital types. *Obstet Gynecol* 1992;79:328–337.

Mitchell MF. The natural history of cervical intraepithelial neoplasia. *Clin Consult Obstet Gynecol* 1994;6:31–36.

Mitchell MF, Hittelman WK, Lotan R, et al. Chemoprevention trials and surrogate endpoint biomarkers in the cervix. *Cancer* 1995;76:1956–1977.

Mitchell MF, Schottenfeld D, Tortolero-Luna G, Cantor SB, Richards-Kortum R. Colposcopy for the diagnosis of squamous intraepithelial lesions: a meta-analysis. *Obstet Gynecol* 1998;91:626–631.

Mitchell MF, Tortolero-Luna G, Cook E, Whittaker L, Rhodes-Morris H, Silva E. A randomized clinical trial of cryotherapy, laser vaporization, and loop electro-surgical excision for treatment of squamous intraepithelial lesions of the cervix. *Obstet Gynecol* 1998;92:737–744.

Mitchell MF, Tortolero-Luna G, Wright T, et al. Cervical human papillomavirus infection and intraepithelial neoplasia: a review. *J Natl Cancer Inst Monogr* 1996;21:17–25.

Morbidity and Mortality Weekly Report. *Results from the National Breast and Cervical Cancer Early Detection Program, October 31, 1991–September 30, 1993.* Centers for Disease Control and Prevention. 1994;43:530–534.

Mor-Yosef S, Lopes A, Pearson S, Monaghan JM. Loop diathermy cone biopsy. *Obstet Gynecol* 1990;75:884–886.

Munoz N, Bosch FX. Epidemiology of cervical cancer. *IARC Sci Publ* 1989;94:9–39.

Nasiell K, Nasiell M, Vaclavinkova V. Behavior of moderate cervical dysplasia during long-term follow-up. *Obstet Gynecol* 1983;61:609–614.

Nasiell K, Roger V, Nasiell M. Behavior of mild cervical dysplasia during long-term follow-up. *Obstet Gynecol* 1986;67:665–669.

Parkin DM, Pisani P, Ferlay J. Estimates of the worldwide incidence of eighteen major cancers in 1985. *Int J Cancer* 1993;54:594–606.

Prendiville W, Cullimore J, Norman S. Large loop excision of the transformation zone (LLETZ). A new method of management for women with cervical intraepithelial neoplasia. *Br J Obstet Gynaecol* 1989;96:1054–1060.

Schiffman MH, Bauer HM, Hoover RN, et al. Epidemiologic evidence showing that human papillomavirus infection causes most cervical intraepithelial neoplasia. *J Natl Cancer Inst* 1993;85:958–964.

Whiteley PF, Olah KS. Treatment of cervical intraepithelial neoplasia: experience with the low-voltage diathermy loop. *Am J Obstet Gynecol* 1990;162:1272–1277.

Wolcott HD, Gallup DG. Wide local excision in the treatment of vulvar carcinoma in situ: a reappraisal. *Am J Obstet Gynecol* 1984;150:695–698.

4 SELECTED TOPICS IN GYNECOLOGIC PATHOLOGY

Anais Malpica, Michael T. Deavers,
and Elvio G. Silva

CHAPTER OUTLINE

CHAPTER OVERVIEW

In this chapter, updated information about a selected group of gynecologic pathology topics is presented. For the most part, the selection of these topics was guided by the availability of new information that has provided a better understanding of previously described entities. A minority of the issues discussed herein reflect our own experience.

The following topics are covered:

- Vulvar intraepithelial neoplasia, simplex type, which has distinct clinicopathologic features and an apparently marked potential for progression to invasive squamous carcinoma
- The role of p16 immunostaining in the evaluation of cervical intraepithelial neoplasia associated with high-risk human papillomavirus
- Large cell neuroendocrine carcinoma, a type of high-grade neuroendocrine carcinoma with an aggressive clinical course that can

be mistaken histologically for poorly differentiated squamous carcinoma or adenocarcinoma

• The role of immunohistochemical studies in the differentiation of an adenocarcinoma arising in the endocervix from one arising in the endometrium

• The current approach to endometrial hyperplasia and proposed changes

• The concept of dedifferentiation in endometrioid adenocarcinoma and the importance of its recognition from the clinical standpoint

• A 2-tier system for grading ovarian serous carcinoma that facilitates accuracy, in addition to being prognostically significant

• Proposed·changes to the diagnostic criteria for invasive implants of ovarian serous tumors of low malignant potential

• Ovarian mucinous tumors: an up-to-date review

• Cellular fibroma, an ovarian tumor revisited.

VULVAR INTRAEPITHELIAL NEOPLASIA, SIMPLEX TYPE

Although the simplex type of vulvar intraepithelial neoplasia (VIN) was first described in the 1960s by Abell and coworkers, the literature on this form of highly differentiated vulvar carcinoma in situ is limited. Recent studies have shown that simplex, or differentiated, VIN displays clinical and pathologic features that differ from those of the classic type of VIN.

VIN simplex represents 2% to 10% of cases of VIN and affects mostly postmenopausal patients. The mean age at diagnosis is 67 years. Approximately 25% of the patients have a history of cigarette smoking. VIN simplex is not commonly associated with multicentric lower genital tract intraepithelial squamous neoplasia, and human papillomavirus (HPV) is almost always absent.

VIN simplex produces less bulky lesions than does classic VIN, and the lesions frequently arise in association with lichen sclerosus or squamous hyperplasia. Histologically, VIN simplex is characterized by a thickened epithelium that tends to have elongated and branching rete ridges. The cardinal feature is the presence of abnormal squamous cells in the lower third of the epithelium (Figure 4–1). These cells have enlarged nuclei with prominent nucleoli and abundant eosinophilic cytoplasm. Immunostaining for p53 aids in the recognition of VIN simplex in difficult cases; in most cases, this marker is expressed by the majority of the cells in the lower third of the epithelium. Immunostaining for p16, a cyclin-dependent kinase inhibitor, yields negative results in VIN simplex, in contrast to the p16 positivity frequently seen in classic VIN.

VIN simplex appears to have a greater potential for progression to invasive squamous carcinoma than classic VIN. Yang and Hart (2000) have reported that up to 58% of cases of VIN simplex are associated with a prior, synchronous, or subsequent invasive squamous carcinoma.

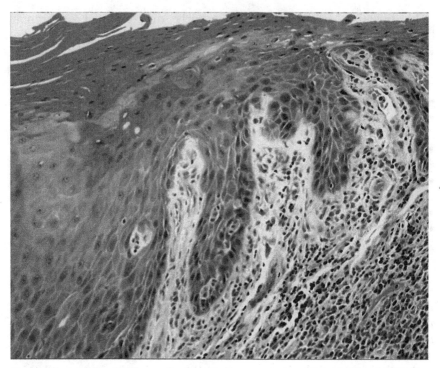

Figure 4–1. VIN simplex with elongated rete ridges and keratinization in the lower third of the epithelium.

P16 IN CERVICAL INTRAEPITHELIAL NEOPLASIA

Accurate grading of cervical intraepithelial neoplasia (CIN) is important in guiding therapy but can be difficult in some cases. The accepted gold standard for the diagnosis of CIN is histologic examination, in spite of intra- and interobserver variability. Ancillary techniques, like HPV testing using Hybrid Capture 2 (Digene Corporation, Gaithersburg, MD) or Ki-67 (a proliferation marker) immunostaining, have been found to be sensitive but not specific for CIN.

High-grade CIN, associated with high-risk HPV, is treated because it carries a significant risk of progression to invasive carcinoma. In contrast, low-grade CIN, associated with both low- and high-risk HPV, is only followed because most cases will regress. A simple test to identify the type of HPV present in these lesions could be important in helping to distinguish between low-grade and high-grade CIN in equivocal cases.

Most of the techniques used to identify the virus associated with CIN are difficult to perform and therefore not practical for routine use; however, recent studies have suggested that p16 may be a useful biomarker for high-risk HPV. Although increased expression of p16 is not direct proof of HPV infection, it does correlate well with HPV DNA identification using in situ hybridization. p16 expression is positive in 35% to 50% of CIN I cases and in 70% to 100% of CIN II and CIN III cases. Because p16 overexpression correlates well with the presence of high-risk HPV, histologically indeterminate cases of CIN that are negative for p16 likely are associated with low-risk HPV or are negative for HPV infection; therefore, these cases may be managed with surveillance only. p16 may also help in the interpretation of Ki-67 immunostaining results because p16 is frequently negative in cases of reactive and atypical lesions that can be positive for Ki-67. Although p16 may be a useful tool in the diagnosis of CIN, it is not intended to replace histologic examination.

LARGE CELL NEUROENDOCRINE CARCINOMA OF THE CERVIX

Currently, neuroendocrine tumors are divided into low, intermediate, and high grade (carcinoid, atypical carcinoid, and high-grade neuroendocrine carcinoma, respectively). The incidences of these different types of neuroendocrine tumors in the uterine cervix are different from those observed in other organs. In the cervix, almost all of the neuroendocrine tumors are high-grade carcinomas, and cases of low- and intermediate-grade tumors are rare.

High-grade neuroendocrine carcinomas are subdivided into small and large cell types. The recognition of the former is relatively easy, and its differential diagnosis includes other small blue cell tumors such as lymphoma, rhabdomyosarcoma, and melanoma. However, the accurate diagnosis of large cell neuroendocrine carcinoma can be challenging because this type of tumor can share histologic features with other poorly differentiated large cell carcinomas of the uterine cervix (i.e., adenocarcinoma or squamous carcinoma). Additionally, large cell neuroendocrine carcinoma sometimes occurs with invasive squamous carcinoma, adenocarcinoma, or adenocarcinoma in situ, which can lead to misdiagnosis.

The correct identification of large cell neuroendocrine carcinoma is important for treatment and prognosis. Most patients with large cell neuroendocrine carcinoma of the cervix have a recurrence in less than 4 years and die of the disease. In addition, this type of tumor appears to be more resistant to radiotherapy than squamous carcinoma or adenocarcinoma of the cervix.

Histologic features that could indicate possible neuroendocrine differentiation in a large cell carcinoma include a trabecular or insular pattern, numerous mitoses, numerous apoptotic bodies, and geographic necrosis. Immunohistochemically, chromogranin, synaptophysin, and more recently, CD56 have been shown to be useful markers of neuroendocrine differentiation (Figure 4–2).

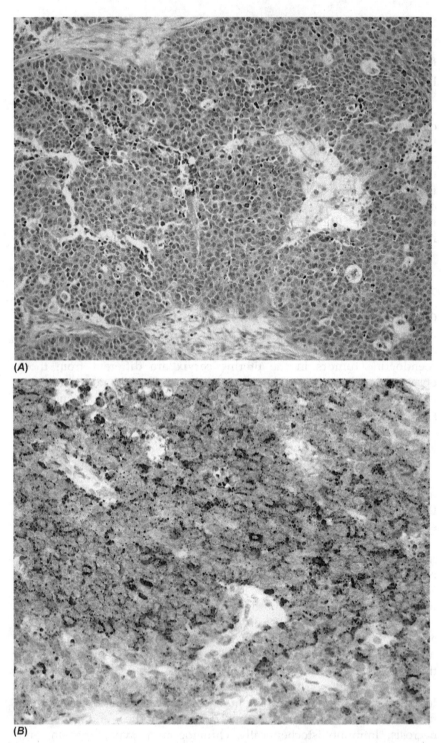

Figure 4–2. (A) Large cell neuroendocrine carcinoma. (B) Positive chromogranin immunostain.

Large cell neuroendocrine carcinomas are associated with HPV 16 and 18, and it has been postulated that they originate from neuroendocrine cells that are normally present in 1% to 20% of uterine cervices.

ENDOCERVICAL ADENOCARCINOMA VERSUS ENDOMETRIAL ADENOCARCINOMA

Distinguishing endocervical adenocarcinoma from endometrial adenocarcinoma is important for therapy, but in some cases the histologic distinction between these 2 neoplasms can be extremely difficult to ascertain. Tumors arising in the endocervix can have an endometrioid appearance (Figure 4–3A), and conversely, tumors arising in the endometrium can have an endocervical appearance.

Immunoperoxidase studies have been used to assist in making this distinction in problematic cases. It has been recognized that the majority of endocervical adenocarcinomas are positive for carcinoembryonic antigen and negative for vimentin (Figure 4–3B). The opposite pattern characterizes the majority of endometrial adenocarcinomas; however, these 2 stains are helpful in only 70% to 80% of cases, and the results can depend upon the histologic type of the adenocarcinoma. For example, mucinous carcinoma involving either the endocervix or the endometrium may be positive for carcinoembryonic antigen.

Recently, the use of p16 as a marker for endocervical adenocarcinoma has been proposed. Overexpression of p16 has been observed in cervical intraepithelial lesions and in invasive carcinomas associated with high-risk HPV types. p16 is not a direct marker of HPV infection; however, there is excellent correlation between immunohistochemical expression of p16 and in situ hybridization for HPV DNA. In endocervical adenocarcinoma, 75% to 100% of the tumor cells are positive for p16, and in 90% of the cases analyzed, the stain is moderately to strongly positive. In endometrial adenocarcinoma, fewer than 75% of the cells are positive for p16, and in 40% of the cases the staining is weak.

Other markers that are helpful in distinguishing between endocervical and endometrial adenocarcinoma are hormone receptors. In endometrial adenocarcinoma, approximately 70% of the cases are positive for both estrogen and progesterone receptors. In endocervical adenocarcinoma, only approximately 20% of the cases are positive for both estrogen and progesterone receptors. In the normal endocervix, the glandular cells and stromal cells are estrogen receptor positive; however, in malignant endocervical glandular cells, this positivity is lost, and the expression of estrogen receptors in the stromal cells adjacent to invasive carcinoma also decreases.

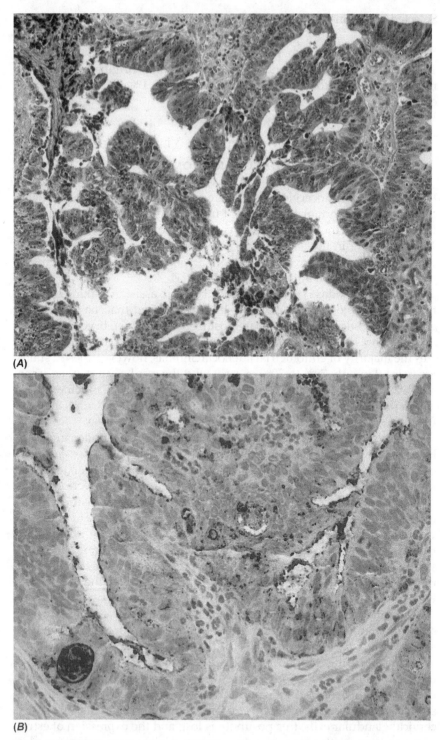

Figure 4–3. (*A*) Endocervical adenocarcinoma with endometrioid features. (*B*) Positive immunostain for carcinoembryonic antigen.

ENDOMETRIAL HYPERPLASIA AND CARCINOMA

In 1900, Cullen described endometrial lesions that could be considered precursors of endometrial carcinoma owing to their proximity to areas of malignancy. In 1952, Speert introduced the term "adenomatous atypical hyperplasia" to designate these premalignant lesions. Ten years later, Gore and Hertig agreed with the use of this term and its meaning. Since then, several studies have analyzed endometrial hyperplasia and its relationship to endometrial adenocarcinoma.

The first study establishing reproducible criteria for differentiating endometrial hyperplasia from well-differentiated endometrioid adeno-carcinoma was published in 1982 by Kurman and Norris. According to these authors, stromal invasion in an endometrial biopsy specimen was the main histologic parameter correlating with adenocarcinoma in the subsequent hysterectomy specimen. Stromal invasion is identified by the presence of desmoplastic changes, confluent glandular growth, or an extensive papillary pattern. Any of these features must involve half (2.1 mm) of a low-power field (4.2 mm in diameter) to have value in pre-dicting the presence of a biologically significant carcinoma in the uterus. Currently, these criteria are still used, despite the fact that when stromal invasion is identified in an endometrial biopsy or curettage specimen, residual adenocarcinoma is found in only 50% of the subsequent hys-terectomy specimens, and when stromal invasion is not identified, ade-nocarcinoma is still found in 17% of the subsequent hysterectomy specimens. The current World Health Organization classification of endometrial hyperplasia was adopted in 1994 and is based on the evalu-ation of architectural and cytologic features. According to this scheme, hyperplasias are divided into simple or complex type, with or without atypia. Although this classification has been widely accepted, its repro-ducibility is far from optimal. This poor reproducibility, together with poor interobserver agreement in differentiating endometrial hyperplasia from adenocarcinoma, has prompted the proposal of a new model for pre-malignant endometrial disease that would integrate molecular, genetic, histomorphometric, and clinical data to identify premalignant lesions in the endometrium.

In this new model, premalignant endometrial disease is designated "endometrial intraepithelial neoplasia," and its diagnosis requires the existence of architectural changes (glandular proliferation resulting in the glands occupying more than 50% of the total tissue volume), cyto-logic alterations (in the areas of glandular crowding distinct from the glandular epithelium in the background), and a size larger than 1 mm². At a molecular level, these glands show a loss of *PTEN*, a tumor suppres-sor gene mutated in many endometrioid adenocarcinomas. The clinical relevance of this model has yet to be determined.

DEDIFFERENTIATED ENDOMETRIOID ADENOCARCINOMA

The existence of dedifferentiation in sarcomas is well known, but a similar phenomenon in carcinomas is less well recognized. Currently, only a few reports of dedifferentiated carcinomas in the head and neck, prostate, and lung have been published. In some of these cases the "dedifferentiated neoplasm" was a sarcoma. No reports of this phenomenon in the gynecologic tract have been published thus far.

In general, endometrioid adenocarcinomas of the endometrium and ovary and those associated with endometriosis maintain the same degree of differentiation throughout the course of the disease. However, in rare cases low-grade endometrioid adenocarcinoma (International Federation of Gynecology and Obstetrics grades 1 and 2) can dedifferentiate into a highly malignant neoplasm that retains some features of carcinoma, which we designate as "undifferentiated carcinoma" (Figure 4–4). We have studied several cases of low-grade endometrial endometrioid adenocarcinoma

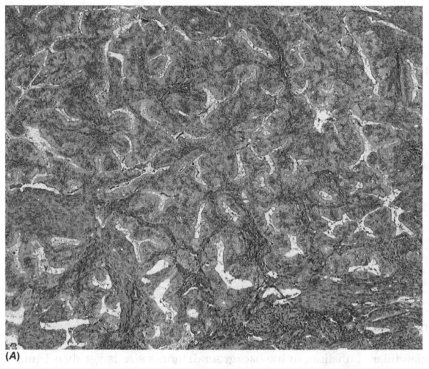

(A)

Figure 4–4. Dedifferentiated endometrioid adenocarcinoma. (A) Area displaying a well-differentiated endometrioid adenocarcinoma. (*Continued*)

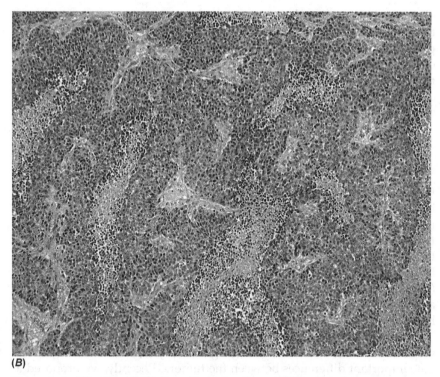

(B)

Figure 4–4. (*Continued*) (*B*) Area displaying the undifferentiated carcinoma component of the tumor.

with areas of undifferentiated carcinoma and have found that the latter component is characterized by any of 3 different histologic patterns: (1) solid with well-demarcated groups of undifferentiated cells, (2) sheets of undifferentiated cells with rhabdoid features (a pattern well recognized in other anaplastic neoplasms), and (3) groups of undifferentiated cells with foci of abrupt squamous differentiation. In most cases, the undifferentiated component is intimately associated with the glands of the low-grade endometrioid adenocarcinoma. In some instances, however, the dedifferentiated carcinoma is found only in metastases at the time of initial surgery or several months to years after the initial surgery. We have not found any clinical, pathologic, or immunohistochemical features that are unique to these cases or that separate them from cases of typical low-grade endometrioid adenocarcinoma without dedifferentiation.

The prognosis of patients with dedifferentiated carcinoma is dismal. Most patients experience progressive disease and die within 24 months after the dedifferentiated carcinoma is detected. Dedifferentiation should be suspected clinically whenever an alleged low-grade endometrioid adenocarcinoma progresses rapidly or has lymph node metastases in the absence of deep myometrial invasion or cervical involvement. For the pathologist, it is important to carefully examine solid areas in an endometrioid adenocarcinoma to rule out an undifferentiated carcinoma component. The experience accumulated thus far indicates that undifferentiated carcinoma is associated with rapid progression and therefore warrants aggressive therapy.

GRADING OF OVARIAN SEROUS CARCINOMA

Histologic grading has been found to be of prognostic significance in ovarian carcinoma; however, there is no universally accepted system for grading these tumors. The most commonly used systems are the International Federation of Gynecology and Obstetrics system, which is based on architectural features, and the World Health Organization system, which is based on both architectural and cytologic features. Recently, Shimizu et al (1998) proposed a grading system based on architecture, cytologic atypia, and mitotic index to be applied to all ovarian carcinomas, regardless of histologic type.

In our opinion, the different histologic types of ovarian carcinoma represent different diseases, and a single grading system may not accommodate important differences between the tumors. Recently, we proposed a 2-tier grading system for ovarian serous carcinoma that appears to be useful for prognosis and relatively easy to apply. This grading system is based primarily on nuclear atypia and uses mitotic index as a secondary feature. Carcinomas are classified into 2 categories: high-grade, which is characterized by the presence of marked cytologic atypia, and low-grade, which shows mild to moderate atypia (Figure 4–5). As a secondary feature, high-grade carcinomas tend to have more than 12 mitoses per 10 high-power fields, and low-grade carcinomas tend to have up to 12 mitoses per 10 high-power fields. Of interest, low-grade carcinomas generally have multiple calcifications and may have foci of intracellular mucin, whereas high-grade carcinomas have calcifications in fewer than 50% of cases and rarely have mucin. Most tumors of both grades are papillary, although glandular and solid areas can be found in either.

It is also important to note that up to 60% of low-grade serous carcinomas of the ovary are associated with areas of serous neoplasm of low malignant potential, which in many cases have a micropapillary/cribriform pattern. This association is very rare in ovarian high-grade serous carcinoma and appears to suggest differences in the pathogenesis of low- and high-grade serous carcinoma.

Using this grading system, the 5- and 10-year survival rates are 40% and 20% for low-grade carcinomas and 10% and 5% for high-grade carcinomas, respectively.

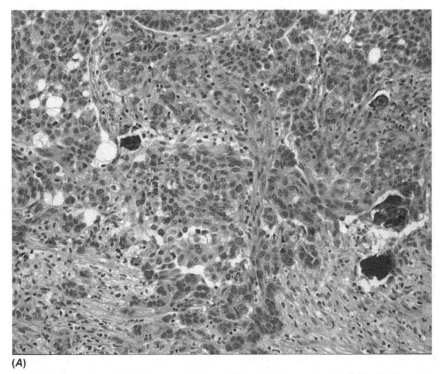

(A)

Figure 4–5. (*A*) Low-grade ovarian serous carcinoma consisting of uniform cells with regular oval or rounded nuclei having evenly distributed chromatin and inconspicuous mitotic activity. (*Continued*)

INVASIVE IMPLANTS OF OVARIAN SEROUS BORDERLINE TUMORS

Stage of disease and the type of implant are the most important prognostic indicators in cases of ovarian serous borderline tumors. Advanced-stage cases have a recurrence rate ranging from 8% to 30%, in contrast to a recurrence rate of 1.8% to 15% for stage I cases. A recent meta-analysis of the literature on advanced-stage cases of serous borderline tumors reported that the overall survival rate for tumors with noninvasive serous implants was 95.3%, while the survival rate in cases with invasive implants decreased to 66%. Currently, there is nearly unanimous agreement that patients with invasive implants have recurrences more frequently and within a shorter interval than do patients with noninvasive implants. However, the criteria used to differentiate invasive from noninvasive implants vary among investigators. Traditionally, a diagnosis of invasive implants is made when invasion of underlying nonneoplastic tissue is identified, but this approach has been challenged by a proposed expansion of the diagnostic criteria for invasion to also include cases that

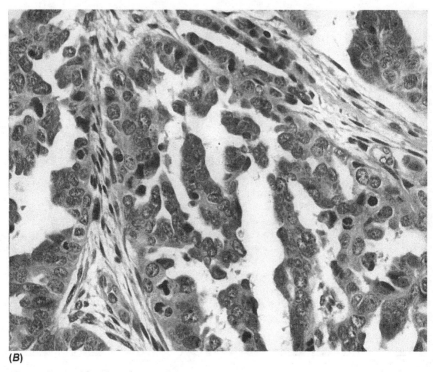

(B)

Figure 4–5. (*Continued*) (*B*) High-grade ovarian serous carcinoma with nuclear pleomorphism and numerous mitotic figures.

have either nests of cells surrounded by a clear space or cleft or micropapillary architecture. Preliminary data appear to indicate that these newly proposed criteria could be useful in identifying cases with a poor prognosis. However, larger studies with long-term follow-up are necessary to confirm these findings.

MUCINOUS TUMORS OF THE OVARY

Approximately 15% of all ovarian epithelial tumors are mucinous, with 90% of these being either benign or borderline. Primary mucinous carcinomas in the ovary are rare, representing fewer than 5% of all ovarian carcinomas. During the past 5 years, the criteria used for the diagnosis of these tumors have been redefined. Currently, mucinous carcinomas of the ovary are divided into noninvasive (intraepithelial, intraglandular) and invasive types. Noninvasive mucinous carcinomas are characterized by the presence of marked cytologic atypia in the epithelium, regardless of the number of epithelial layers. Invasive mucinous carcinomas are subdivided into 2 types, those with an expansile (confluent) pattern of invasion (Figure 4–6) and those with an infiltrative pattern of invasion. The expansile pattern is characterized by an area, at least 5 mm in greatest dimension, with a confluent glandular pattern and little intervening stroma. The infiltrative pattern of invasion has ragged glands or clusters of cells occupying an area of at least 5 mm in greatest dimension.

A review of the literature shows that the mortality rate for stage I mucinous intraepithelial carcinoma is 6.2%. Invasive mucinous carcinomas with an expansile (confluent) pattern have a very low recurrence rate, which reflects a more indolent behavior pattern than that of the stage I mucinous carcinomas with an infiltrative pattern, which have a recurrence rate of 10% to 15%. However, rare cases of stage I ovarian mucinous carcinoma with an expansile pattern have had a rapidly fatal course.

An important problem regarding mucinous tumors of the ovary is the differentiation of these neoplasms from metastatic adenocarcinomas. The latter are associated with the following features: bilaterality, small size of the mucinous tumor in the ovary, involvement of the ovarian surface, a nodular pattern of invasion into the ovarian parenchyma, or an extensive infiltrative pattern. Histologically, some metastatic mucinous carcinomas, especially those from the pancreaticobiliary tract or cervix, can be very difficult to differentiate from an ovarian primary tumor.

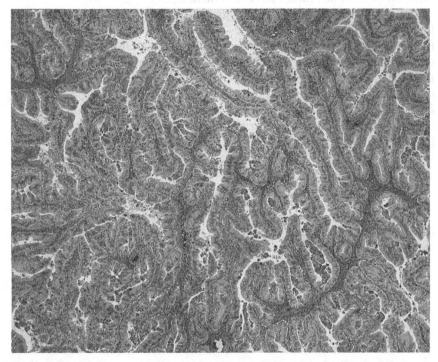

Figure 4–6. Mucinous carcinoma with an expansile (confluent) pattern of invasion.

CELLULAR FIBROMA OF THE OVARY

Ten percent of ovarian fibromas are characterized by dense cellularity that warrants the designation "cellular fibroma." In contrast to regular fibromas, these tumors tend to have more conspicuous mitotic activity, with an average mitotic index of 3 mitoses per 10 high-power fields. In the 1980s it was postulated that a mitotic index of 4 mitoses or more per 10 high-power fields was the main diagnostic feature that separated cellular fibromas from fibrosarcomas. However, during the past 20 years it has become evident that cellular fibromas may have more than 4 mitoses per 10 high-power fields and still not recur. In a recent review of 21 cases of cellular fibroma with 4 or more mitoses per 10 high-power fields (Alkushi et al, 2004), the patients had a median age of 33 years. All of the tumors were stage I, the mitotic index reached up to 19 mitoses per 10 high-power fields, and there was no significant cytologic atypia. The follow-up of these patients revealed no recurrences.

From an investigational standpoint, attempts have been made to distinguish cellular fibromas from fibrosarcomas by detecting chromosomal aberrations. These studies were initiated because of reports of trisomy 12 in stromal tumors of the ovary. Some authors have found trisomy 8 in cases of fibrosarcoma but not in cellular fibroma. Currently, however, these chromosomal studies have no practical use.

Cellular fibromas are considered tumors of uncertain malignant potential because a total of 3 recurrences have been reported thus far. In 2 of those cases, there were problems during the original surgery: in 1, the ovarian tumor ruptured, and in the other, the tumor was incompletely removed owing to adherence to the pelvic wall. A single reported case of ovarian cellular fibroma without adhesions or rupture has been associated with an alleged implant in the cul de sac. At this point, however, the actual recurrence rate of cellular fibroma is not known. Until it is known, long-term follow-up of patients is recommended.

KEY PRACTICE POINTS

- VIN, simplex type, is a distinct clinicopathologic entity that is not commonly associated with multicentric lower genital tract intraepithelial squamous neoplasia.

- p53 immunostaining is a useful tool to identify difficult cases of VIN, simplex type, which apparently has a marked tendency for progression to invasive squamous carcinoma.

- Histologic examination still represents the gold standard for the diagnosis of CIN; however, the expression of p16 correlates well with the presence of high-risk HPV types.

- The diagnosis of large cell neuroendocrine carcinoma of the uterine cervix may constitute a challenge because it can share histologic features with other types of poorly differentiated carcinomas (i.e., squamous carcinoma or adenocarcinoma).

- Immunohistochemical studies such as CD56, chromogranin, and synaptophysin are useful for identifying large cell neuroendocrine carcinoma.

- The histologic and clinical distinction between endocervical adenocarcinoma and endometrial adenocarcinoma can be extremely difficult, but the use of immunohistochemical studies can be helpful.

- A new model for endometrial premalignant disease has been proposed in which this entity is designated "endometrial intraepithelial neoplasia" and diagnosed on the basis of architectural changes and cytologic features in an area greater than 1 mm^2.

- Dedifferentiated endometrioid adenocarcinoma appears to be aggressive and may require aggressive therapy.

- We have proposed a 2-tier system for grading ovarian serous carcinoma that is based primarily on nuclear atypia and uses the mitotic index as a secondary feature.

- Recently, the presence of a micropapillary architecture or small nests of cells surrounded by a space or cleft within the implant has been proposed to designate an implant of ovarian serous borderline tumor as invasive. The validity of these criteria has not yet been confirmed.

- Among mucinous carcinomas of the ovary, stage I intraepithelial carcinomas and invasive carcinomas with an expansile pattern have a more indolent behavior than do stage I carcinomas with an infiltrative pattern of invasion.

- Cellular fibromas, which are characterized by dense cellularity and a tendency to have conspicuous mitotic activity, are considered tumors of uncertain malignant potential owing to rare cases associated with recurrence.

SUGGESTED READINGS

Abell MR. Intraepithelial carcinomas of epidermis and squamous mucosa of vulva and perineum. *Surg Clin North Am* 1965;45:1179–1198.

Agoff SN, Morihara J, Mao C, Kiviat NB, Koutsky LA. p16^{ink4a} expression correlates with degree of cervical neoplasia: a comparison with Ki-67 expression and detection of high-risk HPV types. *Mod Pathol* 2003;16:665–673.

Alkushi A, Young RH, Clement PB. Cellular fibroma of the ovary: a study of 62 cases including 21 with ≥ 4 mitoses per 10 HPFs. *Mod Pathol* 2004;17:189A.

Ansari-Lari MA, Staebler A, Zaino R, Shah KV, Ronnett B. Distinction of endocervical and endometrial adenocarcinomas. *Am J Surg Pathol* 2004;28:160–167.

Bell DA, Longacre TA, Prat J, et al. Serous borderline (low malignant potential, atypical proliferative) ovarian tumors: workshop perspectives. *Hum Pathol* 2004;35:934–948.

Bell DA, Weinstock MA, Scully RE. Peritoneal implants of ovarian serous borderline tumors. Histologic features and prognosis. *Cancer* 1988;62:2212–2222.

Brawn PN. The dedifferentiation of prostate carcinoma. *Cancer* 1983;52:246–251.

Carey MS, Dembo AJ, Simm JE, et al. Testing the validity of a prognostic classification in patients with surgically optimal ovarian carcinoma: a 15 year review. *Int J Gynecol Cancer* 1993;3:24–35.

Cullen TS. *Cancer of the Uterus*. New York, NY: D. Appleton & Co; 1900.

Deavers MT, Malpica A, Liu JS, Broaddus R, Silva EG. Large cell neuroendocrine carcinoma of the uterine cervix. *Mod Pathol* 2004;17:196A.

Gershenson DM, Silva EG, Tortolero-Luna G, Levenback C, Morris M, Tornos C. Serous borderline tumors of the ovary with noninvasive peritoneal implants. *Cancer* 1998;83:2157–2163.

Gilks CB, Young RH, Gersell DJ, Clement PB. Large cell neuroendocrine carcinoma of the uterine cervix: a clinicopathologic study of 12 cases. *Am J Surg Pathol* 1997;21:905–914.

Gore H, Hertig AT. Premalignant lesions of the endometrium. *Clin Obstet Gynecol* 1962;5:1148.

Gosling JRG, Abell MR, Drolette BM, Loughrin TD. Infiltrative squamous cell (epidermoid) carcinoma of vulva. *Cancer* 1961;14:330–343.

Grayson W, Rhemtula HA, Taylor LF, Allard U, Tiltman AJ. Detection of human papillomavirus in large cell neuroendocrine carcinoma of the uterine cervix: a study of 12 cases. *J Clin Pathol* 2002;55:108–114.

Henley JD, Geary WA, Jackson CL, Wu CD, Gnepp DR. Dedifferentiated acinic cell carcinoma of the parotid gland: a distinct rarely described entity. *Hum Pathol* 1997;28:869–873.

Kamoi S, AlJuboury MI, Akin MR, Silverberg SG. Immunohistochemical staining in the distinction between primary endometrial and endocervical adenocarcinomas: another viewpoint. *Int J Gynecol Pathol* 2002;21:217–223.

Klaes R, Friedrich T, Spitkovsky D, et al. Overexpression of p16^{ink4a} as a specific marker for dysplastic and neoplastic epithelial cells of the cervix uteri. *Int J Cancer* 2001;92:276–284.

Kurman R, Norris H. Evaluation of criteria for distinguishing atypical endometrial hyperplasia from well-differentiated carcinoma. *Cancer* 1982;49:2547–2559.

Lee KR, Scully RE. Mucinous tumors of the ovary. *Am J Surg Pathol* 2000;24:1447–1464.

Lee KR, Young RH. The distinction between primary and metastatic mucinous carcinomas of the ovary: gross and histologic findings in 50 cases. *Am J Surg Pathol* 2003;27:281–292.

Ludwig CL, Gilks CB, Haziji H, Clement PB. Aggressive behavior of stage I ovarian mucinous tumors without destructive stromal invasion. *Mod Pathol* 2004;17(Suppl 1):205A.

Malpica A, Deavers MT, Lu K, et al. Grading ovarian serous carcinoma using a two-tier system. *Am J Surg Pathol* 2004;28:496–504.

McCusker ME, Cote TR, Cleg LX, Tavassoli FJ. Endocrine tumors of the uterine cervix: incidence, demographics, and survival with comparison to squamous cell carcinoma. *Gynecol Oncol* 2003;88:333–339.

Miyagi J, Tsuhako K, Kinjo T, Iwamasa T, Hashimoto H, Ishikawa S. Rhabdoid tumour of the lung is a dedifferentiated phenotype of pulmonary adenocarcinoma. *Histopathology* 2000;37:37-44.

Norris H, Tavassoli FA, Kurman R. Endometrial hyperplasia and carcinoma. *Am J Surg Pathol* 1983;8:839–847.

Prat J, de Nictolis M. Serous borderline tumors of the ovary. A long-term follow-up study of 137 cases, including 18 with a micropapillary pattern and 20 with microinvasion. *Am J Surg Pathol* 2002;26:1111–1128.

Prat J, Scully RE. Cellular fibromas and fibrosarcomas of the ovary: a comparative clinicopathologic analysis of seventeen cases. *Cancer* 1981;47:2663–2670.

Riopel MA, Ronnett BM, Kurman RJ. Evaluation of diagnostic criteria and behavior of ovarian intestinal-type mucinous tumors: atypical proliferative (borderline) tumors and intraepithelial, microinvasive, invasive, and metastatic carcinomas. *Am J Surg Pathol* 1999;23:617–635.

Rodriguez I, Prat J. Mucinous tumors of the ovary. *Am J Surg Pathol* 2002;26:139–152.

Santos M, Montagut C, Mellado B, et al. Immunohistochemical staining for p16 and p53 in premalignant and malignant epithelial lesions of the vulva. *Int J Gynecol Pathol* 2004;23:206–214.

Sato Y, Shimamoto T, Amada S, Asada Y, Hayashi T. Large cell neuroendocrine carcinoma of the uterine cervix: a clinicopathological study of six cases. *Int J Gynecol Pathol* 2003;22:226–230.

Seidman JD, Kurman RJ. Ovarian serous borderline tumors: a critical review of the literature with emphasis on prognostic indicators. *Hum Pathol* 2000;31:539–557.

Seidman JD, Kurman RJ, Ronnett BM. Primary and metastatic mucinous adenocarcinomas in the ovaries: incidence in routine practice with a new approach to improve intraoperative diagnosis. *Am J Surg Pathol* 2003;27:985–993.

Shimizu Y, Kamoi S, Amada S, et al. Toward the development of a universal grading system for ovarian epithelial carcinoma. I. Prognostic significance of histopathologic features—problems involved in the architectural grading system. *Gynecol Oncol* 1998;70:2–12.

Silverberg SG, Kurman RJ, Nogales F, Mutter GL, Kubik-Huch RA, Tavassoli FA. Tumors of the uterine corpus. Epithelial tumors and related lesions. In: Tavassoli FA, Devilee P, eds. *World Health Organization Classification of Tumors.*

Pathology and Genetics of Tumors of the Breast and Female Genital Organs. Lyon: IARC Press; 2002:221–232.

Speert H. The premalignant phase of endometrial carcinoma. *Cancer* 1952;5:927.

Staebler A, Sherman ME, Zaino R, Ronnett B. Hormone receptor immunohisto-chemistry and human papillomavirus in situ hybridization are useful for dis-tinguishing endocervical and endometrial adenocarcinomas. *Am J Surg Pathol* 2002;26:998–1006.

Tsuji T, Kawauchi S, Utsunomiya T, Nagata Y, Tsuneyoshi M. Fibrosarcoma versus cellular fibroma of the ovary. *Am J Surg Pathol* 1997;21:52–59.

Yang B, Hart WR. Vulvar intraepithelial neoplasia of the simplex (differentiated) type. A clinicopathologic study including analysis of HPV and p53 expression. *Am J Surg Pathol* 2000;24:429–441.

5 IMAGING OF GYNECOLOGIC MALIGNANCIES

Revathy Iyer

CHAPTER OUTLINE

CHAPTER OVERVIEW

Imaging studies are used to help in the diagnosis, initial staging, and follow-up of patients with gynecologic malignancies, including cervical, endometrial, and ovarian cancer. The imaging modalities currently used for evaluating patients with gynecologic cancer include pelvic ultrasonography, computed tomography (CT), magnetic resonance imaging (MRI), and positron emission tomography using 2-[^{18}F]fluoro-2-deoxy-D-glucose (FDG-PET). There are advantages and disadvantages to each of these modalities. Ultrasonography and MRI use no ionizing radiation. CT and MRI provide excellent anatomic detail. FDG-PET provides total body coverage and physiologic information, which is particularly valuable when evaluating for the presence of metastatic disease.

The clinical staging of cervical cancer can be difficult in some patients. Imaging can be used to supplement clinical findings, and MRI, with its superior soft tissue resolution, is probably best suited for imaging cervical cancer and local spread in the pelvis. Endometrial cancer is a disease of postmenopausal women and the most common gynecologic malignancy in women. Given that many patients present with dysfunctional uterine bleeding, which is an early sign of the disease, imaging studies are often not performed before surgical staging once the diagnosis has been established. Imaging techniques such as sonohysterography can be helpful, however, for guiding interventional diagnostic procedures. Also, imaging can be used to determine the extent of disease in patients with more advanced disease. Ovarian cancer has the highest mortality rate among gynecologic cancers. Imaging procedures can help confirm the presence of a pelvic mass and determine whether it is ovarian in origin. Characterization of ovarian lesions is important, and pelvic ultrasonography is particularly helpful in this regard. Features on imaging that are suggestive of malignancy include complex cystic masses, which have soft tissue thickening or nodularity, and solid masses. MRI can be used to evaluate sonographically indeterminate masses. Once a diagnosis of ovarian cancer is made, imaging can be used to assist in staging the disease. Surgical staging remains essential, but imaging studies such as CT can provide additional useful baseline information. Ascites, lymphadenopathy, and peritoneal deposits of disease, as well as hematogenous metastases to other organs, can be seen on imaging studies. CT is probably the most widely used imaging technique for staging ovarian cancer.

INTRODUCTION

The evolution of imaging techniques over the past few decades has occurred at an astounding pace, and we now have an armamentarium of imaging studies with which to examine the human body. These imaging techniques may be used as tools in the diagnosis, staging, and follow-up of oncology patients. The ever-increasing complexity of diagnostic radiology challenges radiologists and oncologists to use these tools in a clinically efficient and cost-effective manner, with the ultimate goal being a safe and effective examination that provides clinically relevant information for the treatment of an individual patient. Imaging modalities that are presently being used to evaluate patients with gynecologic cancers include ultrasonography (US), computed tomography (CT), magnetic resonance imaging (MRI), and positron emission tomography (PET). This chapter will provide an overview of clinically available imaging techniques and their relative strengths and weaknesses and also discuss the roles of specific imaging techniques in the diagnosis and management of common gynecologic malignancies such as cervical cancer, endometrial cancer, and ovarian cancer.

IMAGING MODALITIES

US

US relies on the piezoelectric effect, which is produced when energy is applied to a piezoelectric crystal, resulting in mechanical vibration of the crystal and production of sound waves that are transmitted through tissues and detected on US imaging. The development of high-frequency US probes with excellent resolution has improved the diagnostic accuracy of demonstrating both normal anatomy and pathologic states in the female pelvis. US is both widely available and cost-effective and therefore is typically the initial imaging modality used in evaluating patients with a pelvic mass. Doppler imaging techniques, especially color Doppler, may be used to assess the vascularity of the pelvis and pelvic masses. Three-dimensional US is now available and can reliably measure the volume of ovarian and endometrial tumors (Pretorius et al, 2001).

When a pelvic mass is found by US, it may be characterized by its size, location (uterine or extrauterine), external contour (well-defined versus ill-defined or irregular), and internal consistency (cystic, solid, or complex). Although a specific diagnosis cannot be made in many instances, a more limited differential diagnosis may be given.

Standard transabdominal US is performed with the patient's urinary bladder distended. The bladder provides an acoustic window through which to view the pelvic organs and serves as an internal standard for evaluating cystic structures in the pelvis. The distended bladder also displaces bowel loops out of the pelvis. Typically, 3.5-MHz transducers are used for transabdominal US. Imaging of the uterus and adnexa is performed in both the sagittal and transverse planes. Transabdominal US of the pelvis is limited in patients who are unable to fill the bladder, in obese patients, and in patients with a retroverted uterus in whom the fundus is located beyond the focal zone of the transducer.

Transvaginal US is performed with the patient's urinary bladder empty so that the pelvic organs are in the focal zone of the transvaginal probe. Transvaginal transducers are higher in frequency than those used for transabdominal US, typically 5 to 7.5 MHz. Transvaginal US provides superior resolution of pelvic structures and greater detail of the characteristics of pelvic masses. The main disadvantage of transvaginal US is the limited field of view allowed by the transducer, making large masses or masses high in the pelvis difficult to evaluate.

Sonohysterography is performed by first instilling fluid to distend the endometrial cavity and then using transvaginal US to image the endometrial lining. This technique may be used to more optimally image and define endometrial pathology and thereby guide decisions regarding interventions such as hysteroscopy and endometrial biopsy or curettage (Laing et al, 2001).

CT

Helical CT images are obtained as the movements of the CT table and radiation exposure occur simultaneously, resulting in the creation of a helical or spiral data set. These data are then interpolated to reconstruct transaxial slices. High-quality reformations in other two-dimensional planes, such as the sagittal or coronal plane, may then be produced. Three-dimensional reformations can also be produced (Brink, 1995). The advent of helical scanners, which allow very rapid, high-resolution imaging of the body in the span of a single breath-hold, has revolutionized CT imaging. For example, the entire abdomen and pelvis can now be scanned in 30 seconds or less.

For imaging pelvic malignancies, helical CT is usually performed after the oral and rectal administration of contrast material to outline large and small bowel loops. Iodinated intravenous contrast is necessary for the adequate delineation of abdominal and pelvic structures. CT scans are obtained approximately 50 seconds after intravenous contrast is administered to allow for maximum opacification of pelvic organs. Scans are typically obtained with a collimation or slice thickness of 5 mm or less and reconstruction intervals of 5 mm (Pannu et al, 2001).

The disadvantages of CT are the cost, the radiation exposure, and the inability to use this modality in patients in whom iodinated contrast material is contraindicated because of allergy or renal insufficiency.

MRI

MRI is an extremely useful tool for imaging the female pelvis because it does not require ionizing radiation and provides superior soft tissue contrast resolution. Images can be obtained using a body coil or a phased array coil, which usually provides superior images because of its higher signal-to-noise ratio. Images are obtained in coronal, axial, and sagittal planes. Off-axis imaging also can be performed for better evaluation of specific pelvic structures. T1- and T2-weighted images are typically obtained, with T2-weighted images providing excellent soft tissue definition of normal anatomy and disease in the pelvis. Intravenous gadolinium contrast may be used to further delineate specific disease states.

Patients with pacemakers or other devices and certain metallic implants cannot undergo MRI. Patients with severe claustrophobia and those unable to remain still for an extended period may require sedation before MRI can be performed.

PET

PET is a metabolic imaging technique and therefore differs from cross-sectional imaging modalities such as US, CT, and MRI that primarily provide morphologic information. Increased glucose metabolism in tumors has been observed, and the glucose analogue 2-[^{18}F]fluoro-2-deoxy-D-glucose (FDG) is the most commonly used agent for PET imaging. FDG is widely available and has a favorable half-life of 110 minutes. There is also high uptake of FDG in most cancers. Malignant cells have enhanced glycolysis, and once taken up by tumor cells and phosphorylated, FDG becomes trapped in the cell. Glucose-6-phosphatase, which mediates dephosphorylation, has a low concentration in many tumors. Factors that increase FDG uptake include the following: intact vascular supply, high mitotic rate, high number of tumor cells or high volume of tumor, tumor hypoxia, and a lesser degree of cellular differentiation. Patient preparation is important before performing FDG-labeled PET scans. Patients must fast for at least 6 hours, and their last meal should be high in protein and low in carbohydrates. Diabetics must have well-controlled blood sugar levels. Because PET provides information about metabolic activity rather than morphology, it can be valuable for assessing both primary and metastatic tumors.

CERVICAL CANCER

Cancer of the uterine cervix ranks as the third most common gynecologic malignancy and is associated with significant morbidity and mortality (Jemal et al, 2002). Once a diagnosis of invasive cervical cancer is made, accurate staging is of great importance for treatment planning. Clinical staging relies primarily on physical examination, which may be difficult in some patients, such as those with advanced disease. Imaging is used to supplement clinical examination, especially in patients who are difficult to examine clinically.

US is of limited use in the staging of cervical malignancies because its low-contrast-resolution images do not allow reliable distinction of the tumor from surrounding normal tissues. Endoluminal US probes, such as transvaginal or transrectal probes, have been used to assess local disease spread but are considered inadequate for detecting nodal and pelvic side-wall involvement. CT has a role in the evaluation of advanced cervical disease and nodal involvement and in surveillance for distant metastasis; however, in general, CT is considered to inaccurately define cervical and uterine disease (Subak et al, 1995).

MRI, with its superior soft tissue contrast resolution and multiplanar capabilities, is well suited for imaging cervical cancer. The overall accuracy of MRI in the staging of cervical cancer is reported to be about 90% (Hricak et al, 1988; Subak et al, 1995). Currently, MRI is recommended for imaging of cervical cancer in the following cases: (1) tumors with a transverse diameter greater than 2 cm on physical examination, (2) endocervical or infiltrative tumors that cannot be accurately evaluated clinically, and (3) patients in whom clinical examination is difficult, such as those who have other uterine lesions such as leiomyomas or who are pregnant (Ascher et al, 2001).

T2-weighted MRI images, obtained without a contrast agent, provide excellent detail of normal uterine and cervical anatomy and clearly define the primary tumor and its extent (Figure 5–1). The overall reported accuracy of T2-weighted MRI in predicting tumor size is 93% (Subak et al, 1995). On T2-weighted images, cervical tumors typically have a higher signal intensity than the surrounding stroma. Parametrial invasion by a cervical tumor is an important factor in determining whether a patient will be a candidate for surgery. The negative predictive value of MRI in the identification of parametrial invasion is reported to be about 95% (Subak et al, 1995). When the fibrocervical stroma surrounding the tumor are seen to be intact on imaging, parametrial spread is easily excluded. On the other hand, the positive predictive value of MRI in the identification of parametrial invasion is considerably lower because peritumoral reactive changes cannot be easily distinguished from invasive tumor by imaging (Ascher et al, 2001). Endocervical tumors may be difficult to evaluate

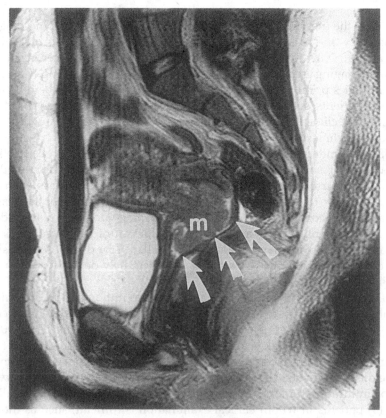

Figure 5–1. Sagittal T2-weighted MRI of stage IB2 cervical cancer in a 21-year-old woman. The tumor (m) is exophytic and protrudes into the vagina (arrows).

clinically, but they are clearly identifiable on MRI. Stromal invasion by the primary tumor is also well delineated by MRI, especially when the primary tumor is covered by normal-appearing epithelium (Ascher et al, 2001).

It is not yet clear whether the use of a contrast agent, such as gadolinium, with MRI for the staging of cervical cancer is advantageous. Most radiologists agree that delayed-contrast-enhanced images provide little advantage over non-contrast-enhanced images, except when invasion of an adjacent organ is suspected. Dynamic gadolinium-enhanced images may be useful for defining small cervical lesions, detecting or confirming the invasion of adjacent organs, and identifying fistulous tracts. The overall accuracy of MRI for determining bladder wall invasion is greater than 90% (Kim and Han, 1997). Dynamic gadolinium-enhanced imaging may also be useful for determining the degree of tumor microcirculation and perfusion, which could help predict which tumors will be more responsive to therapy (Yamashita et al, 2000).

MRI has been shown to be a cost-effective method of staging cervical cancer. In a study by Hricak et al (1996), patients with cervical cancer who underwent MRI as the initial imaging procedure for staging required fewer subsequent tests and procedures than did those who underwent standard clinical staging. As a result, the cost of treating the patients who underwent MRI was significantly less, not only because fewer procedures were required but also because the patients' overall treatment was modified on the basis of the MRI findings.

In summary, MRI has been shown to facilitate the accurate determination of cervical tumor size or volume and stage, especially in cases of advanced disease.

PET findings have been shown to be a better predictor of survival than CT scans in patients with carcinoma of the cervix (Grigsby et al, 2001). Grigsby et al found that the 2-year progression-free survival rate was 64% in patients who had negative CT and PET scans, 18% in patients who had a negative CT scan but a positive PET scan, and 14% in patients who had positive CT and PET scans. FDG-PET is not particularly helpful in evaluating primary disease in the pelvis but has been used successfully to detect metastatic lymphadenopathy in patients with advanced cervical cancer.

ENDOMETRIAL CANCER

Endometrial cancer is the most common invasive gynecologic malignancy, afflicting more than 30,000 women a year (Jemal et al, 2002). Most patients present with dysfunctional postmenopausal uterine bleeding, which is an early sign of the disease; overall, more than 75% of patients have stage I disease at presentation. Surgery is the primary method of staging for endometrial cancer, and organ-confined disease is typically treated with surgical resection. Radiation therapy and chemotherapy are used to treat patients with inoperable disease, and imaging can play a role in defining the extent of the tumor in these patients (Hawner, 1998).

Transvaginal US is frequently used to determine the presence of endometrial thickening in patients with postmenopausal bleeding and thereby select patients for interventional diagnostic procedures such as dilatation and curettage. The appearance of endometrial thickening on transvaginal US is not specific to the diagnosis of endometrial cancer; differential diagnoses that must be considered in a patient with endometrial thickening include endometrial polyps, hyperplasia, and carcinoma (Hulka et al, 1994). Imaging findings that are suggestive of malignancy are (1) diffuse endometrial thickening, (2) endometrial thickening with a heterogeneous echotexture and irregular or poorly defined margins, and (3) a heterogeneous mass-like lesion (Reinhold and Khalili, 2002). Doppler blood flow measurements are sometimes used to distinguish between benign and malignant causes of endometrial thickening, but the technique is considered by most radiologists to have poor specificity (Flam et al, 1995).

On sonohysterography, endometrial cancer typically appears as a broad-based mass. The overall sensitivity, specificity, positive predictive value, and negative predictive value of sonohysterography in patients with endometrial cancer are 89%, 46%, 16%, and 97%, respectively (Dubinsky et al, 1999). Direct extension of endometrial tumor into the myometrium is an important prognostic factor, and the depth of tumor infiltration assessed using transvaginal US correlates with histologic findings in about 85% of cases (Weber et al, 1995). On sonohysterographic images, an intact subendometrium is suggestive of localized disease, whereas extension of heterogeneity and increased echogenicity in the myometrium are suggestive of invasive endometrial carcinoma (Karlsson et al, 1995). The assessment of tumor extension beyond the uterus and evaluation of pelvic lymph nodes are suboptimal with US.

CT with intravenous contrast typically shows endometrial cancers as hypodense lesions in the endometrial cavity or myometrium. Tumors may obstruct the endocervical canal and appear as a fluid-filled uterus. In some cases, contrast-enhanced lesions within the myometrium may be seen. Cervical enlargement, suggesting tumor extension into the cervix, may also be seen on CT (Hawner, 1998). The overall accuracy of conventional CT in the identification of stage I or II endometrial disease is about 76% (Dore et al, 1987). CT is considered more useful for imaging advanced disease that extends beyond the uterus and associated adenopathy in the pelvis and retroperitoneum. The limitations of CT in the imaging of endometrial cancer are (1) it is difficult to differentiate small leiomyomas from uterine carcinoma, (2) the extent of myometrial invasion, especially in elderly women with atrophic myometrium, cannot be reliably determined, and (3) microscopic tumor extending beyond the uterus or within the lymph nodes cannot be detected (Hawner, 1998).

MRI is similar to US and CT in that a diagnosis of endometrial cancer cannot be made on the basis of the appearance of abnormal endometrial thickening alone. MRI is appropriate when a histologic diagnosis has been made and the tumor is of high grade, when there is a clinical suspicion of advanced disease, or when the patient is considered a poor candidate for surgery and the imaging findings may affect treatment (Hawner, 1998). T2-weighted images can estimate the depth of myometrial invasion with an overall accuracy of up to 85% (Hricak et al, 1991). Overestimation of myometrial invasion is responsible for more errors than underestimation (Hawner, 1998). The use of dynamic gadolinium-enhanced imaging allows for the distinction between viable tumor and necrotic or hemorrhagic debris in the endometrial cavity and improves the differentiation between tumor and normal myometrium, with a reported accuracy of up to 92% (Joja et al, 1996). MRI can also demonstrate disease extension beyond the uterus and associated lymphadenopathy. MRI is therefore probably at present the most accurate modality for the pretreatment evaluation of patients with endometrial cancer.

Ovarian Cancer

Ovarian cancer accounts for approximately 4% of all cancers in women and is the most common cause of death from gynecologic malignancy (Jemal et al, 2002). Surgical exploration is typically performed in patients with ovarian cancer to confirm the histologic diagnosis and disease stage and to debulk the tumor. Adjuvant chemotherapy may be administered to treat residual disease. The presence of bulky disease at some sites may preclude adequate debulking, and 1 of the major challenges in oncologic imaging today is the accurate detection and delineation of the extent of ovarian malignancy. Imaging is important in the management of ovarian cancer because it allows for the characterization of ovarian masses, the identification of metastatic disease to prevent understaging of disease, and the identification of patients who may be candidates for neoadjuvant chemotherapy (Coakley, 2002).

Imaging plays a role in confirming the presence of a pelvic mass, determining its site of origin, and characterizing the mass. Transvaginal US is often the first modality used to determine the origin and characteristics of a pelvic mass. Most ovarian malignancies are epithelial in origin and appear as cystic adnexal masses with irregular internal solid components (Coakley, 2002). The sonographic features suggestive of malignancy are a homogeneous solid mass, a complex cystic or solid mass, soft tissue thickening or nodularity extending from the walls of a cystic mass, and the presence of ascites or peritoneal nodules (Sohaid et al, 1998; Coakley,

2002). Although these features are useful, absolute characterization of malignancy and accurate prediction of tumor histology are not possible with US or any other imaging technique. Color flow Doppler techniques have been used to complement the morphologic information provided by grayscale US and to demonstrate tumor vascularity, although there is some overlap between the flow characteristics of benign and malignant lesions (Brown et al, 1994). Once a diagnosis of ovarian malignancy is confirmed, staging is difficult with US, and the reported accuracy is 60% or less (Khan et al, 1986).

The appearance of ovarian tumors on CT varies according to the histology of the tumor. The overall accuracy of CT for the detection of ovarian masses approaches 95%, while the specificity of CT in distinguishing benign versus malignant lesions ranges between 66% and 94% (Buy et al, 1991; Johnson, 1993). As with US, morphologic findings on CT such as cystic masses with septations, nodules, vegetations, or papillary projections and necrosis within solid masses suggest malignancy; however, the features of ovarian masses on CT are also not entirely specific (Sohaid et al, 1998).

CT is probably the most widely used imaging technique for staging of ovarian cancer (Figure 5–2). Opacification of the gastrointestinal tract is essential to distinguish peritoneal implants from the bowel and to determine the presence of bowel invasion. Intravenous contrast is important in defining the solid viscera in the abdomen and pelvis as well as more clearly delineating peritoneal deposits. Ascites and lymphadenopathy in the pelvis and retroperitoneum are well demonstrated by CT. The detection of peritoneal tumor deposits is largely dependent on their location, their size, and the presence of ascites or calcification, which increases their conspicuity (Sohaid et al, 1998). The overall sensitivity of conventional CT in the diagnosis of peritoneal metastases in ovarian cancer is on the order of 63% to 79%, with a reported specificity approaching 100% (Buy et al, 1988; Jacquet et al, 1993). Recent studies suggest that the use of helical CT improves the lesion detection rate to about 90%, which may be owing to technical considerations such as the thinner sections that can be obtained with the helical technique (Coakley, 2002). Lesions measuring 1 cm or less are still difficult to detect, however.

MRI is often used to characterize adnexal masses that have an indeterminate appearance on US and CT. The presence of fat or hemorrhaging in benign ovarian masses such as teratomas or hemorrhagic cysts is easily confirmed with MRI. The overall accuracy of MRI in distinguishing benign from malignant ovarian masses ranges between 60% and 90% (Outwater and Dunton, 1995).

In patients with a diagnosis of ovarian cancer, extraovarian spread of tumor within the pelvis is well characterized by MRI. However, MRI is used less frequently than CT for the evaluation of abdominal metastasis because CT is less expensive and more widely available. Peritoneal

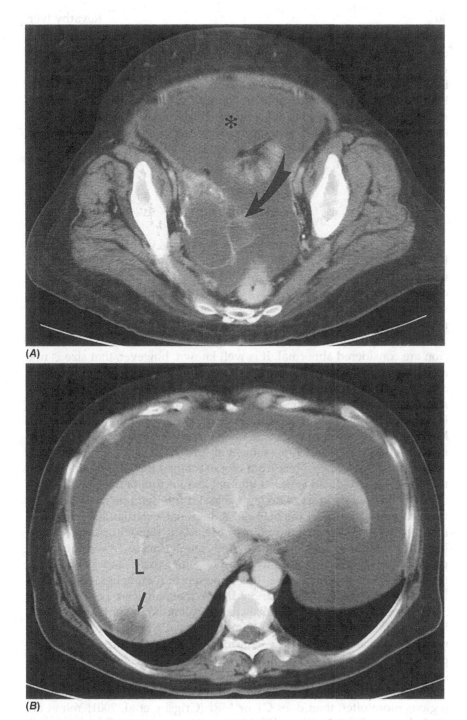

Figure 5–2. Axial CT images of stage IIIC serous carcinoma of the ovary in a 59-year-old woman. (*A*) The primary tumor in the pelvis (curved arrow) and ascites (*). (*B*) Perihepatic implant (arrow) at the dome of the liver (L).

deposits larger than 1 cm can be detected with MRI if optimal technique is used, including oral and intravenous contrast agents to define the bowel, fat suppression, and fast sequences that may be performed with breath-holding. Mesenteric and bowel wall implants are still probably more readily detected with CT, and calcified deposits are more clearly seen on CT than on MRI. Given its wider availability and greater ease of performance, CT is considered the modality of choice for staging ovarian cancer (Sohaid et al, 1998).

LYMPHADENOPATHY

The presence of lymph node metastasis in patients with a known gyneco-logic malignancy often affects treatment decisions. For example, nodal metastases are not incorporated into the clinical staging system for cervi-cal cancer, but they are very important in determining prognosis. Cross-sectional imaging techniques such as CT and MRI use nodal size as the primary criterion for determining the presence of metastatic disease within a lymph node. Nodes that are larger than 1 cm in short-axis dimen-sion are considered abnormal. It is well known, however, that size is not an ideal criterion for determining the presence or absence of tumor within a node. Enlarged nodes may be hyperplastic, and nodes smaller than 1 cm may contain tumor. The presence of central necrosis within a lymph node is a useful predictor of metastatic disease. The overall accuracy of both MRI and CT in determining lymph node metastases in cervical carcinoma ranges between 85% and 90% (Yang et al, 2000).

Lymphangiography differs from cross-sectional imaging modalities in that it allows visualization of the internal architecture of opacified lymph nodes. Iodinated contrast material is injected into lymphatic channels in the feet, which transport the material to inguinal, external iliac, common iliac, and retroperitoneal lymph nodes. Metastatic tumor appears as a fill-ing defect within an opacified node. Both the performance and the inter-pretation of lymphangiography require time, skill, and experience. Because very few centers have this experience, lymphangiography has largely been replaced by CT and MRI. A meta-analysis performed by Scheidler et al (1997) suggests that the overall accuracy of CT, MRI, and lymphangiography in the evaluation of metastatic disease in the lymph nodes is similar. These authors consider CT and MRI superior to lym-phangiography for lymph node evaluation, however, because these stud-ies are less invasive.

Some studies have shown that PET detects abnormal lymph node regions more often than does CT or MRI (Grigsby et al, 2001; Yeh et al, 2002; Lin et al, 2003). Since FDG-PET relies on detection of increased metabolic activity within metastatic lymph nodes, it can help detect dis-ease in lymph nodes that are considered normal in size on CT or MRI.

KEY PRACTICE POINTS

- US is typically the initial imaging modality used in evaluating patients with a pelvic mass. When a pelvic mass is found on US, it may be characterized by its size, location, external contour, and internal consistency.

- When a diagnosis of cervical cancer has been made, MRI has been shown to accurately assess tumor volume and stage, especially in cases of advanced disease. MRI is recommended for patients with cervical cancer in the following cases: (1) tumors with a transverse diameter greater than 2 cm on physical examination, (2) endocervical or infiltrative tumors that cannot be accurately evaluated clinically, and (3) patients in whom clinical examination is difficult, such as those who have other uterine lesions such as leiomyomas or who are pregnant.

- Dynamic gadolinium-enhanced MRI differentiates between invasive endometrial tumor and normal myometrium more accurately than US or CT. MRI can also demonstrate disease extension beyond the uterus and associated lymphadenopathy. Therefore, MRI is the best modality for the pretreatment evaluation of endometrial cancer.

- CT is probably the most widely used imaging technique for the staging of ovarian cancer. Metastatic implants from ovarian cancer measuring 1 cm or less are still difficult to detect by any imaging modality, however.

- Cross-sectional imaging techniques such as CT and MRI rely on nodal size as the primary criterion for determining the presence of metastatic disease within lymph nodes. The overall accuracy of CT and MRI in the detection of metastatic disease in lymph nodes is reported to be about 85%. Metabolic imaging with PET is also useful for detecting metastatic lymph nodes in patients with pelvic malignancies.

SUGGESTED READINGS

Ascher SM, Takahama J, Jha RC. Staging of gynecologic malignancies. *Top Magn Reson Imaging* 2001;12:105–129.

Brink JA. Technical aspects of helical (spiral) CT. *Radiol Clin North Am* 1995;33:825–841.

Brown DL, Frates MC, Laing FC, et al. Ovarian masses: can benign and malignant lesions be differentiated with color and pulsed Doppler US? *Radiology* 1994;190:333–336.

Buy JN, Ghossain MA, Sciot C, et al. Epithelial tumors of the ovary: CT findings and correlation with US. *Radiology* 1991;178:811–818.

Buy JN, Moss AA, Ghossain MA, et al. Peritoneal implants from ovarian tumors: CT findings. *Radiology* 1988;169:691–694.

Coakley FV. Staging ovarian cancer: role of imaging. *Radiol Clin N Am* 2002;40:609–636.

Dore R, Moro G, D'Andrea F, et al. CT evaluation of myometrial invasion in endometrial carcinoma. *J Comput Assist Tomogr* 1987;11:282–289.

Dubinsky TJ, Stroehlein K, Abu-Ghazzeh Y, Parvey HR, Maklad N. Prediction of benign and malignant endometrial disease: hysterosonographic-pathologic correlation. *Radiology* 1999;210:393–397.

Flam F, Almstrom H, Hellstrom AC, Moberger B. Value of uterine artery Doppler in endometrial cancer. *Acta Oncol* 1995;34:779–782.

Grigsby PW, Siegel BA, Dehdashti F. Lymph node staging by positron emission tomography in patients with carcinoma of the cervix. *J Clin Oncol* 2001;19:3745–3749.

Hawner J. Uterine and cervical tumors. In: Husband JES, Reznek RH, eds. *Imaging in Oncology*. 1st ed. Oxford, UK: Isis Medical Media Ltd.; 1998:309–328.

Hricak H, Lacey CG, Sandles LG, et al. Invasive cervical carcinoma: comparison of MR imaging and surgical findings. *Radiology* 1988;166:623–631.

Hricak H, Powell CB, Yu KK, et al. Invasive cervical carcinoma: role of MR imaging in pretreatment work-up-cost minimization and diagnostic efficacy analysis. *Radiology* 1996;198:403–409.

Hricak H, Rubinstein LV, Gherman GM, et al. MR imaging evaluation of endometrial carcinoma: results of an NCI co-operative study. *Radiology* 1991;179:829–832.

Hulka CA, Hall DA, McCarthy K, et al. Endometrial polyps, hyperplasia and carcinoma in post-menopausal women: differentiation with endovaginal sonography. *Radiology* 1994;191:755–758.

Jacquet P, Jelinek JS, Steves MA, et al. Evaluation of computed tomography in patients with peritoneal carcinomatosis. *Cancer* 1993;72:1631–1636.

Jemal A, Thomas A, Murray T, Thun M. Cancer statistics, 2002. *CA Cancer J Clin* 2002;52:23–47.

Johnson RJ. Radiology in the management of ovarian cancer (review). *Clin Radiol* 1993;48:75–82.

Joja K, Asakawa M, Asakawa T, et al. Endometrial carcinoma: dynamic MRI with Turbo-FLASH technique. *J Comput Assist Tomogr* 1996;20:878–887.

Karlsson B, Gransberg S, Wikland M, et al. Transvaginal ultrasonography of the endometrium in women with postmenopausal bleeding: a Nordic multicenter study. *Am J Obstet Gynecol* 1995;172:1488–1494.

Khan O, Cosgrove DO, Fried AM, et al. Ovarian carcinoma follow-up: US versus laparotomy. *Radiology* 1986;159:111–113.

Kim SH, Han MC. Invasion of the urinary bladder by uterine cervical carcinoma: evaluation with MR imaging. *AJR Am J Roentgenol* 1997;168:393–397.

Laing FC, Brown DL, DiSalvo DN. Gynecologic ultrasound. *Radiol Clin North Am* 2001;39:523–540.

Lin WC, Hung YC, Yeh LS, et al. Usefulness of (18)F-fluorodeoxyglucose positron emission tomography to detect para-aortic lymph nodal metastasis in advanced cervical cancer with negative computed tomography findings. *Gynecol Oncol* 2003;89:73–76.

Outwater EK, Dunton CJ. Imaging of the ovary and adnexa: clinical issues and application of MR imaging [review]. *Radiology* 1995;194:1–18.

Pannu HK, Corl FM, Fishman EK. CT evaluation of cervical cancer: spectrum of disease. *Radiographics* 2001;21:1155–1168.

Pretorius DH, Borok NN, Coffler MS, Nelson TR. Three-dimensional ultrasound in obstetrics and gynecology. *Radiol Clin North Am* 2001;39:499–521.

Reinhold C, Khalili I. Postmenopausal bleeding: value of imaging. *Radiol Clin North Am* 2002;40:527–562.

Scheidler J, Hricak H, Yu KK, Subak L, Segal MR. Radiological evaluation of lymph node metastases in patients with cervical cancer: a meta-analysis. *JAMA* 1997;278:1096–1101.

Sohaid S, Reznek R, Husband J. Ovarian cancer. In: Husband JES, Reznek RH, eds. *Imaging in Oncology.* 1st ed. Oxford, UK: Isis Medical Media Ltd.; 1998:277–308.

Subak LL, Hricak H, Powell CB, et al. Cervical carcinoma: computed tomography and magnetic resonance imaging for preoperative staging. *Obstet Gynecol* 1995;86:43–50.

Weber G, Merz E, Bahlmann F, et al. Assessment of myometrial infiltration and preoperative staging by transvaginal ultrasound in patients with endometrial carcinoma. *Ultrasound Obstet Gynecol* 1995;6:362–367.

Yamashita Y, Baba T, Baba Y, et al. Dynamic contrast-enhanced MR imaging of uterine cervical cancer: pharmacokinetic analysis with histopathologic correlation and its importance in predicting the outcome of radiation therapy. *Radiology* 2000;216:803–809.

Yang WT, Lam WWM, Yu MY, et al. Comparison of dynamic helical CT and dynamic MR imaging in the evaluation of pelvic lymph nodes in cervical carcinoma. *AJR Am J Roentgenol* 2000;175:759–768.

Yeh LS, Hung YC, Shen YY, et al. Detecting para-aortic lymph nodal metastasis by positron emission tomography of 18F-fluorodeoxyglucose in advanced cervical cancer with negative magnetic resonance imaging findings. *Oncol Rep* 2002;9:1289–1292.

6 CONTEMPORARY TREATMENT OF VAGINAL AND VULVAR CANCERS

Patricia J. Eifel and Thomas W. Burke

CHAPTER OUTLINE

CHAPTER OVERVIEW

Vaginal and vulvar cancers are very rare neoplasms, occurring in fewer than 2 women per 100,000 annually. These cancers are most effectively treated by a multidisciplinary team with expertise in the specialized surgical and radiotherapeutic techniques needed to achieve high rates of local control and cure with minimal morbidity.

Very small superficial vaginal cancers, particularly those involving the apical vagina, may be treated successfully with surgical excision alone. However, definitive organ-sparing surgery is rarely possible for more advanced lesions; these are usually treated with radiation therapy alone. Radiation therapy fields include the primary tumor site and regional lymph nodes. If tumor involves the distal third of the vagina, the inguinal lymph nodes should be included in the treatment fields. The radiation dose to the primary tumor site is supplemented with 1 of a variety of intracavitary or interstitial radiation therapy techniques or with conformal external-beam therapy; careful treatment planning is required to assure adequate tumor coverage. At M. D. Anderson Cancer Center, 10-year tumor control rates of 70% to 80% for stage I and II and 40% to 50% for stage III disease have been achieved with radiation therapy alone. Today, high-risk cases are sometimes treated with concurrent chemoradiation, on the basis of the improved survival rates achieved with this approach in patients with cervical cancer.

For patients with vulvar carcinomas, the selection of locoregional treatment is based on the extent of disease in the vulva and in the regional lymph nodes. Vulvar intraepithelial neoplasia can usually be treated with local excision or laser ablation if invasion has been ruled out. Minimally invasive T1a tumors may be treated with local excision alone. All other tumors require inguinal lymph node dissection or radiation therapy as well as definitive treatment of the vulva. T1 and some small T2 tumors are effectively treated with radical wide excision and inguinal lymph node dissection. Today we recommend dissection of the superficial and medial femoral lymph nodes; simple excision of enlarged nodes may be preferred if postoperative radiation therapy is planned, as this may reduce the morbidity of combined therapy in the groin.

Patients who have positive lymph nodes or whose vulvar cancers cannot be widely resected (i.e., resected with 2-cm tumor-free margins) without compromising bowel or bladder function require radiation therapy. Postoperative radiation therapy improves regional disease control and survival in patients with positive inguinal lymph nodes. Advanced vulvar cancers that involve or are immediately adjacent to the anus or urethra are usually treated with radiation therapy, preferably with concurrent chemotherapy. In most cases, a total dose of 60 to 65 Gy is sufficient to achieve local disease control; however, patients are followed up closely to ensure timely detection of local recurrences that may be successfully treated with surgical resection. Although the groin may also be treated effectively with radiation alone when there are no enlarged lymph nodes on computed tomographic imaging, bulky lymph nodes may require combined-modality treatment for optimal regional control.

INTRODUCTION

Vaginal and vulvar cancers are rare neoplasms. Cancers that originate in these sites are frequently curable, but the most effective treatments often require highly specialized techniques and close multidisciplinary cooperation. Although vaginal and vulvar cancers are usually locoregionally confined at diagnosis, regional spread may occur in patients with relatively small tumors, a risk that must be addressed in treatment planning. Although extensive involvement of the bladder, urethra, rectum, or anus is uncommon, the proximity of these structures to the vagina and vulva necessitates careful multidisciplinary cooperation to achieve functional organ sparing without compromising tumor control.

EPIDEMIOLOGY

There are fewer than 2 new cases of vaginal and vulvar cancer per 100,000 women annually in the United States (Eifel et al, 2005). These tumors tend to occur in postmenopausal women older than 60 years. The peak incidence of vulvar carcinomas is in women older than 70 to 75 years. However, intraepithelial vulvar lesions tend to occur in younger women, and invasive cancers—particularly those associated with human papillomavirus (HPV)—tend to occur in younger, premenopausal women, occasionally in women younger than 30 years.

HPV appears to play a role in many vaginal and vulvar cancers. Most vulvar intraepithelial lesions are HPV positive, although only about 30% to 40% of invasive vulvar cancers are HPV positive. Women with HPV-positive vulvar cancers tend to have risk factors similar to those associated with cervical cancer. Younger women with vulvar cancer are more likely than older women with the disease to have condylomata or other evidence of HPV infection. Smoking and immunosuppression also appear to be more common in young patients than in those diagnosed at an older age. HPV-negative cancers tend to occur in older women and are often associated with *p53* mutations.

ANATOMY AND PATTERNS OF SPREAD

Vaginal intraepithelial neoplasia (VAIN) and small invasive vaginal cancers may be detected as a result of abnormal findings on a Papanicolaou test. VAIN is rare and is more frequently diagnosed in patients with a history of cervical intraepithelial neoplasia. The vagina should be carefully examined during pelvic examinations, and in any patient who has an unexplained finding of cancer on a cytologic screening test, the vagina should be colposcopically evaluated. Early vaginal cancers can easily be missed if they are hidden by the blades of a speculum. Care must be taken to visualize the entire vagina. Vulvar intraepithelial neoplasia (VIN) may arise anywhere on the vulva or perineum and usually presents as an asymptomatic raised area on the vulva; some lesions are associated with pruritis or pain.

Despite their accessible location, vaginal and vulvar cancers sometimes present as very advanced lesions. The most common presenting symptom for women with invasive vaginal cancers is postmenopausal bleeding. Vulvar cancers usually present as asymptomatic or pruritic lesions noted on pelvic examination or, in more advanced cases, with vulvar pruritis, pain, and an abnormal mass in the vulva.

Vaginal cancers can arise anywhere in the vaginal mucosa. Invasive carcinomas typically infiltrate the subvaginal tissues beneath the site of mucosal origin; tumors may also exhibit an exophytic growth pattern. Although tumors originating in the vagina can spread superiorly to invade the cervix, tumors that involve both sites are conventionally classified as cervical cancers. For this reason, vaginal cancers that involve the upper vagina are frequently diagnosed in women who have had a hysterectomy. Cancers that involve both the vulva and vagina are usually classified as vulvar cancers unless there is extensive vaginal disease with minimal vulvar involvement. Large anterior vaginal cancers may invade the bladder, and although direct invasion of the rectal mucosa is uncommon, infiltration of the rectovaginal septum from posterior lesions can produce particularly challenging problems with respect to organ preservation during treatment.

Depending on the location and extent of the primary tumor, vaginal cancers can spread to involve any of the nodal groups in the pelvis. The external and internal iliac nodes are most commonly involved, but vaginal cancers can also spread to common iliac or presacral nodes or, with involvement of the rectovaginal septum, to perirectal lymph nodes. Invasive lesions involving the distal third of the vagina can metastasize directly to the inguino-femoral lymph nodes.

Locally, vulvar cancers can spread from the clitoris, labia, or perineum to involve the vagina, distal urethra, or anus. Modern multidisciplinary management emphasizes techniques and treatments that control and sterilize disease while preserving these adjacent structures. Very extensive tumors may invade the proximal urethra or bladder, rectum, perineal muscles, or bone. In advanced cases, invasion of subdermal lymphatics can result in inflammatory skin involvement with satellite lesions involving the skin of the lower abdominal wall or medial thighs.

The vulva is richly supplied with lymphatics, and regional spread of vulvar cancers is common. Tumors that invade less than 1 mm rarely involve lymphatics, but even relatively superficial lesions that invade only 2 to 3 mm frequently involve lymphatics. More than 50% of cancers that invade more than 8 to 10 mm involve regional lymph nodes. The primary site of regional spread from the vulva is to the superficial inguinal and medial femoral lymph nodes. From there, cancer can spread to the deep inguinal and pelvic lymph nodes. Although pelvic lymph node involvement is rare when the inguino-femoral lymph nodes are free of cancer, occasionally cancers (particularly those involving the periclitoral region) may spread directly to the deep inguinal or even obturator lymph nodes.

The lungs are the most common site of hematogenous metastasis from vaginal and vulvar cancers.

CLINICAL EVALUATION AND STAGING

In some cases, vaginal or vulvar carcinoma may occur in the context of extensive condylomata or dysplasia, making it difficult to identify the best site for biopsy. When faced with a lesion suggestive of vaginal or vulvar cancer, we usually proceed directly to colposcopy-directed biopsies under local anesthesia. Punch biopsies should include sufficient underlying stroma to permit assessment of the depth of tumor penetration. We emphasize the importance of prompt and adequate biopsy of suspicious lesions to prevent unnecessary delays in diagnosis.

Pelvic examination continues to be the most important tool for evaluating the local extent of vaginal and vulvar cancers. The location, gross morphology, sites of involvement, and dimensions of the visible and palpable tumor should be carefully recorded and illustrated with a tumor diagram or photograph. The proximity of the tumor to midline structures should be noted.

Relatively superficial lesions are best evaluated by physical examination. However, tomographic scans, particularly magnetic resonance imaging, can be used to assess sites of deep infiltration into the bladder, urethra, or subvaginal tissues. Proctoscopy or cysto-urethroscopy should always be performed to confirm radiographic evidence of bladder, proximal urethral, anal, or rectal involvement; biopsies should be done of suspicious lesions to confirm these sites of involvement. Although computed tomography (CT) can be helpful in detecting pelvic or inguinal lymphadenopathy, conventional CT usually yields poor detail with respect to local anatomy.

All patients with vaginal or vulvar cancers should have a careful history and physical examination, chest radiography, complete blood cell count, and biochemical profile as part of their initial evaluation.

Because most vaginal cancers are treated without complete surgical resection, they are staged using the International Federation of Gynecology and Obstetrics (FIGO) staging system, which is based on clinical evaluation and radiographic studies; the rules for staging are the same as those used for cervical cancer (Table 6–1). As with cervical cancer, findings on tomographic studies (e.g., CT and magnetic resonance imaging) cannot be used to alter the FIGO stage, although they may be useful for treatment planning.

In 1988, the FIGO staging system for vulvar cancer was changed to a surgical staging system based on the findings of vulvar excision and inguinal

Table 6–1. International Federation of Gynecology and Obstetrics Clinical Staging of Carcinoma of the Vagina

Stage 0	Carcinoma in situ, intraepithelial carcinoma.
Stage I	The carcinoma is limited to the vaginal wall.
Stage II	The carcinoma has involved the subvaginal tissues but has not extended onto the pelvic wall.
Stage III	The carcinoma has extended onto the pelvic wall.
Stage IV	The carcinoma has extended beyond the true pelvis or has clinically involved the mucosa of the bladder or rectum. Bullous edema as such does not permit a case to be allotted to stage IV.
Stage IVA	Spread of the growth to adjacent organs and/or direct extension beyond the true pelvis.
Stage IVB	Spread to distant organs.

Reprinted with permission from Benedet et al (2000).

lymph node dissection (Table 6–2) (Benedet et al, 2000). This system provides the most robust information about sites of involvement for patients who are treated with a primary surgical approach and can be applied to patients who have surgical evaluation of lymph nodes before treatment with radiation or chemoradiation to the primary tumor. As discussed below, some patients with vulvar cancer who have locally advanced primary lesions and clinically disease-free groins (by CT or magnetic resonance imaging) may be successfully treated with radiation alone to the inguinal regions. In these cases, the groins must be classified as "NX."

Prognostic Factors

The outcome for women with vaginal cancers is related to the extent of local disease—specifically tumor size and stage (Table 6–3). Most investigators have reported correlations between the recurrence rate and the location of the vaginal lesion, although the details of their findings have been inconsistent. Relapse rates for lesions occurring in various sites may depend somewhat on the treatment techniques available at different centers. At M. D. Anderson, tumors involving the proximal third of the vagina have been associated with a somewhat better prognosis than those involving the distal two thirds. The influence of regional involvement on prognosis is poorly understood because most reports have not included consistent evaluation of the pelvic lymph nodes.

In 1991, Rutledge et al reviewed the relationship between clinical features and recurrence in 365 patients with vulvar carcinoma (Table 6–4). Most of the patients in their series (283; 77%) had surgery as their only locoregional treatment; 21 had radiation therapy only, and 61 had surgery plus irradiation of the vulva or lymph nodes. Tumor size, stage, and the

Table 6–2. International Federation of Gynecology and Obstetrics Staging of Carcinoma of the Vulva

Stage I	Lesions 2 cm or less in size confined to the vulva or perineum (T1).*
	No nodal metastases (N0).
Stage IA	Lesions 2 cm or less in size confined to the vulva or perineum and with stromal invasion no greater than 1 mm.†
	No nodal metastases (N0).
Stage IB	Lesions 2 cm or less in size confined to the vulva or perineum and with stromal invasion greater than 1 mm.†
	No nodal metastases (N0).
Stage II	Tumor confined to the vulva or perineum and more than 2 cm in the greatest dimension (T2).
	No nodal metastases (N0).
Stage III	Tumor of any size with:
	Adjacent spread to the lower urethra and/or the vagina, or the anus (T3) or unilateral regional node metastasis (N1).
Stage IVA	Tumor invasion of any of the following: upper urethra, bladder mucosa, rectal mucosa, pelvic bone (T4); or bilateral regional node metastasis (N2).
Stage IVB	Any distant metastasis, including pelvic lymph nodes (M1).

*Equivalent TNM groupings according to the TNM Committee of the International Union Against Cancer are indicated in parentheses.
†The depth of invasion is defined as the measurement of the tumor from the epithelial-stromal junction of the adjacent most superficial dermal papilla to the deepest point of invasion.
Reprinted with permission from Benedet et al (2000).

status of the inguinal and pelvic lymph nodes were the most powerful predictors of outcome in that study. Most authors have reported higher rates of locoregional recurrence and death in patients whose tumors are deeply invasive, are high grade, have a high mitotic rate, or are associated with lymph-vascular space invasion. However, a recent review of data from M. D. Anderson (Katz et al, 2003) suggests that the more frequent use of combined-modality treatment in recent years may have reduced the influence of some of these factors on prognosis. Postoperative radiation therapy has reduced recurrence and death rates for patients with positive inguinal lymph nodes. Although patients with pelvic lymph node involvement are generally considered to have a dismal prognosis, these data were collected from patients who underwent pelvic lymph node dissection before the mid-1980s. Today, routine pelvic dissections are rarely performed. Instead, patients with inguinal metastases have postoperative radiation therapy with fields that include the pelvic nodes. Because the presence or absence of microscopic pelvic involvement is rarely documented before radiation therapy, the influence of modern combined-modality treatment on the prognosis of patients with pelvic lymph node metastases is unknown.

Table 6–3. Patient, Tumor, and Treatment Characteristics and Correlation with Outcome for 193 Patients with Squamous Cell Carcinoma of the Vagina Treated with Radiation Therapy at M. D. Anderson Cancer Center

Characteristic	No. of Patients (%)	PDC Rate	P	DSS Rate	P
Stage			.027		.0013*
I	50 (26)	86		85	
II	96 (50)	84		77	
III or IVA	47 (24)	72		58	
III	40 (21)	65			
IVA	7 (3)	86			
Tumor size			.015		.0001*
≤ 4 cm	129 (67)	85		82	
> 4 cm	64 (33)	75		60	
Tumor site			.71		.13
Apex	28 (14)	87		82	
Upper 2/3	94 (49)	81		77	
Lower 1/3	42 (22)	77		73	
Whole vagina	29 (15)	83		58	
Circumferential location			.81		.49
Anterior	33 (17)	87		84	
Posterior	48 (25)	74		67	
Lateral	41 (22)	84		77	
Circumferential	43 (22)	79		68	
Previous hysterectomy			.70		.75
Yes	121 (63)	83		74	
No	72 (39)	79		75	

Abbreviations: PDC = pelvic disease control (at 5 years); DSS = disease-specific survival (at 5 years).
*Significant in multivariate analysis ($P < 0.01$).
Modified from Frank et al (2005). Reprinted with permission.

TREATMENT OF VAGINAL CARCINOMAS

VAIN

VAIN can be successfully treated with a variety of techniques, including excisional biopsy, CO_2 laser ablation, and topical 5-fluorouracil. Surgical excision should be considered for lesions with colposcopic or cytologic findings suggestive of invasion. Topical 5-fluorouracil therapy may be advantageous in women with extensive or multifocal lesions and women who develop VAIN after irradiation. The success rates for any therapeutic option approach 85% to 90%. All patients require careful surveillance after treatment.

Stage I Tumors

Stage I tumors are those defined by FIGO as "limited to the vaginal wall." In practice, this distinction is difficult to make on clinical grounds. Except

Table 6–4. Predictors of Relapse for Patients with Invasive Carcinoma of the Vulva Treated at M. D. Anderson Cancer Center between 1944 and 1990. Summary of Cox Proportional Hazards Model

	Relative Hazard (± 95% C.I.)		P
Tumor size (cm)			
0–2	1.00		.009
3–4	1.10	(0.66–1.82)	
5–6	1.99	(1.16–3.38)	
>6	2.08	(1.13–3.82)	
Tumor grade			.202
I	1.00		
II	0.79	(0.49–1.24)	
III	1.18	(0.73–1.92)	
FIGO stage (pre 1988)			.000
I	1.00		
II	1.94	(0.88–4.25)	
III	4.22	(2.01–8.84)	
IV	12.00	(5.16–27.88)	
Therapy aim			.000
Curative	1.00		
Palliative	4.16	(2.43–7.12)	
Groin nodes			.000
Bilaterally negative	1.00		
Unilaterally positive	2.52	(1.54–4.10)	
Bilaterally positive	7.37	(4.25–12.75)	
Pelvic nodes			.000
Bilaterally negative	1.00		
Unilaterally positive	4.25	(2.10–8.57)	
Bilaterally positive	12.83	(2.96–55.60)	
Cloquet's nodes			.9305*
Negative	1.00		
Positive	0.94	(0.22–3.91)	
Deep surgical margins			.0438†
Negative	1.00		
Invasive	4.31	(1.37–13.57)	
Vaginal surgical margins			.878‡
Negative	1.00		
Invasive	4.31	(0.34–3.45)	
Lateral surgical margins			.090§
Negative	1.00		
Invasive	3.26	(1.03–10.35)	
Age, years			.573
<41	1.00		
41–60	0.91	(0.45–1.82)	
61–80	0.96	(0.49–1.89)	
>80	1.54	(0.64–3.72)	

(Continued)

Table 6–4. (*Continued*) Predictors of Relapse for Patients with Invasive Carcinoma of the Vulva Treated at M. D. Anderson Cancer Center between 1944 and 1990. Summary of Cox Proportional Hazards Model

	Relative Hazard (± 95% C.I.)		P
Site of lesion			.128
Clitoris or mons	1.00		
Labia	3.55	(0.48–26.39)	
Gross appearance			.869
Other	1.00		
Ulcerative	0.97	(0.67–1.39)	
Clinical stage (tumor)			.000
T1	1.00		
T2	1.93	(1.00–3.74)	
T3	3.40	(1.78–6.51)	
T4	4.20	(0.54–32.94)	
Clinical stage (nodes)			.000
N0	1.00		
N1	1.15	(0.69–1.94)	
N2	2.02	(1.30–3.16)	
N3	6.06	(3.47–10.57)	
Clinical stage (metastasis)			.006‖
M0	1.00		
M1A or M1B	8.65	(2.68–27.94)	
Medical status			.190
No illness	1.00		
Obesity	1.10	(0.53–2.25)	
Diabetes	0.48	(0.12–1.99)	
Hypertension	1.28	(0.79–2.08)	
Cardiovascular disease	1.78	(1.02–3.13)	

Abbreviation: FIGO, International Federation of Gynecology and Obstetrics.
*Of the 134 patients with Cloquet's nodes evaluated, only 10 had positive nodes.
†Of the 333 patients with deep surgical margins evaluated, only 4 had invasive carcinoma.
‡Of the 327 patients with vaginal surgical margins evaluated, only 8 had invasive carcinoma.
§Of the 331 patients with lateral surgical margins reported, only 6 had invasive carcinoma.
‖Of 365 patients, there were only 5 with M1A or M1B disease.
Modified from Rutledge et al (1991). Reprinted with permission from Elsevier.

in the region of the pouch of Douglas, the vagina lacks a serosa and generally has little anatomical barrier to submucosal spread. The submucosal muscularis and adventitia are thin, and their penetration may be difficult to appreciate on clinical examination. For this reason, clinicians' criteria for labeling a lesion as "stage I" or "stage II" probably vary widely. However, we believe that rare tumors that have little or no palpable substance, that are small and appear purely exophytic, or that have been excised revealing no invasion beyond the muscularis can be appropriately classified as stage I. The true risk of regional involvement from such lesions is unclear but may be small.

Highly selected stage I tumors that are small and minimally invasive may be adequately treated with local excision alone. Small, superficial lesions of the apical vagina are particularly amenable to this approach. However, we rarely attempt curative resection of a palpable lesion unless it appears to be purely exophytic. Even very superficial tumors can be difficult to resect with adequate margins without compromising bladder or rectal function. Partial excision or excision that leaves a positive margin often complicates subsequent radiation therapy planning; the site of residual disease may be poorly defined and frequently lies beyond the reach of intracavitary radiation treatment, necessitating the use of more complex interstitial or external-beam techniques to achieve an adequate dose.

Stage I tumors can be treated with radiation alone, which results in local control and survival rates that approach 100% with appropriate management. Only very superficial tumors may be treated with brachytherapy alone. At M. D. Anderson, a Delclos dome cylinder is usually used to treat superficial carcinomas of the vaginal apex, whereas interstitial therapy is emphasized for more distal lesions. Pelvic external-beam irradiation is added for tumors that are believed to invade more than 1 mm.

Stage II Tumors

Unless the patient has already received radiation therapy for another reason, stage II disease is almost always treated with radiation therapy. In some cases, larger tumors may be treated with concurrent chemoradiation, on the basis of the results of studies in patients with cervical cancer.

Stage II disease is usually treated with an initial course of external-beam radiation therapy to sterilize regional disease and to reduce the volume of gross disease in the vagina. Radiation fields encompass the regional lymph nodes (as discussed in the section "Regional Management" below) and the primary lesion, with at least a 4-cm margin on the most distal disease. If the vulva must be treated to accomplish this, the patient is treated in an open-leg position to minimize the vulvar skin reaction. We usually treat this volume to an initial total dose of 40 to 45 Gy. Depending on the primary tumor response and the distribution of disease, an additional 5 to 10 Gy may be delivered to the central tumor using smaller external-beam fields, bringing the total dose of external-beam irradiation to the primary tumor site to 40 to 50 Gy.

A variety of approaches may be used to increase the radiation dose to the primary tumor site. The approach selected depends on the site and size of the tumor and on the pattern and extent of tumor response. The extent of involvement from bulky tumors may be difficult to clearly define at the time of initial evaluation; we find that it is important to examine patients several times during external-beam radiation therapy to define the volume that will need to receive additional treatment and the best approach to delivering that treatment. Each of these rare tumors is different, and relatively small differences in disease distribution can warrant radically different approaches.

Apical tumors can be treated with intracavitary radiation therapy if the cervix is still present (permitting placement of an intrauterine tandem) or if there has been an excellent response in a patient who has had a hysterectomy. In the latter case, we use intracavitary radiation therapy only if the residual disease is no more than 3 to 5 mm from the vaginal surface. This is because the dose from a vaginal cylinder falls off very rapidly with increasing distance from the vaginal surface. For patients with deeper lesions, we prefer to treat with an interstitial implant, which is inserted using a vaginal template under laparoscopic guidance; the needles are inserted until they tent or even protrude beyond the vaginal apex and are then separated from the small bowel with a flap of omentum that is secured to the pelvic floor. A total dose of 75 to 85 Gy (including previous external-beam irradiation) is given, balancing the risks of tumor recurrence and normal tissue complications. If the patient is not deemed to be a candidate for this procedure, we treat the tumor with an external-beam irradiation boost rather than attempting to use inadequate intracavitary therapy. Although the dose of radiation is necessarily lower with external-beam treatment, a dose of 60 to 70 Gy may be given using conformal treatment and daily catheterization to achieve consistent bladder filling.

Although superficial tumors that involve the middle third of the vagina can be treated with intracavitary radiation therapy, this approach treats the entire circumference of the vagina to a uniform dose; we usually prefer to use a combination of intracavitary and interstitial brachytherapy, adding interstitial needles loaded with iridium 192 to increase the dose to the site of gross tumor involvement. Lateral-wall and anterior-wall lesions are particularly amenable to interstitial therapy. However, interstitial implants are rarely used to treat posterior lesions of the mid-vagina because the risk of damage to the thin rectovaginal septum is excessive. If a small posterior tumor responds well to initial external-beam therapy, additional treatment may be given using a cylinder fitted with shielding to protect the anterior vagina with a vaginal mold. Larger tumors, particularly those that circumferentially involve the vagina, are often best treated with conformal external-beam techniques.

Tumors involving the distal third of the vagina are usually treated most effectively with an interstitial radiation therapy boost. For tumors of the midvagina and distal vagina, we use a freehand technique (Figure 6–1) that allows us to space individual needles within the tumor and to monitor their location by vaginal and rectal examination. We find that this technique permits more accurate needle placement than techniques that use a perineal template.

Stage III–IVA Tumors

Most stage III tumors are large tumors that involve most of the vagina and are fixed to the pelvic wall. Intracavitary therapy is never appropriate for such tumors. Although some relatively localized tumors can be treated

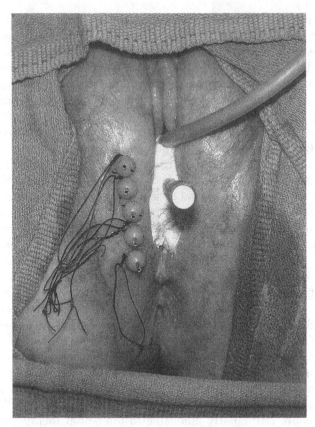

Figure 6–1. Interstitial implant used to boost the radiation dose to the lateral vaginal wall in a patient with squamous cell carcinoma of the vagina. Needles are inserted transperineally and are sutured to the perineum. Iridium 192 is inserted into the needles after the implant has been placed. Treatment is usually delivered over 48 to 72 hours, after which the needles are removed.

with an interstitial therapy boost, we prefer to boost most tumors with conformal external-beam fields rather than to treat these large volumes with brachytherapy. Intensity-modulated radiation therapy may be particularly well suited to treat these tumors. Magnetic resonance imaging before and after external-beam therapy may be used to help define the extent of disease. Ideally, the patient should have a full bladder during treatment. However, this may be difficult toward the end of the treatment course if the patient is having diarrhea. If the tumor involves the upper vagina, it is often wise to confirm that there is no change in the target volume with variations in bladder filling.

    Fortunately, stage IVA tumors are rare. When they occur, they may present with a tumor fistula of the vesicovaginal or rectovaginal septum. If a fistula is not present, one frequently develops as the tumor responds to treatment. Occasionally, even fixed tumors are cured with radiation therapy or chemoradiation alone, so treatment with curative intent is usually indicated. Selected stage IVA tumors that are not fixed and do not have evidence of regional involvement may be treatable with a combination of radiation and exenteration.

Regional Management

Possible sites of regional involvement by vaginal cancers vary with the site and extent of local disease. However, vaginal cancers can spread to nearly every lymph node group in the pelvis. For tumors involving the upper two thirds of the vagina, we usually treat the internal, external, common iliac, and presacral lymph nodes; the upper border of the treatment fields is usually at the L4-L5 or L5-S1 interspace. Tumors that involve the rectovaginal septum are particularly prone to spread to perirectal lymph nodes, which must be included in the treatment fields. If the distal third of the vagina is involved, the inguinal lymph nodes must be included in the treatment field. When a small tumor is confined to the distal third of the vagina and the nodes are clinically negative, we may reduce the upper extent of the radiation field to the S1-S2 interspace.

TREATMENT OF VULVAR CARCINOMAS

In recent years, treatment of vulvar carcinoma has moved toward a more individualized, multidisciplinary approach. The classical radical vulvectomy and bilateral inguinal dissection is rarely performed today. Greater emphasis is placed on organ- and tissue-sparing surgical procedures that are intended to reduce the morbidity of treatment without compromising cure rates. The benefit of radiation therapy in achieving locoregional control and improved survival of patients with advanced lesions has been clearly demonstrated, and the role of concurrent chemoradiation is being explored in selected patients.

VIN

VIN progresses to invasion less frequently than was once believed. Low-grade dysplasia (VIN I) can be followed with periodic colposcopy if the lesions do not change. Many low-grade lesions regress spontaneously. Higher-grade lesions (VIN II or III) should be excised or treated with laser ablation. Laser treatment tends to be preferred in younger women with multifocal lesions because it produces less deformity than excision; however, it is appropriate only if a careful colposcopic examination has not demonstrated features suggestive of invasion. In older women, the risk of invasion is greater, and excisional biopsy is usually preferred because it permits careful histologic examination of the lesion. Skinning vulvectomy with a skin graft is occasionally used for older women who have very extensive multifocal disease, but because of the poor cosmetic result, this approach should be reserved for women who cannot be treated with more limited excisions or a combination of biopsy and laser therapy.

T1a Tumors

The rich lymphatic supply of the vulva facilitates early regional spread from relatively small vulvar carcinomas. However, many series have now demonstrated that the risk of lymph node metastasis is less than 1% for patients with tumors that invade no more than 1 mm (Eifel et al, 2005). These are the only cases that can safely be approached without dissection or other treatment of the inguinal nodes. Wide local excision should be performed with a 1-cm margin of normal tissue. The surgical specimen must be carefully examined to rule out deeper invasion that would require greater attention to the inguinal nodes. Although many patients will be cured with this procedure, the risk of recurrent invasive cancer (often from a new primary lesion) is significant. Thus, patients should be followed up at least twice a year with careful examinations; colposcopy and directed biopsy should be performed when an abnormality is noted.

T1b–T2 Tumors

Although traditional radical vulvectomy plus bilateral groin dissection achieves high rates of local control for patients with T1b–T2 tumors, the less than ideal functional outcomes with this approach—a poor cosmetic result and high rates of wound complications, lymphedema, and other complications—led clinicians to explore more conservative surgical procedures for this group of patients. Today at M. D. Anderson, the goal of the primary surgery is to obtain a wide excision that extends to the perineal fascia with a 2-cm margin of uninvolved tissue. In most cases, this does not require resection of the entire vulva. For patients with lateralized T1 and smaller T2 tumors, vulvar appearance and function are usually very good after this procedure.

Most T1 and T2 tumors are treated with initial resection with wide margins (1 to 2 cm). However, when cancers are close to the urethra or anus, it may be impossible to achieve adequate tumor-free margins without compromising organ function. In those cases, a multidisciplinary treatment plan may achieve the best overall result. Some very large T2 tumors that lie immediately adjacent to the urethra or anus may be treated with radiation or chemoradiation in a manner similar to the approach described below for T3 tumors.

Even the smallest T1b tumors are associated with a risk of regional metastases of at least 15% to 20%. Regional surgery or radiation therapy is almost always indicated, as discussed below in the section "Regional Management."

T3–T4a Tumors

T3–T4a tumors involve the urethra, bladder, anus, rectum, or vagina. Although they are sometimes curable with ultraradical surgical procedures, current treatment policies at M. D. Anderson emphasize multidisciplinary organ-sparing approaches. In most cases, radiation therapy is used alone or in combination with chemotherapy or surgery. To achieve optimal results, close multidisciplinary cooperation is required from the time of the patient's initial evaluation.

If the tumor can be removed without compromising urethral or anal function and with negative margins, initial surgery may be sufficient. However, initial surgery is usually performed with the expectation that the urethral or anal margins will be less than 5 mm and that postoperative radiation therapy will be necessary. In this case, radiation therapy should be started within 6 weeks of surgery; we have found that longer intervals tend to be associated with disease recurrence. Most patients who require radiation therapy to the primary tumor site also receive radiation therapy to regional nodes. Initial fields are designed to treat the vulva, inguinal lymph nodes, and distal pelvic lymph nodes to a dose of 40 to 45 Gy. The treatment fields are usually designed using CT-based treatment planning to cover these sites completely while minimizing the dose to the hips and other critical structures (Figure 6–2). After this dose has been delivered to the entire region at risk, reduced fields are used to supplement the dose to the vulva and involved lymph nodes. Although a variety of techniques have been used to supplement the dose to the vulva, we prefer to use appositional electron-beam fields that are applied to the perineum with the patient in the frog-leg or lithotomy position (Figure 6–3). Through several field reductions, the region of the close or positive margin is treated to 54 to 66 Gy depending on the level of risk.

If the surgeon believes that organ-sparing resection would be likely to leave tumor at the resection margins, we prefer to treat the patient initially with radiation therapy or chemoradiation; surgical resection is reserved as an option if the tumor fails to respond completely to radiation therapy. Because the dose required to sterilize microscopically positive surgical margins is similar to the dose needed to control gross disease, incomplete resection tends to add to morbidity without clearly improving the likelihood of local control. When patients are treated with initial radiation therapy, the radiation treatment fields are similar to those used for postoperative treatment; gross disease on the vulva is usually treated to a total dose of 60 to 66 Gy using electron-beam fields as described in the preceding paragraph. The patient is followed up closely over the next 6 to 12 weeks; if by the end of this time the tumor has not responded completely to treatment, surgical resection of residual disease is considered.

The role of concurrent chemoradiation has not been firmly established in patients with locoregionally advanced vulvar cancer. Clinicians have been encouraged by the favorable results of chemoradiation for cervical

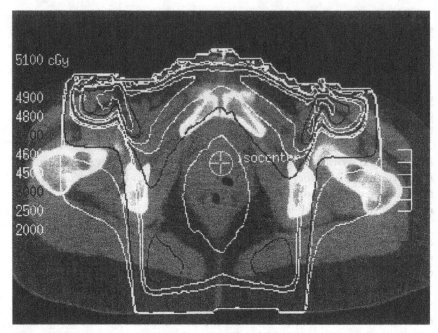

Figure 6–2. Several techniques have been developed to deliver external-beam radiation therapy to the inguinal and pelvic lymph nodes without excessively irradiating the femoral heads. In this case, the anterior radiation field was wide, encompassing all the pelvic and inguino-femoral lymph nodes. A narrower posterior field covered the pelvic and medial inguinal lymph nodes; 2 superficial electron-beam fields were used to supplement the areas not covered by the posterior fields. This technique requires careful planning but delivers 45 to 50 Gy to the targeted areas while keeping the dose to the femoral head to less than 35 Gy.

and anal cancers. However, there have been no phase III trials of concurrent chemoradiation in women with vulvar cancer. Elderly vulvar cancer patients may be more prone to chemotherapy-related complications than are cervical cancer patients, who tend to be much younger. A number of phase II clinical experiences have suggested that vulvar cancers respond well to chemoradiation; we have seen many dramatic responses to chemoradiation, although we have also seen favorable responses to radiation therapy alone. At M. D. Anderson, concurrent chemotherapy is usually offered to women who have locoregionally advanced disease and a good performance status, although we inform the patient that there is less support for combined-modality therapy in their situation than for combined-modality therapy in patients with anal or cervical cancer.

The acute side effects of vulvar irradiation can be daunting, and close attention to care of the treated area is required. We warn patients that they will have 3 to 4 weeks of moderately severe skin reactions. We prescribe

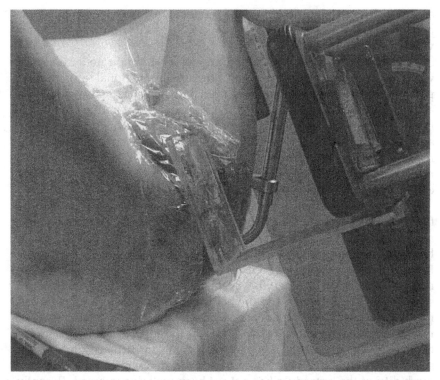

Figure 6–3. When the vulva requires a dose of radiation higher than 45 Gy, we supplement the area using an appositional field of electrons. The patient is treated in a lithotomy position, and a Lucite compression device is gently positioned against the vulva to improve the homogeneity of the radiation dose.

sitz baths from the beginning of treatment and watch closely for evidence of fungal or bacterial superinfection. Most patients develop a candidal infection by the third or fourth week of treatment; we have found that treatment with fluconazole usually produces a prompt improvement in vulvar erythema and pain. Satellite lesions or an expanding margin of erythema that extends outside the treatment field suggest a bacterial infection; in such cases, culture and immediate treatment with antibiotics are indicated. We have found that patients who receive careful education and aggressive care of the treated region rarely require a break during treatment. Healing progresses rapidly once treatment is completed.

Regional Management

Numerous studies have demonstrated that patients who have inguinal metastases from vulvar cancer frequently can be cured if their regional disease is eliminated with appropriate treatment. It is critical that this be accomplished at the time of initial treatment because fewer than 20% of patients survive 5 years after an inguinal recurrence of previously treated vulvar cancer.

Before the mid-1980s, radical inguino-femoral lymph node dissection was the standard diagnostic and therapeutic regional approach to patients with inguinal metastases from vulvar cancer. Classically, this approach involved en bloc resection of the superficial and deep inguinal lymph nodes with removal of the cribriform fascia. This procedure was associated with a very low rate of disease recurrence in the groin if all the nodes were negative for metastases. However, acute and late morbidity rates were high: wound complications, lymphocyst formation, and lower-extremity lymphedema were common.

More recently, surgeons have sought to define less radical procedures that still offer the diagnostic benefits of radical lymphadenectomy. Initial reports (Stehman et al, 1992a; Burke et al, 1995) suggested that superficial lymphadenectomy might be sufficient. As usually described, this operation involves the removal of 8 to 10 nodes from the superficial compartment bounded by the inguinal ligament superiorly, the border of the sartorius muscle laterally, and the border of the adductor longus muscle medially. More recent experience suggests that it may be necessary to remove the medial femoral nodes as well as the superficial inguinal nodes to achieve an acceptably low rate of regional recurrence; this can be achieved without removing the entire cribriform fascia, but the long-term morbidity of the procedure has not yet been well documented. Recently, there has been a growing literature on the use of lymphatic mapping and sentinel lymph node biopsy to guide limited groin dissections. Preliminary studies indicate that sentinel nodes can be identified in most cases; sentinel node identification may be more difficult in cases of midline lesions or when an excisional biopsy was performed before the mapping procedure (Table 6–5). These results are encouraging but need to

Table 6–5.   Successful Groin Sentinel Node Identification by Site of Primary Tumor

Location	Yes/Total	%
Lateral	22/25	88
Left labium	11/13	85
Right labium	9/9	100
Bartholin's gland	2/3	67
Midline	35/51	69
Clitoris	18/26	69
Perineum	8/14	57
Fourchette	9/11	82
Total	57/76	75

Reprinted from Levenback et al (2001), with permission from Elsevier.

be followed by large series with mature follow-up to confirm the role of lymphatic mapping in treatment.

When lymph node dissection reveals inguinal metastases, postoperative radiation therapy is given to prevent groin recurrence. In a 1986 study of patients who had positive inguinal nodes after radical vulvectomy and lymphadenectomy, Homesley et al demonstrated that postoperative radiation therapy (versus pelvic and inguinal lymphadenectomy alone) reduced the rate of groin recurrence (3 of 59 with radiation therapy versus 13 of 55 without) and significantly improved the survival rate. A retrospective review of the M. D. Anderson experience (Katz et al, 2003) revealed 3 inguinal recurrences in 35 patients who had postoperative radiation therapy because of inguinal metastases (7% recurrence rate at 5 years). All 3 recurrences occurred in patients whose radiation therapy was begun more than 50 days after lymph node dissection, suggesting that prompt referral and treatment may be important. When the patient is known to have lymph node metastases before surgery, we have found that simple excision of enlarged nodes plus carefully planned radiation therapy achieves a high rate of regional control; this approach minimizes wound complications that might delay radiation therapy. When postoperative radiation therapy is indicated, we recommend a total dose of at least 45 to 50 Gy to the pelvis and inguinal regions. If there is evidence of extracapsular extension or residual disease in the groin, the treatment is usually supplemented to a dose of 60 to 70 Gy using small fields of electron-beam irradiation. In all cases, CT-based treatment planning should be used to confirm that the operative bed will be adequately treated without overexposing the femoral heads to radiation.

For patients who are treated initially with radiation therapy for locally extensive disease, we sometimes elect to treat clinically negative lymph nodes with radiation alone. In 1992, a randomized Gynecologic Oncology Group study (Stehman et al, 1992b) comparing lymph node dissection versus radiation therapy for clinically negative inguinal lymph nodes was closed early because there were 5 inguinal recurrences in the first 25 patients in the group treated with radiation alone. However, the patients in this trial did not have tomographic diagnostic studies to rule out enlarged nodes that may have been missed on physical examination; more importantly, many of the patients were treated with low-energy electron-beam fields that are now known to be inadequate to cover the desired clinical target volume in the groin and distal pelvis. Retrospective studies (Petereit et al, 1993; Katz et al, 2003) suggest that very high rates of regional control can be achieved with radiation therapy alone in properly selected patients who are treated with techniques that deliver an adequate dose to the superficial and deep inguinal lymph nodes and the distal pelvic lymph nodes.

KEY PRACTICE POINTS

- Vaginal and vulvar carcinomas are rare and are best treated in a center that can offer a multidisciplinary team of radiation oncologists and gynecologic oncologists who are experienced in specialized surgical and radiation therapy techniques.

- Because they are located in close proximity to the bladder and rectum, most vaginal cancers are treated with radiation therapy, although surgical excision may be adequate for very small superficial lesions. Treatment is individualized according to the site and extent of local disease; a combination of external-beam radiation therapy and intracavitary or interstitial brachytherapy may be required to achieve the best results.

- Although the classical treatment of vulvar cancer included radical surgical resection and lymphadenectomy for most patients, in recent years treatment has moved to a more individualized, multidisciplinary approach. Treatments often include a combination of surgery and radiation therapy selected to obtain maximum tumor control rates with as few serious side effects as possible.

- Radical vulvectomy has been replaced by more selective wide local excision of the primary lesion. Primary radiation therapy or combined primary radiation therapy and surgery may be used to control lesions that approach or involve critical structures.

- Regional recurrences of vulvar cancer are rarely curable and should be prevented whenever possible. In patients who have gross or multiple lymph node metastases, postoperative radiation therapy is required to achieve acceptable regional control rates. Lymphatic mapping and sentinel lymph node biopsy is increasingly being used to improve the diagnostic accuracy of modified lymph node dissections.

- The success of concurrent chemoradiation in patients with cervical and anal cancer has encouraged clinicians to use similar treatments in patients with vulvar and vaginal cancer; however, the role of chemotherapy has not yet been well defined in this population.

SUGGESTED READINGS

American Joint Committee on Cancer. *Cancer Staging Manual*. Greene FL, Page DL, Fleming ID, et al, eds. New York, NY: Springer; 2002:241–300.

Benedet JL, Bender H, Jones H 3rd, Ngan HY, Pecorelli S. FIGO staging classifications and clinical practice guidelines in the management of gynecologic cancers. FIGO Committee on Gynecologic Oncology. *Int J Gynaecol Obstet* 2000;70:209–262.

Burke TW, Levenback C, Coleman RL, et al. Surgical therapy of T1 and T2 vulvar carcinoma: further experience with radical wide excision and selective inguinal lymphadenectomy. *Gynecol Oncol* 1995;57:215–220.

Chyle V, Zagars GK, Wheeler JA, et al. Definitive radiotherapy for carcinoma of the vagina: outcome and prognostic factors. *Int J Radiat Oncol Biol Phys* 1996;35:891–905.

Eifel PJ, Berek JS, Markman MA. Cancer of the cervix, vagina, and vulva. In: DeVita VT, Hellman S, Rosenberg SA, eds. *Cancer Principles and Practice.* Philadelphia, Pa: Lippincott Williams & Wilkins; 2005:1295–1341.

Faul C, Mirmow D, Gerszten K, et al. Isolated local recurrence in carcinoma of the vulva: prognosis and implications for treatment. *Int J Gynecol Cancer* 1998;8:409–414.

Faul CM, Mirmow D, Huang Q, et al. Adjuvant radiation for vulvar carcinoma: improved local control. *Int J Radiat Oncol Biol Phys* 1997;38:381–389.

Frank SJ, Jhingran A, Levenback C, et al. Definitive radiation therapy for squamous cell carcinoma of the vagina. *Int J Radiat Oncol Biol Phys* 2005;62:138–147.

Homesley HD, Bundy BN, Sedlis A, et al. Radiation therapy versus pelvic node resection for carcinoma of the vulva with positive groin nodes. *Obstet Gynecol* 1986;68:733–740.

Homesley HD, Bundy BN, Sedlis A, et al. Prognostic factors for groin node metastasis in squamous cell carcinoma of the vulva (a Gynecologic Oncology Group study). *Gynecol Oncol* 1993;49:279–283.

Katz A, Eifel PJ, Jhingran A, Levenback CF. The role of radiation therapy in preventing regional recurrences of invasive squamous cell carcinoma of the vulva. *Int J Radiat Oncol Biol Phys* 2003;57:409–418.

Kirkbride P, Fyles A, Rawlings GA, et al. Carcinoma of the vagina—experience at the Princess Margaret Hospital (1974–1989). *Gynecol Oncol* 1995;56:435–443.

Koh WJ, Chiu M, Stelzer KJ, et al. Femoral vessel depth and the implications for groin node radiation. *Int J Radiat Oncol Biol Phys* 1993;27:969–974.

Kucera H, Vavra N. Radiation management of primary carcinoma of the vagina: clinical and histopathological variables associated with survival. *Gynecol Oncol* 1991;40:12–16.

Kuppers V, Stiller M, Somville T, et al. Risk factors for recurrent VIN. Role of multifocality and grade of disease. *J Reprod Med* 1997;42:140–144.

Levenback C, Coleman RL, Burke TW, et al. Intraoperative lymphatic mapping and sentinel node identification with blue dye in patients with vulvar cancer. *Gynecol Oncol* 2001;83:276–281.

Levenback C, Morris M, Burke TW, et al. Groin dissection practices among gynecologic oncologists treating early vulvar cancer. *Gynecol Oncol* 1996;62:73–77.

Montana GS, Thomas GM, Moore DH, et al. Preoperative chemo-radiation for carcinoma of the vulva with N2/N3 nodes: a Gynecologic Oncology Group study. *Int J Radiat Oncol Biol Phys* 2000;48:1007–1013.

Moore DH, Thomas GM, Montana GS, et al. Preoperative chemoradiation for advanced vulvar cancer: a phase II study of the Gynecologic Oncology Group. *Int J Radiat Oncol Biol Phys* 1998;42:79–85.

Perez CA, Grigsby PW, Garipagaoglu M, et al. Factors affecting long-term outcome of irradiation in carcinoma of the vagina. *Int J Radiat Oncol Biol Phys* 1999;44:37–45.

Petereit DG, Mehta MP, Buchler DA, et al. A retrospective review of nodal treatment for vulvar cancer. *Am J Clin Oncol* 1993;16:38–42.

Rutledge FN, Mitchell MF, Munsell MF, et al. Prognostic indicators for invasive carcinoma of the vulva. *Gynecol Oncol* 1991;42:239–244.

Stehman FB, Bundy BN, Dvoretsky PM, et al. Early stage I carcinoma of the vulva treated with ipsilateral superficial inguinal lymphadenectomy and modified radical hemivulvectomy: a prospective study of the Gynecologic Oncology Group. *Obstet Gynecol* 1992a;79:490–497.

Stehman FB, Bundy BN, Thomas G, et al. Groin dissection versus groin radiation in carcinoma of the vulva: a Gynecologic Oncology Group study. *Int J Radiat Oncol Biol Phys* 1992b;24:389–396.

Stock RG, Chen ASJ, Seski J. A 30-year experience in the management of primary carcinoma of the vagina: analysis of prognostic factors and treatment modalities. *Gynecol Oncol* 1995;56:45–52.

7 TREATMENT OF EARLY CERVICAL CANCER

Charles F. Levenback

CHAPTER OUTLINE

CHAPTER OVERVIEW

Early-stage cervical cancer is a highly curable condition when patients are well staged and treatment planning is appropriate. Both surgery and radiotherapy are treatment options. Multiple factors, including age, comorbidities, tumor size, resource availability, and patient preference, should be considered in the treatment planning process. New, less-invasive approaches, including sentinel node biopsy, laparoscopy, and radical trachelectomy, hold promise for selected patients.

INTRODUCTION

The purpose of this chapter is to outline the typical care of patients with early cervical cancer at M. D. Anderson Cancer Center. At the outset, it is important to emphasize that the care of patients is multidisciplinary and individualized on the basis of physical findings, imaging studies, performance status, and patient preferences. The etiology, epidemiology, and risk factors for cervical cancer have been discussed in earlier chapters. In this chapter, we will focus on clinical presentation, clinical assessment, and treatment modalities, with an emphasis on treatment selection. In this chapter, "early cervical cancer" will refer to stage I disease (cancer confined to the uterus).

Treatment of early cervical cancer is a challenge for gynecologic oncologists and gynecologic radiation oncologists. The disease occurs in patients over a very wide age range. Depending on the age of the patient, issues such as preservation of fertility, preservation of ovarian function, comorbid conditions, and the risk of complications may play a major role in treatment recommendations. Treatment recommendations may also depend on the resources available in a community. Most obstetrician-gynecologists understand that radical pelvic surgery for cervical cancer requires referral to a gynecologic oncologist, even though this means that the patient must leave the local medical community. Since the subspecialty of gynecologic radiation oncology does not exist outside of a few major centers like M. D. Anderson, it is common for patients with cervical cancer to be treated by radiation oncologists with very little experience treating gynecologic cancers. It has been documented by multiple Patterns of Care studies that patients treated by radiation oncologists with a low volume of cervical cancer patients have worse outcomes than patients treated at higher-volume centers. We believe that all patients with invasive cervical cancer should be offered at least a consultation with a gynecologic oncologist and, when appropriate, a radiation oncologist with broad experience treating this disease.

CLINICAL PRESENTATION

Many patients with early invasive cervical cancer are asymptomatic. Typically in these patients the lesion is not visible and is detected during routine cytologic screening. Discharge and bleeding are the most common symptoms in patients with a visible lesion. The bleeding may be postcoital. Premenopausal patients with small lesions continue to have regular menstrual bleeding. Pain is rare in patients with early cervical cancer. Bleeding and discharge may be worse with an exophytic tumor, whereas endophytic and endocervical tumors can grow with minimal symptoms.

Because of their appearance, small invasive cervical cancers can easily be confused with benign conditions, including a broad transformation zone and cervicitis. It cannot be repeated often enough for primary care physicians that a cervix with changes suggestive of cervical cancer should be biopsied. Too often, clinicians rely on a Papanicolaou test to detect an invasive cervical cancer. Pap tests have a high false-negative rate in this setting because blood and debris from the tumor can obscure the malignant cells on the slide. Biopsy can result in bleeding; therefore, the office suite should be appropriately equipped with silver nitrate sticks, gauze for packing, and ferric subsulfate solution (Monsel's solution). It is rare that pressure and application of these simple compounds cannot stop bleeding from a punch biopsy site.

HISTORY AND PHYSICAL EXAMINATION

A gynecologic oncologist evaluates each patient with a newly diagnosed cervical cancer referred to M. D. Anderson for treatment. A complete history is obtained. This includes a detailed obstetric and gynecologic history, including specific questions regarding sexual history, sexually transmitted diseases, and previous Pap test findings; a smoking history; and a complete family history. Some of these factors do not influence treatment planning; however, they are important elements of future epidemiologic and health services research studies. A complete physical examination is performed, including a speculum examination and digital vaginal and rectal examinations. The importance of these latter elements cannot be overstated. A sure sign of low-quality care of a patient with cervical cancer is failure to perform a rectal examination. The cervix should be completely visualized with the aid of an adequate speculum, usually a medium Graves' speculum. The location of the lesion on the cervix, the size of the visible lesion, and any extension to the upper vagina should be recorded in the medical record. Careful palpation of the parametrium and pelvic sidewall on digital examination is also vital. Physical examination, blood work, and chest radiography may be the only staging procedures performed in a patient with early invasive cervical cancer.

STAGING

The staging system for cervical cancer is shown in Table 7–1. The primary staging procedure is physical examination, as previously described. The staging procedures allowed by the International Federation of Gynecology and Obstetrics (FIGO) include options that are widely available throughout the world. In patients who have small lesions and no physical findings suggestive of metastases, treatment is selected after

Table 7–1. International Federation of Gynecology and Obstetrics (FIGO) Staging of Cervical Cancer

0	Carcinoma in situ
I	Cervical carcinoma confined to uterus (extension to corpus should be disregarded)
IA	Invasive carcinoma, diagnosed only by microscopy. All macroscopically visible lesions—even with superficial invasion—are stage IB/T1b. Stromal invasion with a maximum depth of 5 mm measured from the base of the epithelium and horizontal spread of 7 mm or less. Vascular space involvement, venous or lymphatic, does not affect classification.
IA_1	Measured stromal invasion 3 mm or less and 7 mm or less in horizontal spread
IA_2	Measured stromal invasion more than 3 mm and not more than 5 mm with a horizontal spread of 7 mm or less
IB	Clearly visible lesion confined to the cervix or microscopic lesion greater than T1a2/IA_2
IB_1	Clearly visible lesion 4 cm or less in greatest dimension
IB_2	Clearly visible lesion more than 4 cm in greatest dimension
II	Cervical carcinoma invades beyond uterus but not to pelvic wall or to the lower third of vagina
IIA	Tumor without parametrial invasion
IIB	Tumor with parametrial invasion
III	Cervical carcinoma extends to the pelvic wall and/or involves lower third of vagina or causes hydronephrosis or nonfunctioning kidney
IIIA	Tumor involves lower third of the vagina, no extension to pelvic wall
IIIB	Tumor extends to pelvic wall or causes hydronephrosis or nonfunctioning kidney
IVA	Tumor invades mucosa of bladder or rectum and/or extends beyond true pelvis
IVB	Distant metastasis

Reprinted with permission from Benedet et al (2000).

minimal evaluation: blood work and chest radiography. Patients who will undergo radiation therapy require some sort of imaging to ensure that they do not have a pelvic kidney that would be in a planned radiation field.

Patients at M. D. Anderson who have visible lesions and a significant risk of nodal metastases undergo cross-sectional imaging with computed tomography (CT) or magnetic resonance imaging (MRI). For many years we relied on lymphangiography for evaluation of regional nodes; however, the expertise required to accurately interpret lymphangiograms has declined while the interpretive expertise and technical capacity for the cross-sectional modalities have advanced. We now primarily use MRI, as it provides more detailed images of the primary tumor than does CT (Table 7–2).

Table 7–2. Evaluation of New Patients with Cervical Cancer

Review of medical records

Complete history and physical examination

Histologic confirmation of cancer

Complete blood cell count; laboratory studies to measure liver and renal function

Chest radiography

Magnetic resonance image from pelvis to kidneys when appropriate

Another promising technology is positron emission tomography (PET), which is becoming more popular with the Department of Gynecologic Oncology. PET is a form of molecular imaging that detects altered glucose metabolism associated with tumors. In the past, PET use was limited because of its high cost, poor availability, and inability to provide detailed images of the cervical anatomy. As PET and combined PET and CT become more widely available and Medicare and insurance reimbursement improves, I anticipate that we will use PET more frequently. The promise of PET is that it can detect lymph node metastases that are smaller than those detected by CT or MRI.

Although we meticulously stage patients with early cervical cancer, there are some practical problems with the FIGO classification that make its use for treatment planning difficult, especially for early cervical cancer. In 1985, FIGO created stage IA for lesions that are diagnosed by microscopy only. The category was further subdivided into stage IA$_1$ and stage IA$_2$. The distinction is based on both depth of invasion and extent of lateral spread. Measurement of depth is easy and reproducible, and depth is universally reported by pathologists in North America. In contrast, measurement of lateral spread is more difficult and less reproducible, and lateral spread is usually not reported by pathologists. For this and other reasons, the stage IA categories have never gained widespread clinical acceptance at M. D. Anderson or in the rest of North America.

On the other hand, the Society of Gynecologic Oncologists (SGO) definition of microinvasion is widely used in clinical decision-making. Microinvasion is defined as squamous carcinoma with less than 3 mm invasion, negative cone margins, and no lymph-vascular space invasion (LVSI). Retrospective reviews have confirmed that lymph node metastases are extremely rare with such disease and that the risk of relapse after conization or simple hysterectomy is extremely low. The SGO definition is used at M. D. Anderson to guide treatment planning for patients with early cervical cancer.

What about a visible lesion that meets the SGO criteria for microinvasion? For years we have considered all patients with visible lesions to have stage IB$_1$ disease and have recommended that such patients undergo radical hysterectomy. At present, we will do a cone biopsy in patients with what appears to be a small superficially invasive visible lesion to determine depth of invasion and LVSI if the patient wishes to preserve fertility.

IMPACT OF HISTOLOGIC SUBTYPE ON TREATMENT PLANNING

Squamous Carcinoma

Squamous carcinomas account for the majority of cervical cancers. Because the depth of invasion and LVSI are much more powerful predictors of lymph node metastases than grade in patients with squamous carcinoma, treatment planning for such patients is conducted without much regard to grade. Patients who are surgical candidates with small tumors but have comorbid conditions that preclude surgery can usually be treated with brachytherapy only. Patients with microinvasive squamous carcinomas of the cervix can be treated with conization or simple hysterectomy. The choice depends largely on the patient's preference regarding preservation of fertility. We have been using this approach since the late 1980s with a high degree of safety.

There are some low-grade variants of squamous carcinoma of the cervix, notably verrucous carcinoma, that require specialized treatment planning. The sensitivity of these tumors to radiotherapy has been debated over the years. In general, if complete surgical removal with negative margins can be achieved, this is the preferred management.

Adenocarcinoma

Treatment planning for patients with adenocarcinoma of the cervix is more complicated than treatment planning for patients with squamous carcinoma for several reasons. The first is the difficulty of accurate distinction between preinvasive and invasive disease. Our own data suggest that cone biopsy margins for adenocarcinomas are not as predictive of the adequacy of lesion resection as are cone biopsy margins for squamous carcinomas. In our retrospective review (Wolf et al, 1996), we found patients who had adenocarcinoma in situ with negative margins on a cone biopsy but persistent atypia, in situ disease, or even invasive disease in the hysterectomy specimen. However, several other investigators using a similar study design could not reproduce our findings. At present, the weight of the evidence supports a view that cone biopsy margins have the same significance for both adenocarcinomas and squamous carcinomas.

The second important issue in treatment planning for patients with adenocarcinoma of the cervix is accurate measurement of the depth of invasion. For many years it was said that depth could not be accurately measured, and therefore, we recommended radical hysterectomy for all patients with adenocarcinoma. Recent experience, however, has suggested that depth can be accurately measured and has the same clinical significance as it has in patients with squamous carcinomas. Recently, we have begun offering fertility-sparing cone biopsy or simple hysterectomy to selected patients with microinvasive adenocarcinoma of the cervix.

The third important issue in treatment planning for patients with adenocarcinoma is grade. Grade is much more important in treatment planning for patients with adenocarcinoma than in treatment planning for patients with the other histologic types. It is our belief that the biological behavior of a high-grade adenocarcinoma is closer to that of a neuroendocrine tumor than that of a well-differentiated adenocarcinoma. We consider chemoradiation for patients with a small, poorly differentiated adenocarcinoma of the cervix, even in the presence of normal findings on CT or MRI with no evidence of nodal metastases.

Neuroendocrine Tumors

Special mention should be made of neuroendocrine cancers of the cervix. The terminology used to describe these tumors continues to evolve. Small-cell carcinomas are the most aggressive subset of neuroendocrine tumors. Non-small-cell neuroendocrine tumors should also be considered aggressive. A poorly differentiated adenocarcinoma or undifferentiated cancer of the cervix can be confused with a neuroendocrine tumor. If there is a suspicion of neuroendocrine differentiation, it is appropriate for the clinician to request that the pathologist perform special staining.

Patients with neuroendocrine tumors should undergo more extensive pretreatment assessment, including a bone scan and brain imaging, as bone and brain are much more common sites of metastatic disease in patients with neuroendocrine than in those with nonneuroendocrine tumors. Our group has not been able to reach a consensus on the best treatment for early neuroendocrine tumors of the cervix except to say that multimodality treatment, including chemotherapy, radiotherapy, and surgery, should be considered for all patients.

TREATMENT RECOMMENDATIONS FOR MICROINVASIVE CERVICAL CANCER

Patients with squamous carcinomas with less than 3 mm invasion, no LVSI, and negative cone margins who wish to preserve their reproductive options are advised that cone biopsy alone is acceptable treatment. We follow these patients every 3 to 4 months for 2 years with Pap tests and occasional endocervical curettage. The follow-up interval after 2 years is usually 6 months. Once a patient successfully completes childbearing, consideration should be given to hysterectomy.

Patients with adenocarcinomas with less than 3 mm invasion, no LVSI, and negative cone margins who wish to preserve their reproductive options are extensively counseled. We believe that the standard of care remains hysterectomy; however, we are in a transition period that might well end with the conclusion that microinvasive adenocarcinomas should be managed the same way as squamous carcinomas. Our comfort level with patients with grade 1 and 2 cancers opting for cone biopsy only is growing; however, we are not comfortable with cone biopsy only for patients with poorly differentiated tumors.

Patients with microinvasive cancers who are ready to proceed with hysterectomy are advised to undergo simple hysterectomy. Our threshold for recommending radical hysterectomy or modified radical hysterectomy is low if there are questions about the status of margins or LVSI.

Extrafascial hysterectomy for microinvasive cervical cancer can be achieved by a number of routes. In recent years the traditional abdominal and vaginal approaches have been augmented by laparoscopic techniques. We now regularly perform laparoscopically assisted vaginal hysterectomy for microinvasive cervical cancer. The route of hysterectomy depends on patient and physician preference, body habitus, and comorbidities.

TREATMENT RECOMMENDATIONS FOR STAGE IB$_1$ DISEASE: SURGERY VERSUS RADIOTHERAPY

Patients with stage IB$_1$ disease by definition have visible lesions up to 4 cm in greatest dimension and are treated with radical hysterectomy or radiotherapy. In general, the medical literature and our own experience indicate that the survival outcomes for patients with stage IB$_1$ disease treated with radical surgery or radiotherapy are the same. For this reason, treatment recommendations are usually based on other factors, including size of the lesion; extent of infiltration of the cervix with tumor; imaging results; histologic subtype; comorbidities; and physician and patient preference. Elements of patient preference include an aversion to one modality or the other, desire to preserve ovarian and/or sexual function, and time required to complete the treatment. Pretreatment counseling should include a discussion of the impact of the treatment modality on sexual function. The medical literature on this subject is limited; however, most gynecologic oncologists believe that radical hysterectomy preserves the caliber and depth of the vagina better than radiotherapy. We are currently engaged in several prospective trials measuring vaginal length and quality of life before and after treatment for stage I cervical cancer.

At M. D. Anderson, a fundamental factor influencing the decision regarding surgery versus radiotherapy for early cervical cancer is the likelihood that surgery would result in a recommendation for postoperative pelvic irradiation due to high-risk factors such as positive nodes, positive margins, or parametrial involvement. Pretreatment counseling should include an estimation of the risk of postoperative radiotherapy following radical hysterectomy. When the risk goes over 40% to 50%, our recommendation usually shifts towards primary radiotherapy.

The results of Gynecologic Oncology Group (GOG) trial 109 (Sedlis et al, 1999) demonstrated that postoperative radiotherapy significantly reduces the risk of relapse in patients with intermediate risk factors (Tables 7–3 and 7–4). This study essentially expanded the indications for postoperative radiotherapy and has increased the confidence of our clinicians that intermediate-risk patients are not harmed by radical surgery. This study also demonstrated an increase in morbidity for patients treated with radiotherapy. This does not come as a surprise to our group, and it is a factor in our treatment planning. Recently published studies from our group demonstrate a strong correlation between radiotherapy complications and patient characteristics such as smoking, race, and weight (Eifel et al, 2002). These data have nudged some of our clinicians towards radi-

Table 7–3. Eligibility Criteria for Gynecologic Oncology Group Trial 109

CLS	Stromal Invasion	Tumor Size
Positive	Deep 1/3	Any
Positive	Middle 1/3	≥ 2 cm
Positive	Superficial 1/3	≥ 5 cm
Negative	Deep or middle 1/3	≥ 4 cm

Abbreviation: CLS, capillary lymphatic space tumor involvement.
Modified from Sedlis et al (1999). Reprinted with permission from Elsevier.

Table 7–4. Recurrences by Treatment Regimen in Gynecologic Oncology Group Trial 109

Site of Recurrence	Radiation Therapy (N = 137)	No Further Therapy (N = 140)
No evidence of disease	116 (84.7%)	101 (72.1%)
Recurrences	21 (15.3%)	39 (27.9%)
Local	18 (13.1%)	27 (19.3%)
Vagina	2	8
Pelvis	15	17
Vagina and pelvis	1	2
Distal	3 (2.2%)	10 (7.1%)
Abdomen	0	3
Abdomen and pelvis	0	1
Lung	2	2
Lung and pelvis	0	2
Lung and brain	0	1
Bone and supraclavicular lymph node	1	1
Site unknown	0 (0.0%)	2 (1.4%)

Modified from Sedlis et al (1999). Reprinted with permission from Elsevier.

cal surgery in the hope of avoiding radiotherapy completely or at least avoiding brachytherapy, with its very high local dose and associated risk of fistula. Others in our practice interpret the increased risk of late radiation morbidity in GOG 109 as more evidence against combining surgery with radiotherapy.

Our gynecologic oncologists exhibit a range of practice patterns in patients with stage IB_1 cervical cancer. Some believe that radical surgery should be reserved for patients with a very low risk of requiring postoperative radiotherapy due to deep infiltration, positive margins, or positive lymph nodes. Other faculty members are willing to perform radical surgery in patients with a higher risk of postoperative radiotherapy in the hope of avoiding radiotherapy altogether. Some clinicians use arbitrary limits on age or weight to determine which patients they will recommend surgery to, whereas others have more elastic guidelines. Some of our clinicians will abort a radical hysterectomy if microscopic disease is detected on intraoperative frozen section examination of a pelvic lymph node, whereas others do not order frozen section examination of clinically suspicious nodes and complete the operation unless there are unresectable lymph nodes. This range of practice patterns is a departure from previous years, when the predominant pattern was a very conservative approach in which surgery was recommended only to patients with the most favorable disease features.

A critical element influencing the treatment biases displayed by the gynecologic oncology and radiation oncology staff at M. D. Anderson regards our experience with radiotherapy complications. All of our faculty, and probably most gynecologic oncologists, have had patients who require a colostomy because of a rectovaginal fistula or who can no longer have sexual intercourse because of vaginal stenosis. It is difficult to compare these very serious radiation-related complications to complications associated with surgery or the combination of surgery and radiotherapy, including bladder atony, radiation enteritis, lymphedema, and chronic constipation. We are focusing increasing energy on trying to better understand the impact of various treatment options on quality of life by conducting studies of quality of life and sexual function in our long-term survivors and inpatients undergoing active treatment.

In general, patients who are good candidates for surgery also make good candidates for radiotherapy. They have vaginal geometry favorable for brachytherapy and have smaller tumors. The risk of radiotherapy complications in this group is low. Patients who are poor candidates for surgery because of vaginal geometry are also at increased risk for radiation-related complications. There are no easy answers for a thoughtful physician and patient trying to determine the best treatment for a patient with a 3- to 4-cm endophytic tumor, slightly enlarged pelvic lymph nodes on imaging studies, and an estimated 30% to 40% risk of requiring postoperative radiotherapy.

Treatment Recommendations for Stage IB$_2$ Disease

Gynecologic oncologists at M. D. Anderson have rarely recommended radical surgery for patients with stage IB$_2$ cervical cancer. The prevailing opinion of the faculty is that the outcomes with radiotherapy are excellent and that surgery in addition to radiotherapy does not improve survival but may have greater morbidity than either treatment alone. Studies at other institutions have demonstrated that up to 80% of patients with stage IB$_2$ disease treated with radical hysterectomy require postoperative radiotherapy.

Over the years, M. D. Anderson's approach has been challenged by numerous gynecologic oncologists, including many graduates of our fellowship training program. This debate culminated in the design of GOG protocol 201, "Treatment of Patients with Stage IB$_2$ Carcinoma of the Cervix: A Randomized Comparison of Radical Hysterectomy and Tailored Chemo-Radiation versus Chemo-Radiation." Our group considered this a well-designed study, and it was our hope that this study would help answer many of the questions about the management of stage IB$_2$ carcinoma of the cervix. Unfortunately, the study closed because of poor accrual, and the debate over the management of stage IB$_2$ disease continues.

Radical Hysterectomy for Early Cervical Cancer

Radical hysterectomy is one of the most challenging operations performed by gynecologic oncologists. If the surgery is not radical enough, margins and survival will be compromised. If the surgery is overly radical, the patient will be exposed to increased risk of bladder atony and lymphedema. The full extent of the tumor is not totally apparent until the specimen is removed and the uterus dissected. If a close intraoperative margin on the vaginal mucosa is found, an additional margin can be taken; however, it is usually too late to do anything about the lateral margins.

Radical hysterectomy has been divided into several subcategories of radicality. The primary determinant of radicality is the extent of the lateral dissection. Our gynecologic oncologists generally perform a type III radical hysterectomy with resection of the medial parametrium. More extensive lateral resection of the parametrium and paracolpos results in a higher risk of atonic bladder due to trauma to the neural pathways to the bladder, requiring long-term self-catheterization. In addition, if such a radical lateral resection is required to achieve negative margins, the likelihood of postoperative radiotherapy reaches well over 50%.

Choice of Incision

Low transverse incisions offer several advantages for patients undergoing radical hysterectomy. Such incisions provide excellent exposure for the pelvic lymphadenectomy and development of the lateral spaces. The wound heals well, and incisional hernias are rare. Postoperative pain is less than with vertical incisions, and most patients find the cosmetic result superior. The major disadvantage of low transverse incisions is that they make it more difficult to reach the para-aortic lymph nodes. If there are suspicious nodes in this area on preoperative imaging, a vertical incision is preferred. For most other patients, we perform a Maylard or Cherney low transverse incision.

Management of the Ovaries

We recommend removal of the ovaries at the time of radical hysterectomy in all postmenopausal patients. In premenopausal patients, the decision is more complicated, and patient preference is frequently the deciding factor. We inform patients that the risk of ovarian metastases is very low but not zero; that some patients require surgery in the future to remove the ovaries for any of a variety of reasons; and that cervical cancer does not appear to be a hormonally responsive tumor and there is no contraindication for post-operative hormone replacement therapy. We also discuss the relative merits of transposition of the ovaries and the data suggesting that transposition reduces the functional duration of the ovary. We are frequently asked about the impact of oophorectomy on mood and sexual function. These questions are difficult to answer with any meaningful data. We find that some patients can make a very quick decision regarding their ovaries—to leave them in or remove them—whereas others agonize and do not decide until they are in the holding area about to be taken into the operating room.

What to Do First?

There is a long-running debate among gynecologic oncologists regarding the order of procedures during radical surgery for cervical cancer. Some like to do the lymph node dissection first. This offers the opportunity to modify the radicality of the lateral dissection or even abort the operation completely depending on the results of the lymphadenectomy. For example, some gynecologic oncologists reduce the extent of the lateral dissection if there are positive nodes, since positive nodes are already an indication for postoperative radiotherapy.

Other gynecologic oncologists like to perform the radical hysterectomy first. These individuals consider the radical hysterectomy, especially the dissection of the distal ureter, the most difficult part of the operation. Doing the hysterectomy first, before the surgeon becomes tired or bleeding occurs, reduces the risk of complications. These individuals would not abort the operation in the event of positive nodes if they did the lymphadenectomy first.

Laparoscopically Assisted Radical Vaginal Surgery

The laparoscopic approach to radical surgery for cervical cancer is gaining acceptance throughout Europe and North America. The late Dr. Daniel

Dargent of Lyon, France, is generally credited as the driving force behind this procedure, and he trained numerous gynecologic oncologists from around the world. There are 2 laparoscopic procedures of note, radical trachelectomy and radical hysterectomy. Radical trachelectomy allows preservation of fertility for patients with small stage IB_1 cervical cancers. The lymphadenectomy and parametrial dissection are performed laparoscopically and completed vaginally. There are now several series of cases that describe low recurrence rates and high pregnancy rates in patients treated with radical trachelectomy.

When does a new procedure such as radical trachelectomy make the transition from "experimental" to "standard"? The indications for trachelectomy are limited; therefore, the number of cases in the literature remains small, under 300, and the likelihood of any type of randomized study is remote. Each patient and clinician has to reach the answer to this question on his or her own. I believe that in the hands of an experienced surgeon, these procedures can be described as standard. The challenge at M. D. Anderson has been obtaining the requisite experience to provide acceptable outcomes. We are continuing our efforts in this direction on multiple fronts.

Sentinel Node Biopsy

Lymphatic mapping and sentinel node biopsy in patients with vulvar and cervical cancers have been a special interest of ours. The international experience with lymphatic mapping for these cancers is growing, and numerous single-institution case series are in print. Many of these are in patients undergoing laparoscopic surgery, since the sentinel node concept conforms to the laparoscopic surgeon's pursuit of less invasive surgical management. Although the experience is growing and looks promising, we do not think that there are sufficient data to endorse sentinel node biopsy alone as a replacement for pelvic lymphadenectomy at this time. We are awaiting the opening of GOG protocol 206, a validation trial of lymphatic mapping for cervical cancer in the multi-institutional setting. My personal recommendation to patients is to have the lymphatic mapping procedure followed by standard lymphadenectomy since serial sectioning of the sentinel node may increase the chances of finding a micrometastasis.

KEY PRACTICE POINTS

- Biopsy should be performed on any lesion of the cervix that is suggestive of cancer, even if suspicion is low.

- Cone biopsy should be considered only for microinvasive cancer (< 3 mm invasion, no LVSI, negative margins) in patients who wish to preserve fertility.

- High-grade adenocarcinoma and neuroendocrine tumors have a high risk of relapse following surgery alone.

- Postoperative pelvic radiotherapy reduces the risk of relapse in intermediate-risk patients.

- Patient counseling regarding treatment options should include a discussion of sexual function.

- Laparoscopic surgery and sentinel node biopsy hold promise for less invasive surgery with improved outcomes.

SUGGESTED READINGS

Benedet JL, Bender H, Jones H 3rd, Ngan HY, Pecorelli S. FIGO staging classifications and clinical practice guidelines in the management of gynecologic cancers. FIGO Committee on Gynecologic Oncology. *Int J Gynaecol Obstet* 2000;70:209–262.

Burke TW, Hoskins WJ, Heller PB, Shen MC, Weiser EP, Park RC. Clinical patterns of tumor recurrence after radical hysterectomy in stage IB cervical carcinoma. *Obstet Gynecol* 1987;69:382–385.

Copeland LJ, Silva EG, Gershenson DM, Morris M, Young DC, Wharton JT. Superficially invasive squamous cell carcinoma of the cervix. *Gynecol Oncol* 1992;45:307–312.

Eifel PJ. Concurrent chemotherapy and radiation: a major advance for women with cervical cancer [editorial; comment]. *J Clin Oncol* 1999;17:1334–1335.

Eifel PJ, Jhingran A, Bodurka DC, Levenback C, Thames H. Correlation of smoking history and other patient characteristics with major complications of pelvic radiation therapy for cervical cancer. *J Clin Oncol* 2002;20:3651–3657.

Finan MA, DeCesare S, Fiorica JV, et al. Radical hysterectomy for stage IB1 vs IB2 carcinoma of the cervix: does the new staging system predict morbidity and survival? *Gynecol Oncol* 1996;62:139–147.

Grigsby PW, Siegel BA, Dehdashti F, Rader J, Zoberi I. Posttherapy [18F] fluorodeoxyglucose positron emission tomography in carcinoma of the cervix: response and outcome. *J Clin Oncol* 2004;22:2167–2171.

Levenback C, Coleman RL, Burke TW, et al. Lymphatic mapping and sentinel node identification in patients with cervical cancer undergoing radical hysterectomy and pelvic lymphadenectomy. *J Clin Oncol* 2002;20:688–693.

Matthews CM, Burke TW, Tornos C, et al. Stage I cervical adenocarcinoma: prognostic evaluation of surgically treated patients. *Gynecol Oncol* 1993;49:19–23.

Morris M, Eifel PJ, Lu J, et al. Pelvic radiation with concurrent chemotherapy compared with pelvic and para-aortic radiation for high-risk cervical cancer. *N Engl J Med* 1999;340:1137–1143.

Morris M, Mitchell MF, Silva EG, Copeland LJ, Gershenson DM. Cervical conization as definitive therapy for early invasive squamous carcinoma of the cervix. *Gynecol Oncol* 1993;51:193–196.

Ramirez PT, Levenback C, Burke TW, Eifel P, Wolf JK, Gershenson DM. Sigmoid perforation following radiation therapy in patients with cervical cancer. *Gynecol Oncol* 2001;82:150–155.

Roy M, Plante M, Renaud MC, Tetu B. Vaginal radical hysterectomy versus abdominal radical hysterectomy in the treatment of early-stage cervical cancer. *Gynecol Oncol* 1996;62:336–339.

Sedlis A, Bundy BN, Rotman MZ, Lentz SS, Muderspach LI, Zaino RJ. A randomized trial of pelvic radiation therapy versus no further therapy in selected patients with stage IB carcinoma of the cervix after radical hysterectomy and pelvic lymphadenectomy: a Gynecologic Oncology Group Study. *Gynecol Oncol* 1999;73:177–183.

Smiley LM, Burke TW, Silva EG, Morris M, Gershenson DM, Wharton JT. Prognostic factors in stage IB squamous cervical cancer patients with low risk for recurrence. *Obstet Gynecol* 1991;77:271–275.

Wolf JK, Levenback C, Malpica A, Morris M, Burke T, Mitchell MF. Adenocarcinoma in situ of the cervix: significance of cone biopsy margins. *Obstet Gynecol* 1996;88:82–86.

8 TREATMENT OF LOCALLY ADVANCED CERVICAL CANCER

Anuja Jhingran, Patricia J. Eifel,
and Pedro T. Ramirez

CHAPTER OUTLINE

CHAPTER OVERVIEW

Until 1999, radiation therapy was the primary local treatment for most patients with locally advanced cervical cancer (stage IB2 [tumors > 5 cm] or more advanced disease). With radiation therapy alone, 5-year survival rates of 65% to 75%, 35% to 50%, and 15% to 20% have been reported for patients with stage IIB, IIIB, and IVB tumors, respectively. However, both local recurrence and distant metastasis are common in patients with locally advanced disease. In recent studies, the addition of concurrent chemotherapy to radiation therapy (a treatment strategy known as chemoradiation) has been shown to improve pelvic disease control and survival rates. Cisplatin is the chemotherapy agent most commonly combined with radiation therapy in patients with locally advanced cervical cancer. With both external-beam radiation therapy and brachytherapy, technique is very important in achieving excellent local disease control and cure rates without increasing the risk of complications. In this chapter, we will discuss chemoradiation and other treatment approaches for locally advanced cervical cancer that are currently in use at M. D. Anderson Cancer Center.

INTRODUCTION

Cervical cancer is the second-leading cause of cancer death, after breast cancer, in women 20 to 39 years of age. Mortality rates are higher in women 50 years of age or older (7.6 deaths due to cervical cancer per 100,000 women with the disease) than in younger women (1.2 deaths per 100,000 women). Mortality rates are highest among African American women (5.9 per 100,000), intermediate among American Indian women (3.6 per 100,000) and Hispanic women (3.5 per 100,000), and lowest among Caucasian women (2.4 per 100,000). However, with good treatment, including chemotherapy and radiation therapy, survival rates range from 50% to 60% in patients with stage IIIB tumors up to 80% to 85% in patients with stage IB2 tumors.

CLINICAL EVALUATION

Patients with locally advanced cervical cancer should have a thorough physical examination, including a detailed pelvic examination. The pelvic examination should include careful inspection of the external genitals, vagina, and cervix. The pelvic examination should also include a thorough digital vaginal examination during which any vaginal abnormalities are noted and the size and morphology of the cervical tumor are initially assessed. The position (anteverted, axial, or retroverted), flexion (anteflexed or retroflexed), size, and mobility of the uterus should be noted. A thorough rectovaginal examination should be done, and any parametrial or pelvic sidewall involvement should be noted. The size of the cervix should be evaluated by comparing its diameter with the width of the pelvis (usually about 12 cm at the level of the cervix). Paracervical nodularity, pelvic side-wall fixation, and distortion of the normal anatomy should be noted.

Cystoscopy should be performed if there is bulky disease, if there is gross anterior vaginal involvement, or if the patient is having symptoms suggestive of possible bladder or rectal pathology. Suspected bladder involvement identified on magnetic resonance imaging (MRI) or computed tomography (CT) must be confirmed with a biopsy before the patient's International Federation of Obstetrics and Gynecology stage can be increased.

At M. D. Anderson Cancer Center, all patients with locally advanced cervical cancer have either CT or MRI of the abdomen and pelvis.

A biopsy should be performed on lymph nodes larger than 1.0 to 1.5 cm in diameter, which are suggestive of tumor involvement. Unfortunately, although CT is good for identifying large nodes, the accuracy of CT in the detection of positive nodes is compromised by CT's failure to detect small metastases and by the fact that many enlarged nodes are due not to metastases but to inflammation associated with advanced disease. The accuracy of MRI in the detection of positive nodes is similar to that of CT; however, MRI is superior to CT in that it provides more detailed images of the cervix and paracervical tissues. MRI also yields a more objective assessment of the tumor diameter than does a pelvic examination.

Recently, positron emission tomography (PET), a new and increasingly used modality in oncologic imaging, has shown some promise in the detection of cancerous lymph nodes. A number of recent studies have shown that PET scanning may be better than CT or MRI in revealing positive nodes both in the pelvic and para-aortic areas and in the supraclavicular area in patients with cervical cancer (Grisby et al, 2001). However, PET is still an emerging technology in the evaluation of cervical carcinoma.

GENERAL TREATMENT APPROACH

Radiation therapy was the primary local treatment for most patients with locally advanced cervical carcinoma until 1999. Five-year survival rates of approximately 65% to 75%, 35% to 50%, and 15% to 20% have been reported for patients treated with radiation therapy alone for stage IIB, IIIB, and IVB tumors, respectively (Table 8–1). In a French cooperative group study of 1,875 patients who received radiation therapy according to Fletcher's guidelines, 5-year survival rates were 70%, 45%, and 10% in patients with stage IIB, IIIB, and IVA tumors, respectively (Horiot et al, 1988). Both local and distant disease recurrence remain common in patients with locally advanced disease.

Recently, several trials comparing concurrent chemoradiation with radiation therapy alone have demonstrated consistent improvements in survival with chemoradiation, particularly when cisplatin is included in the chemotherapy regimen (Table 8–2). Radiation Therapy Oncology Group (RTOG) trial 90-01 (Eifel et al, 2004) and 2 Gynecologic Oncology Group trials (Keys et al, 1999; Rose et al, 1999) evaluating the use of cisplatin-based chemotherapy in patients with stage IIB–IVA disease demonstrated a significant improvement in local disease control and overall survival with chemoradiation compared with radiation therapy alone. The initial findings of RTOG 90-01, published in 1999 (Morris et al), demonstrated highly significant benefits of chemoradiation among patients with stage IB–IIB disease but no significant difference in overall survival between chemoradiation and radiation therapy alone among

Table 8–1. Pelvic Disease Control and 5-Year Survival Rates after Low-Dose-Rate Brachytherapy and External-Beam Radiation Therapy for Cervical Cancer

Study	FIGO Stage	No. of Patients	Pelvic Disease Control Rate (%)	5-Year Survival Rate (%)	% of Tumors ≥ 6 cm
Coia et al, 1990	IB	168	88	74	
	II	243	73	56	
	III	114	49	33	
Barrillot et al, 1988	I	218	90	89⎫	
	IIA	315	86	82⎭	14.5
	IIB	314	78	70	
	IIIB	482	57	49	
Perez et al, 1992	IB	384	94	90	13.5 (≥ 5 cm)
	IIA	128	88	81	39.1 (≥ 5 cm)
	IIB	353	83	77	
	III	293	64	59	
M. D. Anderson	IB1	524	98	86⎫	
(1980–1994)	IB2	482	81	67⎭	22.8
(unpublished study)	IIA	149	84	67	20.5
	IIB	211	81	54	58.8
	III	328	70	47	
Lowery et al, 1992	IB	130		81	22
	IIA	164		74	5
	IIB	112		64	43

Abbreviation: FIGO, International Federation of Gynecology and Obstetrics.
Reprinted from Eifel PJ. The uterine cervix. In: Cox JD, Ang KK, eds. *Radiation Oncology: Rationale, Technique, Results.* 8th ed. St. Louis: Mosby; 2003:698, with permission from Elsevier.

patients with stage II–IVA disease (5-year survival rates, 63% for chemoradiation vs 57% for radiation therapy alone, $P = .44$). However, a recent update of this study (Eifel et al, 2004) showed a trend towards a benefit of chemoradiation over radiation therapy alone in terms of overall survival (5-year rates, 59% vs 45%, $P = .07$) and disease-specific survival (5-year rates, 62% vs 51%, $P = .05$).

At M. D. Anderson, we treat patients with International Federation of Gynecology and Obstetrics stage IB2 or more advanced cervical carcinoma with a combination of radiation therapy and concurrent chemotherapy—either cisplatin plus 5-fluorouracil or cisplatin alone. Patients who cannot tolerate cisplatin receive radiation therapy alone. The normal course of treatment is 5 weeks of external-beam radiation therapy followed by 2 low-dose-rate radioactive implants. The 2 implants are inserted 2 weeks apart, so the total time period for the therapy is approximately 8 weeks. Patients with positive lymph nodes or pelvic sidewall disease receive an external-beam boost to the positive areas in the period between the 2 implants. Patients receive chemotherapy weekly, concurrent with

Table 8-2. Chemoradiation Trials for Cervical Cancer

Study	Eligibility Criteria	No. of Patients	Chemotherapy in Investigational Arm(s)	Chemotherapy in Control Arm	Relative Risk of Recurrence (90% CI)	P
Rose et al, 1999 (GOG 120)	FIGO IIB–IVA	526	Arm 1: Cisplatin 40 mg/m² /wk (max 6 cycles)	HU 3 g/m² 2x/wk	0.57 (0.42–0.78)	<.001
			Arm 2: Cisplatin 50 mg/m² days 1 and 29; 5-FU 4 g/m² over 96 hr after cisplatin days 1 and 29; HU 2 g/m² 2x/wk for 6 weeks		0.55 (0.40–0.75)	<.001
Eifel et al, 2004 (RTOG 90-01)	FIGO IB–IIA (≥5 cm), IIB–IVA, or positive pelvic nodes	403	Cisplatin 75 mg/m² days 1–5 and 22–26; 5-FU 4 g/m² over 96 hr days 1–5 and 22–26 (3 cycles)	None	0.51 (0.36–0.66)	<.001
Keys et al, 1999 (GOG)	FIGO IB (≥4 cm)	369	Cisplatin 40 mg/m²/wk (max 6 cycles)	None	0.51 (0.34–0.75)	.001
Whitney et al (GOG)	FIGO IIB–IVA	368	Cisplatin 50 mg/m²; 5-FU 4 g/m² over 96 hr (2 cycles)	HU 3 g/m² 2x/wk	0.79 (0.62–0.99)	.03
Peters et al (SWOG/ GOG)	FIGO I–IIA after radical hysterectomy with nodes, margins, or parametrium positive	268	Cisplatin 50 mg/m²; 5-FU 4 g/m² over 96 hr (2 cycles)	None	0.50 (0.29–0.84)	.01

(Continued)

Table 8-2. (*Continued*) Chemoradiation Trials for Cervical Cancer

Study	Eligibility Criteria	No. of Patients	Chemotherapy in Investigational Arm(s)	Chemotherapy in Control Arm	Relative Risk of Recurrence (90% CI)	P
Pearcy et al	FIGO IB–IIA (≥5 cm), IIB–IVA, or positive pelvic nodes	259	Cisplatin 40 mg/m² /wk (max 6 cycles)	None	0.91 (0.62–1.35)	.43
Wong et al	FIGO IB–IIA (>4 cm) or IIB–III	220	Epirubicin 60 mg/m² then 90 mg/m² every 4 wk for 5 more cycles	None	≈0.65	.02
Thomas et al	FIGO IB–IIA	234	5-FU 4 g/m² over 96 hr x 2	None	—	NS
Lorvidhaya et al*	FIGO IB–IVA	926	Mitomycin C 10 mg/m² days 1 and 29; oral 5-FU 300 mg/day days 1–14 and 29–42	None	—	.0001

Abbreviations: GOG, Gynecologic Oncology Group; FIGO, International Federation of Gynecology and Obstetrics; 5-FU, 5-fluorouracil; HU, hydroxyurea; RTOG, Radiation Therapy Oncology Group; SWOG, Southwest Oncology Group.

*This study had four arms: arm 1, conventional radiation therapy (RT); arm 2, conventional RT with adjuvant chemotherapy consisting of 5-FU orally at 200 mg/day given for 3 courses of 4 weeks, with a 2-week rest every 6 weeks; arm 3, conventional RT with concurrent chemotherapy; and arm 4, conventional RT with concurrent and adjuvant chemotherapy. The addition of adjuvant therapy did not affect recurrence, but there was a significant difference in the recurrence rate between the conventional RT and the conventional RT plus concurrent chemotherapy arms.

the radiation therapy. It takes approximately 4 to 5 hours every week to administer the chemotherapy (including hydration, antinausea medications, and chemotherapy), and patients receive up to 5 courses of chemotherapy with external-beam radiation therapy. The last course of chemotherapy is administered while the patient is in the hospital receiving her second implant.

RADIATION THERAPY TECHNIQUE

External-Beam Radiation Therapy

External-beam radiation therapy is used to (1) shrink bulky endocervical tumors to bring them within a higher-dose portion of the intracavitary radiation therapy (ICRT) dose distribution (see the section "Brachytherapy" below), (2) improve tumor geometry by shrinking exocervical tumors that may distort anatomy and prevent optimal brachytherapy, and (3) sterilize disease (paracentral and nodal) that receives an inadequate dose with ICRT. Cervical cancer has a tendency to metastasize in a very orderly fashion. It metastasizes first to the pelvic lymph nodes and then to the para-aortic lymph nodes. It is very rare to find para-aortic metastasis if pelvic nodes are not positive. Therefore, in patients who have clinically negative pelvic nodes or who have clinically positive pelvic nodes and clinically negative para-aortic nodes, we treat the pelvis alone. The pelvic field should include the common iliac, external iliac, internal iliac, obturator, and sacral nodes as well as the primary disease in the cervix (Figure 8–1).

At M. D. Anderson, patients are usually treated with anteroposterior and posteroanterior fields to a total dose of 45 Gy in 25 fractions if chemotherapy will be administered or 40 Gy in 20 fractions if chemotherapy will not be administered. Every attempt is made to complete the treatments within 5 weeks. Studies of patients with cervical cancer treated with radiation have demonstrated a correlation between longer duration of treatment and decreased pelvic disease control rates (treatment times longer than 7 to 8 weeks in duration for external-beam radiation and intracavitary treatments) (Lanciano et al, 1991; Fyles et al, 1992). The top of the field should be placed at the L4-L5 interspace or at the bifurcation of the aorta to cover the common iliac nodes. The bottom of the field is usually 3 to 4 cm below the inferior extent of the disease, which is marked during the pelvic examination using a marker that can be seen on radiography. The lateral borders are usually 1.5 to 2 cm from the pelvic inlet. This allows adequate coverage of the internal and external iliacs (Figure 8–1). High-energy photons (usually 15 MV or 18 MV) are used in all of our treatments. Another option is to use a 4-field technique including anteroposterior, posteroanterior, and 2 lateral fields (Figure 8–1). Some physicians prefer this approach, stating that it spares more of the bladder, rectum, and small bowel than the 2-field technique. However, if

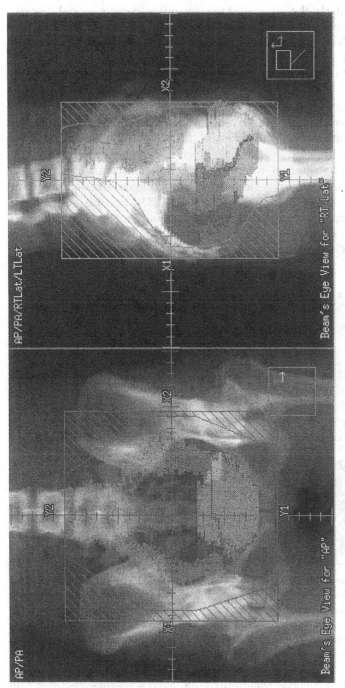

Figure 8–1. An example of the anteroposterior and lateral fields that may be used to treat a patient with cervical cancer. Shading indicates the location of the common, external iliac, and internal iliac lymph nodes and the approximate contour of this patient's 6- to 7-cm endocervical tumor and upper vagina. Lighter shading on the lateral view indicates the contour of the bladder and distal rectum. When lateral fields are used, blocks must be designed to cover the regional lymph nodes and tumor, taking into account the variable position of the uterus and cervix in the pelvis. Reprinted from Eifel PJ. The uterine cervix. In: Cox JD, Ang KK, eds. *Radiation Oncology: Rationale, Technique, Results.* 8th ed. St. Louis: Mosby; 2003:703, with permission from Elsevier.

lateral fields are used, one must be careful not to shield potential sites of disease, particularly the regions at risk for microscopic regional disease: the presacral area and paracardinal ligaments. Also, it is important that the treatment field not underestimate the posterior extent of the central cervical disease in patients who have bulky tumors. If disease involves the lower third of the vagina, the medial inguinal nodes are included in the field. We often place the patient in a frog-leg position to reduce skin damage if we have to flash the vulva to treat the lower vagina.

When a patient has grossly involved nodes on CT or MRI, extracapsular extension, unresected nodal disease, or palpable pelvic-wall disease remaining after 40 to 45 Gy, a boost is given to a total dose of 60 to 62 Gy, including the contribution from ICRT. Nodal boosts are designed to include the nodes with a margin of 1 to 2 cm while not overlapping with the region that receives a high dose from ICRT. The boost is given in the time between the 2 radioactive implants. Intensity-modulated radiation therapy (IMRT) may be used to boost the doses to large pelvic nodes up to a total of 70 Gy to a very tightly defined volume (Figure 8–2).

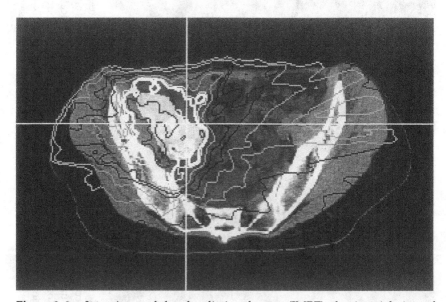

Figure 8–2. Intensity-modulated radiation therapy (IMRT) plan in axial view of a patient treated with an IMRT boost to the gross nodal disease between the 2 brachytherapy treatments. This patient was alive with no evidence of disease at last follow-up, 4 years after completion of initial treatment. The bright mass is the node that was positive. The bright, thick white line that encompasses the mass is the 20-Gy line, and the line immediately adjacent to that is the 18-Gy line. The line surrounding the 18-Gy line is the 15-Gy line. The patient also received 45 Gy of standard external-beam radiation therapy to the pelvis and para-aortic fields with concurrent weekly cisplatin and 2 brachytherapy treatments.

Brachytherapy

The importance of ICRT for cervical cancer should not be underestimated (Table 8–1). Although external-beam radiation therapy plays a critical role in sterilizing pelvic wall disease and improving tumor geometry, too much reliance on external-beam irradiation will compromise the chance for central disease control and increase the risk of complications. Brachytherapy is usually delivered using afterloading applicators that are placed in the uterine cavity and vagina. At M. D. Anderson, we use a variation of the Fletcher-Suit-Delclos low-dose-rate system. In this variation, the intrauterine tandem and vaginal applicators are placed while the patient is under general anesthesia to ensure an optimal relationship between the system and the adjacent tumor and normal tissues (Figure 8–3). The tandem should be placed midway between the bladder and the

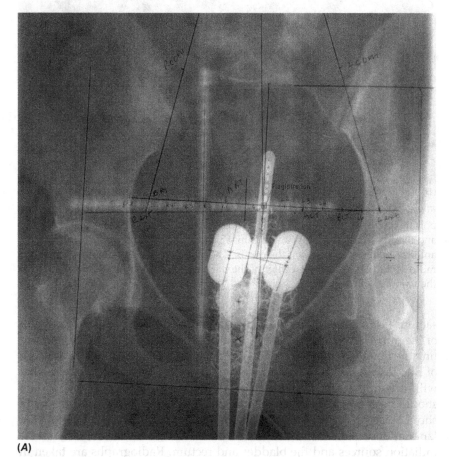

(A)

Figure 8–3. Radiographs of a Fletcher-Suit-Delclos tandem and small (2-cm) colpostats. (*A*) Anteroposterior radiograph. (*Continued*)

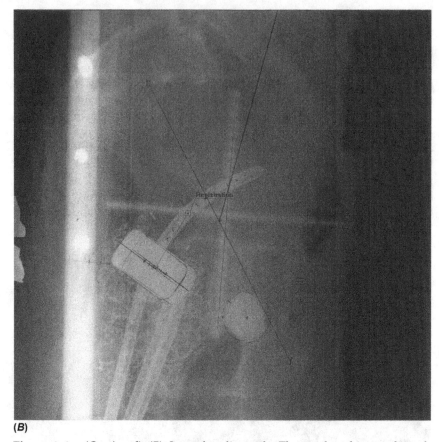

(B)

Figure 8–3. (*Continued*) (*B*) Lateral radiograph. The tandem bisects the colpostats on the lateral view and is in a roughly central position between the sacrum and bladder. The colpostats are within 0.5 cm of the marker seeds inserted in the anterior and posterior lips of the cervix. The vaginal packing (visible because of a radio-opaque thread in the center of the packing) displaces the vagina away from the vaginal sources.

sacrum (ideally one third of the way from the S1-S2 interspace to the tip of the pubis). Also, the ovoids should be separated by 0.5 to 1 cm, admitting the flange (on the tandem) in the space between. To optimize the ratio of the dose at depth to the vaginal mucosal dose, the largest ovoids that will fit comfortably should be used. In addition, the axis of the tandem should be centered between the ovoids on the anterior view and usually should bisect them on the lateral view. Vaginal packing is used to hold the tandem and ovoids in place and to maximize the distance between the radiation sources and the bladder and rectum. Radiographs are taken in the operating room at the time of the insertion, and the system is repositioned and repacked if the original positioning is suboptimal.

Ultrasonography in the operating room may be helpful in determining the position of the tandem in the uterine cavity as well as the relationship between the tandem and the bladder and rectum. Encapsulated radioactive sources consisting of cesium are then inserted into the applicators after the patient has returned to her hospital bed. This practice reduces the radiation exposure of clinical personnel.

Ideal placement of the intrauterine tandem and vaginal ovoids produces a pear-shaped radiation distribution, delivering a high radiation dose to the cervix and paracervical tissues and a reduced dose to the rectum and bladder. Several systems have been used throughout the world to determine dose rates and doses for cervical cancer; there is no inherently correct way to specify the extremely inhomogeneous dose distribution delivered using an intracavitary system. In the United States, the paracentral doses are most frequently expressed as the dose to a single point (point A). Point A is usually placed 2 cm lateral and 2 cm superior to the external os in the central plane of the intracavitary system. This measurement, however, has no consistent relationship with the tumor or target volume but lies approximately where the ureter crosses the uterine artery. Other systems of dose specification include the International Commission on Radiation Units and Measurements (ICRU) reference points based on ICRU Report 38 (International Commission on Radiation Units and Measurements, 1985) and the milligram-hours system. Whichever system of dose specification is used, emphasis should always be placed on optimizing the relationship between the intracavitary applicators and the cervical tumor and other pelvic tissues. Source, strength, and position should be carefully chosen to provide optimal tumor coverage without exceeding safe doses to normal tissue. In patients with bulky central disease, an effort should always be made to deliver at least 85 Gy (using low-dose-rate brachytherapy) to point A. If the intracavitary placement has been optimized, this can usually be accomplished while not exceeding a dose of 70 to 75 Gy to the bladder reference point or 60 to 65 Gy to the rectal reference point, doses that are usually associated with acceptably low risks of major complications. In addition, the dose delivered to the surface of the lateral wall of the apical vagina should not exceed 120 to 140 Gy.

At M. D. Anderson, we deliver ICRT using a low-dose-rate system, which usually delivers 40 to 60 cGy per hour to point A. Several groups, including groups in Japan, Canada, Europe, and the United States, have recently started using a high-dose-rate system to deliver doses greater than 100 cGy per minute to point A. Clinicians have found the high-dose-rate approach attractive because it does not require hospitalization and may be more convenient for patients. However, unless it is heavily fractionated, high-dose-rate brachytherapy loses the radiobiological advantages of low-dose-rate treatment (the ability to recover from sublethal injury in late-reacting normal tissues), potentially narrowing the thera-

Table 8-3. Selected High-Dose-Rate Brachytherapy Regimens and Reported Outcomes

Study	Year	Tumor Description	EBRT Dose (Gy)		HDR Brachytherapy Schedule				No. of Patients	5-yr DSS (%)
			Whole Pelvis	Parametrium	Dose/ Fraction	No. of Fractions	Frequency	Timing		
Kapp et al	1998	<3 cm	44–50.4		4.7–5.3	4	2x/wk	After EBRT	29	96
		3–6 cm	30–60					After EBRT	97	66
		>6 cm	>60					After EBRT	55	28
Petereit et al	1999	IB nonbulky	0	60	9.1–9.9	5	Weekly		52	85
		IB bulky or IIA	20–30	30–40	7.2–8.2	5	Weekly		39	—
		IIB	51	9	3.7–4.9	5	Weekly		50	69
		III	60	—	3.7–4.3	5	Weekly		50	33
Utley et al	1984	I	20	30	5	8–10	2x/wk	Concurrent	29	89
		II	20–30	50	5	8–10	2x/wk	Concurrent	50	58
		IIIB	20–50	50	5	8–10	2x/wk	Concurrent	43	33
Aria et al	1992	IB	0	45	5.8	5	Weekly	Concurrent	147	82
		II (small)	0	50	5.8	5	Weekly	Concurrent	256	62
		II (large)	20	30	5.75	4	Weekly	Concurrent	—	—
		III (small)	20–30	50	5.75	4	Weekly	Concurrent	515	47
		III (large)	20–30	50	5–6	3–4	Weekly	Concurrent	—	—

Abbreviations: EBRT, external-beam radiation therapy; HDR, high-dose-rate; DSS, disease-specific survival.

Reprinted from Eifel PJ. The uterine cervix. In: Cox JD, Ang KK, eds. *Radiation Oncology: Rationale, Technique, Results*. 8th ed. St. Louis: Mosby; 2003:710, with permission from Elsevier.

peutic window for a complication-free cure. In addition, advocates of high-dose-rate treatments disagree about the appropriate number of fractions and the total dose that should be delivered. The most commonly recommended regimen is 600 cGy given in 5 fractions, but this is an area of controversy. High-dose-rate ICRT is not used in standard cases at M. D. Anderson.

Multiple randomized and nonrandomized studies have suggested that survival rates and complication rates with high-dose-rate treatment are similar to those with traditional low-dose-rate treatment. At least 2 studies from the United States have shown similar results with high-dose-rate and low-dose-rate therapy in early-stage disease; however, in stage IIIB disease, the survival rate was lower with high-dose-rate than with low-dose-rate therapy (Table 8–3).

Several groups have advocated the use of interstitial perineal-template brachytherapy in patients with poor anatomy or parametrial or pelvic sidewall disease. These implants are usually placed transperineally, with placement guided by a Lucite template that encourages parallel placement of hollow needles that penetrate the cervix and paracervical spaces and are usually loaded with iridium 192. Advocates state that the advantages of this method are the ease of inserting implants in a patient whose uterus is difficult to probe, the ability to place sources directly into the parametrium, and the relatively homogeneous dose. Local control rates were high in initial reports, but these studies had relatively short follow-up and included few patients. At M. D. Anderson, we do not use interstitial brachytherapy for locally advanced cervical cancer. We are able to probe the uterus without difficulty in the majority of our patients, and if we encounter any difficulty, we are able to resolve it by using ultrasonography in the operating room.

Para-aortic Radiation Therapy

Positive para-aortic lymph nodes can be treated effectively with extended-field external-beam radiation therapy. Five-year survival rates in patients treated this way range from 25% to 50%. A laparoscopy and/or laparotomy dissection of the positive para-aortic nodes using a retroperitoneal approach may enhance control with radiation therapy and help in the design of the treatment field.

At M. D. Anderson, the superior border of extended external-beam radiation therapy portals is usually 3 cm above the highest positive node. If the patient has positive para-aortic nodes, the superior border is at T12, and if the patient has positive common iliac nodes, the superior border is at L2. We treat the pelvis with anteroposterior and posteroanterior fields using a half-beam block for the superior border. This is matched to the fields used to treat the para-aortic region: anteroposterior and posteroanterior fields and right and left lateral fields. Using this 4-field technique for the para-aortic region helps reduce the dose to the spinal cord, kidneys, and small bowel. The match line between the pelvic and para-aortic fields is feathered to eliminate hot and cold spots. Patients seem to tolerate treatment with this technique fairly well (Figure 8–4).

The role of concurrent chemotherapy with extended-field radiation therapy has been evaluated in several phase II studies. In all of these studies, both acute and late toxicity were increased with the addition of chemotherapy. Presently, the RTOG is studying the acute toxicity of extended-field radiation therapy plus weekly cisplatin. If 30% to 50% of the patients experience grade 3 or higher acute side effects, amifostine will be added to see if it reduces the acute toxicity. At M. D. Anderson, we

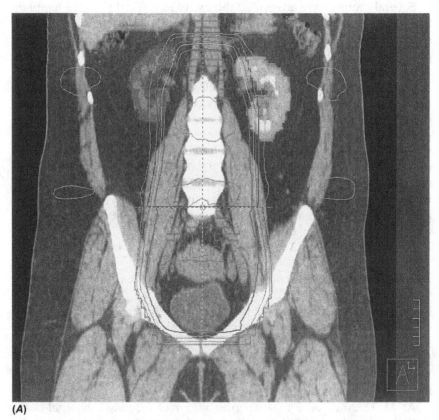

(A)

Figure 8–4. Treatment of extended fields using a split-beam technique that permits different field arrangements above and below the central axis. The pelvis was treated using anteroposterior (AP) and posteroanterior (PA) fields that minimized the amount of bone marrow in the field. The para-aortic nodes were treated using AP, PA, and 2 lateral fields. The match was moved by 0.5 cm once during treatment (not included in plan). (A) Dose distribution in AP direction. (*Continued*)

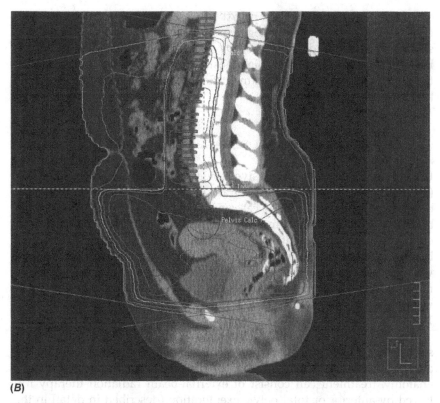

(B)

Figure 8–4. *(Continued)* *(B)* Dose distribution of split-field para-aortic field.

try to enroll patients with positive para-aortic nodes in this RTOG protocol. If a patient refuses or cannot be enrolled for other reasons, we treat
her with extended-field radiation therapy plus weekly cisplatin, which is
the same as the initial phase of the RTOG study.

The value of prophylactic extended-field radiation therapy covering the
para-aortic nodes was tested in 2 randomized trials. In 1 trial, conducted
by the RTOG, 367 patients with stage IB or IIA disease with tumors larger
than 4 cm were randomly assigned to either standard pelvic irradiation or
extended-field radiation therapy (Rotman et al, 1995). Patients who
received extended-field radiation therapy had a better absolute survival
rate than those who were treated with standard pelvic irradiation, but
there was no significant difference in the disease-specific survival rate.
In the second trial, conducted by the European Organization for Research
and Treatment of Cancer, no difference was found between standard
pelvic irradiation and extended-field radiation therapy in terms of local
control or overall survival (Haie et al, 1988). Both studies reported an
increased rate of enteric complications in patients who underwent

extended-field radiation therapy. At M. D. Anderson, for patients with clinically or pathologically negative para-aortic nodes, we administer standard pelvic radiation therapy with concurrent chemotherapy. However, for patients with high positive common iliac nodes, we set the superior border of the treatment fields at L2 or 1 echelon above the highest positive node.

TREATMENT OF STAGE IVA DISEASE

Fewer than 5% of cases of invasive cervical carcinoma are truly stage IVA (i.e., with biopsy-proven bladder or rectal involvement or extension beyond the true pelvis). Most cases of stage IVA disease are so classified because of bladder involvement; rectal involvement is rare at initial presentation. The management of stage IVA disease is particularly challenging because tumors are usually fixed to the pelvic structure and associated with regional metastatic disease. Brachytherapy can often be compromised or impossible to perform because of the development of a vesicovaginal fistula before diagnosis or during treatment. However, at least 10% to 20% of stage IVA tumors are curable with radiation therapy alone.

If a patient has not developed a vesicovaginal fistula or if the fistula is small and the urine stream is diverted, brachytherapy should be attempted. If brachytherapy cannot be delivered because of the patient's anatomy, treatment can consist of external-beam radiation therapy followed by anterior or total pelvic exenteration (described in detail in the next section) or IMRT. Recently, we have been pursuing IMRT in patients who cannot have brachytherapy because of a fistula. We try to deliver a total dose of approximately 60 to 70 Gy. IMRT works in stage IVA disease because either the tumor is very fixed and therefore does not move during treatment or the bladder is totally involved and therefore cannot move the cervix or uterus very much during treatment. We usually deliver chemotherapy concurrently with radiation therapy in patients with stage IVA disease, even though few studies have examined the value of this approach.

TREATMENT OF LOCALLY RECURRENT DISEASE

Following primary management of cervical cancer, a small proportion of patients will present with local-regional failure, and salvage therapy may be contemplated. Multiple factors determine whether salvage therapy is appropriate, including the type of prior therapy, the amount of time since the initial therapy, the site and extent of recurrent disease, and the feasibility of different retreatment techniques. Each case needs to be evaluated individually.

In patients with locally recurrent disease, various features of the recurrent disease have been associated with adverse outcome. These include pelvic sidewall (vs central) location, larger tumor volume, the presence of nodal disease, and nonsquamous (particularly adenocarcinoma) histologic subtype. Another factor associated with adverse outcome is higher International Federation of Gynecology and Obstetrics stage at the time of diagnosis of the primary tumor. Factors whose influence on outcome is controversial include the length of the interval between primary therapy and recurrence and whether the recurrence causes symptoms.

In rare, carefully selected patients initially treated with primary radiation therapy, radical hysterectomy may be a feasible alternative to exenterative surgery. In a small study, Coleman and colleagues (1994) reported 5- and 10-year survival rates of 72% and 60%, respectively, for women treated with radical hysterectomy as salvage treatment for locally recurrent cervical cancer. Factors at the time of radical hysterectomy that were associated with a favorable outcome included tumor size less than 2 cm, lesion confined to the cervix, histologically negative lymph nodes, and normal findings on preoperative intravenous pyelography. Severe complications occurred in 64% of patients, and in 42% of these patients, the complications were permanent. Others also have concluded on the basis of their own experience that radical hysterectomy is an alternative to exenteration in patients with small central recurrent cervical cancer but that this approach should be used only in carefully selected patients.

Pelvic exenteration is a potentially curative procedure for patients who have a central pelvic recurrence or a new primary tumor in the irradiated area after radiation therapy. Patient selection for pelvic exenteration is a challenging task. Pelvic examination and diagnostic images prove inadequate for determining operability in many patients. Despite careful preoperative evaluation and staging, in approximately 30% to 50% of patients in whom an exenteration procedure is started, the procedure is abandoned. The most common reasons reported for abandoning planned salvage pelvic exenteration are peritoneal disease, nodal metastases, and parametrial or pelvic sidewall fixation.

Three types of pelvic exenteration can be performed: anterior, posterior, and total. Anterior exenteration encompasses the uterine adnexa, bladder, urethra, and vagina. This operation is performed in patients with tumors that are significantly anterior, allowing clearance of the rectum, and that do not extend to involve the vaginal apex and posterior vaginal wall. Posterior exenteration includes the uterus, anus, rectum, levator ani muscle, vagina, and adnexa. This procedure is usually performed in patients with lesions confined to the posterior vaginal wall and rectal vaginal septum. A total exenteration includes the uterus, bladder, urethra, vagina, levator ani muscle, rectum, and anus. Total exenteration is usually performed in patients with lesions that are central and involve the upper half of the vagina. Total pelvic exenterations are widely used. At M. D.

Anderson, 448 total exenterations were done between 1955 and 1984, and the 5-year survival rate was between 40% and 50%.

Patients who have an isolated pelvic recurrence after initial treatment with radical hysterectomy can sometimes be cured with radiation therapy. Patients who have an isolated recurrence without pelvic wall fixation or regional metastases can be cured in 60% to 70% of cases with the use of a carefully tailored combination of external-beam radiation therapy and brachytherapy. In patients with pelvic wall involvement, however, the prognosis is much worse: the 5-year survival rate is only 10% to 20% after definitive radiation therapy. There are not enough data available to permit determination of the benefit of concurrent chemotherapy in this situation. However, in patients without contraindications to chemotherapy, we recommend chemoradiation.

Treatment of Stage IVB Disease at Presentation or Recurrence

Stage IVB cervical cancer is rare. Unfortunately, patients with stage IVB disease are usually incurable: 5-year survival rates are less than 10%. Possible rare exceptions include patients with inguinal metastases from lower vaginal involvement and patients with a solitary lung lesion. In some cases, patients with a solitary lung lesion actually have a separate new primary tumor that cannot be distinguished histologically from the original cervical tumor. Most other patients with stage IVB cervical cancer are treated with palliative intent.

At M. D. Anderson, patients with stage IVB disease receive, if they can tolerate this treatment, 30 Gy in 10 fractions to the pelvis followed by a 72-hour ICRT treatment for pelvic disease control. They also receive concurrent chemotherapy and then receive further chemotherapy after radiation therapy is complete. This treatment is very well tolerated and results in very good pelvic disease control rates.

The most active single chemotherapy agent in patients with cervical carcinoma is cisplatin. Cisplatin alone produces response rates of 30% to 50% in patients with stage IVB or recurrent disease. However, median survival duration ranges from 4 to 8 months. Numerous other single agents have been used alone in cervical cancer and have produced response rates of less than 15%. Survival rates have not been improved by adding other drugs to cisplatin. A recent Gynecologic Oncology Group randomized trial (Long, 2004) reported that combining topotecan and cisplatin yielded a response rate superior to that seen with cisplatin alone (27% vs 13%). The median survival duration was 9.4 months for cisplatin and topotecan versus 6.5 months for cisplatin alone.

Two compounds that have been used recently as single agents to treat stage IVB cervical cancer are paclitaxel and irinotecan. In a study of paclitaxel in patients with recurrent disease, paclitaxel produced a response in 9 of 52 patients (McGuire et al, 1996). This has prompted a randomized trial comparing paclitaxel in combination with cisplatin to cisplatin alone. Japanese researchers (Takeuchi et al, 1992) reported that irinotecan produced a response in approximately 24% of patients. Another study (Verschraegen et al, 1997) also showed response rates greater than 20% for irinotecan.

In general, systemic chemotherapy should be given cautiously for both recurrent and metastatic disease. Careful attention should be paid to toxicity and the patient's quality of life. Radiation therapy can provide effective pain relief for patients with localized metastases to bone, brain, lymph nodes, or other sites. Also, new strategies such as molecularly targeted treatments and antiangiogenesis therapies are beginning to be tested.

COMPLICATIONS OF RADIATION THERAPY

Acute side effects are common during pelvic radiation therapy for cervical cancer. Acute side effects can be more severe in patients treated with concurrent chemotherapy—especially nausea and vomiting, which are not generally seen with pelvic radiation therapy alone, and neutropenia. Acute bowel complications occur in 70% of patients and manifest as diarrhea, frequent bowel movements, or abdominal cramping. Usually, these effects begin approximately 2 to 3 weeks into a course of pelvic radiation therapy and last for about 1 to 2 weeks after the completion of such therapy. Enteritis can generally be treated with loperamide hydrochloride (Imodium) or diphenoxylate hydrochloride plus atropine sulfate (Lomotil) plus a low-fiber diet. Other acute side effects of pelvic radiation therapy include burning with urination, burning around the rectum, and fatigue, but these are not as frequent as bowel symptoms.

Life-threatening complications of ICRT are rare. Serious complications that have been reported include pulmonary embolism and deep venous thrombosis; in a large retrospective study of 4,042 patients, only 11 patients were documented to have or suspected of having these complications, and only 4 of these patients died (Jhingran and Eifel, 2000). Less serious complications of ICRT include uterine perforation and vaginal lacerations.

The incidence of late radiation-related complications correlates with tumor extent, patient characteristics, and treatment technique. For patients with cervical carcinoma, overall estimates of the risk of major late complications of radiation therapy usually range between 5% and 15%. The risk of experiencing a late complication is greatest within the first 3 years after treatment; however, there continues to be a small risk of complications throughout the patient's lifetime. In a study from M. D. Anderson of 1,700 patients with stage IB cervical cancer treated with definitive radiation therapy alone (Eifel et al, 1995), the overall incidence of grade 3 to 4 late complications was 14.4% at 20 years. Most complications involved the bladder or bowel. The risk of rectal complications was greatest in the first few years after treatment (2.3% at 5 years), but there was a small continuous risk between 5 and 25 years. The most frequent urinary tract complication was hematuria, which usually resolved with medical management. There was a 2% to 3% incidence of late urinary tract complications. In another study from M. D. Anderson (Eifel et al, 2002), there was a strong correlation between smoking history (smoker vs nonsmoker) and certain ethnicities and increased risk of major gastrointestinal complications, especially in patients who smoked more than 1 pack of cigarettes per day.

Mild to moderate atypical vaginal ulceration or necrosis occurs in 5% to 10% of patients treated with primary radiation therapy for cervical cancer. This complication usually occurs within 12 months after completion of radiation therapy, rarely progresses to fistula formation, and usually heals within 1 to 6 months with appropriate local care, including the use of vaginal estrogen cream or 50% H_2O_2 douches, depending on the severity. Vaginal shortening is another possible side effect. The incidence of vaginal shortening and its influence on sexual interaction is not fully documented. Severe shortening is more common in postmenopausal patients, patients who are not sexually active, and patients with more advanced disease at presentation.

KEY PRACTICE POINTS

- Concurrent chemotherapy and radiation therapy is the primary treatment for most patients with locally advanced cervical cancers.

- Radiation therapy employs a combination of external-beam radiation therapy and brachytherapy.

- Patients with positive para-aortic node disease should be treated with extended-field radiation therapy and have a 5-year survival rate in the range of 25% to 50%.

- Patients with stage IVA tumors have a 5-year survival rate of 10% to 20% with radiation therapy alone.

- In the small proportion of patients with recurrent disease, salvage therapy may be considered. Pelvic exenteration is the primary surgery for patients with disease that recurs after radiation therapy.

- Stage IVB cervical cancer has a 5-year survival rate of less than 10%.

- The incidence of late radiation-related complications correlates with tumor extent, patient characteristics, and treatment technique and is in the range of 5% to 15%.

Suggested Readings

Coleman RL, Keeney ED, Freedman RA, et al. Radical hysterectomy after radiotherapy for recurrent carcinoma of the uterine cervix. *Gynecol Oncol* 1994;55:29–35.

Cunningham MJ, Dunton CJ, Corn B, et al. Extended-field radiation therapy in early-stage cervical carcinoma: survival and complications. *Gynecol Oncol* 1991;43:51–54.

Delclos L, Fletcher GH, Moore EB, Sampiere VA. Minicolpostats, dome cylinders, other additions and improvements of the Fletcher-suit afterloadable system: indications and limitations of their use. *Int J Radiat Oncol Biol Phys* 1980;6:1195–1206.

Eifel PJ, Jhingran A, Bodurka DC, et al. Correlation of smoking history and other patient characteristics with major complications of pelvic radiation therapy for cervical cancer. *J Clin Oncol* 2002;20:3651–3657.

Eifel PJ, Levenback C, Wharton JT, et al. Time course and incidence of late complications in patients treated with radiation therapy for FIGO stage IB carcinoma of the uterine cervix. *Int J Radiat Oncol Biol Phys* 1995;32:1289–1300.

Eifel PJ, Winter K, Morris M, et al. Pelvic irradiation with concurrent chemotherapy versus pelvic and para-aortic irradiation for high-risk cervical cancer: an update of radiation therapy oncology group trial (RTOG) 90-01. *J Clin Oncol* 2004;22:872–880.

Fyles A, Keane TJ, Barton M, et al. The effect of treatment duration in the local control of cervix cancer. *Radiother Oncol* 1992;25:273–279.

Fyles AW, Pintilie M, Kirkbride P, Levin W, Manchul LA, Rawlings GA. Prognostic factors in patients with cervix cancer treated by radiation therapy: results of a multiple regression analysis. *Radiother Oncol* 1995;35:107–117.

Grigsby PW, Siegel BA, Dehdashti F. Lymph node staging by positron emission tomography in patients with carcinoma of the cervix. *J Clin Oncol* 2001;19:3745–3749.

Haie C, Pejovic MH, Gerbaulet A, et al. Is prophylactic para-aortic irradiation worthwhile in the treatment of advanced cervical carcinoma? Results of a controlled clinical trial of the EORTC radiotherapy group. *Radiother Oncol* 1988;11:101–112.

Horiot JC, Pigneux J, Pourquier H, et al. Radiotherapy alone in carcinoma of the intact uterine cervix according to G. H. Fletcher guidelines: a French cooperative study of 1383 cases. *Int J Radiat Oncol Biol Phys* 1988;14:605–611.

International Commission on Radiation Units and Measurements. *Dose and Volume Specification for Reporting Intracavitary Therapy in Gynecology*. Vol. 38. Bethesda, MD: International Commission on Radiation Units and Measurements; 1985.

Jhingran A, Eifel PJ. Perioperative and postoperative complications of intracavitary radiation for FIGO stage I-III carcinoma of the cervix. *Int J Radiat Oncol Biol Phys* 2000;46:1177–1183.

Keys HM, Bundy BN, Stehman FB, et al. Cisplatin, radiation, and adjuvant hysterectomy compared with radiation and adjuvant hysterectomy for bulky stage IB cervical carcinoma. *N Engl J Med* 1999;340:1154–1161.

Lanciano RM, Martz K, Coia LR, et al. Tumor and treatment factors improving outcome in stage III-B cervix cancer. *Int J Radiat Oncol Biol Phys* 1991;20:95–100.

Logsdon MD, Eifel PJ. FIGO IIIB squamous cell carcinoma of the cervix: an analysis of prognostic factors emphasizing the balance between external beam and intracavitary radiation therapy. *Int J Radiat Oncol Biol Phys* 1999;43:763–775.

Long HJ 3rd, Bundy BN, Grendys EC Jr, et al. Randomized phase III trial of cisplatin with or without topotecan in carcinoma of the uterine cervix: a Gynecologic Oncology Group Study. *J Clin Oncol* 2005;23:4626–4633.

McGuire WP, Blessing JA, Moore D, et al. Paclitaxel has moderate activity in squamous cervix cancer. A Gynecologic Oncology Group study. *J Clin Oncol* 1996;14:792–795.

Morris M, Eifel PJ, Lu J, et al. Pelvic radiation with concurrent chemotherapy compared with pelvic and para-aortic radiation for high-risk cervical cancer. *N Engl J Med* 1999;340:1137–1143.

Petereit DG, Sarkaria JN, Potter PM, Schink JC. High-dose-rate versus low-dose-rate brachytherapy in the treatment of cervical cancer: analysis of tumor recurrence—the University of Wisconsin experience. *Int J Radiat Oncol Biol Phys* 1999;45:1267–1274.

Rose PG, Bundy BN, Watkins EB, et al. Concurrent cisplatin-based radiotherapy and chemotherapy for locally advanced cervical cancer. *N Engl J Med* 1999;340:1144–1153.

Rotman M, Pajak TF, Choi K, et al. Prophylactic extended-field irradiation of para-aortic lymph nodes in stages IIB and bulky IB and IIA cervical carcinomas. Ten-year treatment results of RTOG 79-20. *JAMA* 1995;274:387–393.

Takeuchi S, Noda K, Yakushiji M. Late phase II study of CPT-11, topoisomerase 1 inhibitor in advanced cervical carcinoma. *Proc ASCO* 1992;11:224.

Verschraegen CF, Levy T, Kudelka AP, et al. Phase II study of irinotecan in prior chemotherapy-treated squamous cell carcinoma of the cervix. *J Clin Oncol* 1997;15:625–631.

9 UTERINE SARCOMAS

Lois M. Ramondetta, Diane C. Bodurka,
Michael T. Deavers, and Anuja Jhingran

CHAPTER OUTLINE

Chapter Overview

Uterine sarcomas are very rare neoplasms, comprising 1% of all gynecologic malignancies. However, these sarcomas are some of the most aggressive tumors of the gynecologic tract. Sarcoma patients have an overall
survival rate of less than 50%, even when the disease is diagnosed at an
early stage. There is no designated staging system for uterine sarcomas,
and most clinicians use the International Federation of Gynecology and
Obstetrics staging system for endometrial cancer. Although surgical resection is the mainstay of treatment, multidisciplinary teams, including radiation oncology, gynecologic oncology, and sarcoma specialists, are
important. The benefit of surgical lymph node staging is unclear, especially in the setting of uterine leiomyosarcoma. Adjuvant radiation therapy has historically been of little survival value, but palliatively, it can
offer improved quality of life and pain control. Chemotherapy does not
appear to be effective when given adjuvantly but can produce limited
response rates of approximately 17% to 40% when given for recurrences.
Because of the rarity of these tumors, literature on them is scarce, and
reports often cover a broad range of histologic subtypes of sarcoma.

Introduction

This chapter reviews the presentation, evaluation, and treatment of
women with sarcomas of the uterus.

Uterine sarcomas comprise only 1% of all gynecologic malignancies and
fewer than 5% of all cancers of the uterus. However, sarcomas are some of
the most aggressive tumors of the gynecologic tract. Because of the low
incidence of uterine sarcomas and the fact that they lack a preinvasive
stage, there is no established practice for screening for these tumors.

Because of the rare nature of uterine sarcomas and their often aggressive clinical course, the literature on them is scarce. Clinical-trial reports
and literature reviews often include a broad range of histologic subtypes
of sarcoma, which limits interpretation and application of the results.
At M. D. Anderson Cancer Center, we have tried to tailor our approach to
patients with uterine sarcomas by histologic subtype. We do not rely heavily on reported response rates from protocols that have included multiple
subtypes. We believe strongly that patients with uterine sarcomas should
be referred to major academic centers with options for participation in
clinical trials.

Staging

The staging of uterine sarcomas is based on the International Federation of Gynecology and Obstetrics staging system for uterine corpus cancer (see the chapter "Treatment of Endometrial Cancer").

Uterine Malignant Mixed Müllerian Tumors

Epidemiology and Tumor Features

Uterine malignant mixed müllerian tumors (MMMTs) are an uncommon but extremely aggressive subtype of uterine malignancy. These tumors usually present in women over the age of 50 years and peak in incidence during the seventh and eighth decades. MMMTs are more common in African American than in Caucasian patients.

MMMTs of the uterus contain both malignant epithelial and malignant sarcomatous components. Although MMMTs have historically been grouped with all other uterine sarcomas, at M. D. Anderson we believe that MMMTs are actually mixed tumors consisting of both carcinomatous and sarcomatous elements (Figure 9–1). While some authors have suggested renaming these tumors "sarcomatoid carcinomas," we prefer to retain the term "MMMT" to emphasize the mixed components.

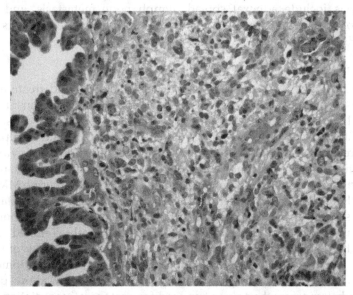

Figure 9–1. Malignant mixed müllerian tumor (MMMT). This MMMT is composed of high-grade serous carcinoma (on the left) and high-grade unclassified sarcoma.

MMMTs are more likely than endometrial stromal sarcomas (ESSs) or leiomyosarcomas (LMSs) to present with postmenopausal bleeding, and the presence of malignancy can usually be determined preoperatively with an endometrial biopsy. Abnormal bleeding usually occurs as a result of the origin of MMMTs in the endometrium rather than in the myometrium. Patients typically present with a bulky polypoid mass extending into and even through the endocervical canal. In contrast with LMS, uterine MMMT quickly metastasizes to pelvic and para-aortic lymph nodes.

The carcinomatous component of uterine MMMTs may be papillary serous, endometrioid, clear cell, squamous, or undifferentiated. The mesenchymal components may be "homologous"—similar to tissues normally present in the uterus, such as smooth muscle or uterine stromal tissue—or "heterologous," resembling tissue foreign to the uterus, such as striated muscle or cartilage. Often the sarcomatous component is consistent with fibrosarcoma, ESS, or rhabdomyosarcoma. The epithelial component, müllerian in origin, has the greatest influence on survival. Typically, recurrences of MMMTs are composed of carcinoma of endometrioid or papillary serous subtype. However, recurrences and distant metastases composed of sarcoma or mixed carcinoma and sarcoma also occur.

The recurrence rate for stage I and II MMMTs is 50%. Distant metastases account for 50% to 80% of all recurrences. The most common sites of metastasis are the lung and omentum. Features associated with poor prognosis include adnexal spread, lymph node metastasis, and high grade of tumor. Unfortunately, the 5-year survival rate for patients with MMMTs is less than 20%.

Surgical Treatment

The M. D. Anderson approach to clinical evaluation and treatment of patients with uterine MMMTs is outlined in Figure 9–2. At our institution, we believe that surgical treatment of MMMTs should consist of exploratory laparotomy, total abdominal hysterectomy, bilateral salpingo-oophorectomy, omentectomy, aspiration of abdominal fluid for cytologic evaluation, pelvic and para-aortic lymph node dissection, and tumor debulking at the time of presentation. Clinical staging of uterine MMMTs is unreliable; tumors are often upstaged after thorough surgical staging. Direct serosal invasion and intraperitoneal metastasis are common. As many as 15% to 40% of tumors with disease clinically confined to the uterus have retroperitoneal lymph node involvement. The risk of nodal spread is proportional to the depth of invasion. As with endometrial cancer, more accurate surgical staging of MMMTs may allow physicians to better assess the value of or need for postoperative radiation therapy or chemotherapy. We always attempt surgical debulking in patients with uterine MMMTs. Patients with minimal residual disease may have

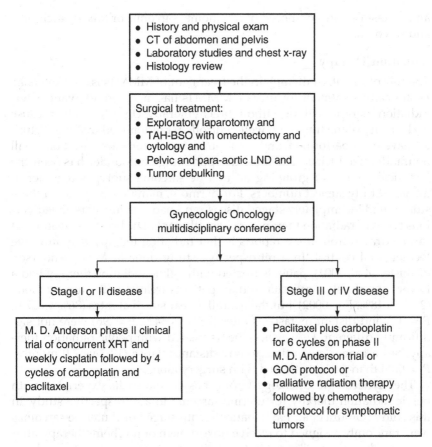

Figure 9–2. Algorithm for clinical evaluation and treatment of patients with malignant mixed müllerian tumors of the uterus. CT, computed tomography; TAH-BSO, total abdominal hysterectomy and bilateral salpingo-oophorectomy; LND, lymph node dissection; XRT, radiation therapy; GOG, Gynecologic Oncology Group.

longer survival than those left with gross residual disease after surgical debulking.

Pathologic Evaluation

Important features of MMMTs that should be evaluated by the pathologist include the depth of myometrial invasion and the presence or absence of extrauterine extension and lymphatic or vascular invasion. At M. D. Anderson, pathologists also estimate the percentages of the primary tumor composed of carcinomatous and sarcomatous components and classify the histologic subtypes present in each component (if they are differentiated enough to classify). Pathologists also state whether recurrences and metastases are composed of carcinoma, sarcoma, or mixed carcinoma and sarcoma.

Radiation Therapy

The role of radiation therapy in the treatment of MMMTs is controversial. Historically, treatment for uterine MMMTs has included adjuvant pelvic radiation therapy with or without brachytherapy. Unfortunately, because of the rarity of the tumor, no well-controlled, randomized treatment studies have been performed, and most published reports are based on small nonrandomized trials. The most disappointing confounder has been the historical pattern of grouping all uterine sarcoma subtypes together to increase study subject numbers. Furthermore, many participants in these studies had incompletely staged disease and had previously received various types of radiation therapy or chemotherapy. The best conclusion that can be drawn from these reports is that radiation therapy may improve locoregional control. In a retrospective study done at M. D. Anderson (Callister et al, 2004), patients treated with pelvic radiation therapy had a lower rate of pelvic recurrence than patients treated with surgery alone (28% vs 48%, P = .0002), but the overall 5-year survival rates (36% vs 27%, P = .10) and distant metastasis rates (57% vs 54%, P = .96) were not significantly different. However, patients treated with pelvic radiation therapy had a longer mean time to any distant relapse (17.3 vs 7.0 months, P = .001) than patients treated with surgery alone.

The Gynecologic Oncology Group has evaluated its experience with pelvic radiation therapy for uterine sarcoma in a retrospective study. In this study (Omura et al, 1985), patients with stage I or II uterine sarcomas were randomly assigned to receive doxorubicin or no chemotherapy after surgery. The use of adjuvant pelvic radiation therapy was not mandated but was left to the discretion of the individual investigator, and the study was not stratified on the basis of use of radiation therapy. In a subset analysis, the authors demonstrated a reduction in pelvic recurrences in patients who received pelvic radiation therapy compared to patients who did not; however, patients who underwent radiation therapy had a higher rate of distant metastasis, and there was no significant difference in the 2-year survival rate between the 2 groups.

Several single-institution studies show that pelvic radiation therapy improves local control, and the results of 2 collaborative trials will be available soon. The European Organization for Research and Treatment of Cancer trial 55874 is an important randomized trial directly addressing the benefit of adjuvant pelvic irradiation. In this study, patients with early-stage uterine sarcomas were randomized to receive either surgery alone or surgery followed by adjuvant radiation therapy. Another study that may help address the question of the importance of radiation therapy is Gynecologic Oncology Group trial 150, which is a phase III randomized study of whole-abdominal radiation therapy versus combination chemotherapy in optimally debulked stage I, II, III, or IV carcinosarcoma of the uterus. This trial has just finished accruing patients, and results are pending.

At M. D. Anderson, patients with stage I or II uterine MMMTs are offered pelvic radiation therapy to improve local control but are clearly told that it may not improve survival. The pelvis is treated adjuvantly with a 4-field technique to a total dose of 45 to 50 Gy. Presently, we are conducting a phase II trial evaluating adjuvant pelvic radiation therapy concurrent with weekly cisplatin followed by 4 courses of carboplatin and paclitaxel in patients with stage I, II, or IIIA uterine MMMTs. In patients with extensive pelvic disease who are poor candidates for surgery, palliative radiation therapy followed by chemotherapy off protocol is also considered.

Chemotherapy

Over the past 2 decades, standard adjuvant treatment of uterine MMMTs at M. D. Anderson has shifted from primarily locoregional radiation therapy to chemotherapy. Unfortunately, chemotherapy has shown only minimal evidence of improved survival. There is no definitive proof for any survival benefit of adjuvant chemotherapy in uterine sarcomas.

Historically, we have treated recurrent MMMTs with platinum-based therapy (cisplatin or carboplatin) in combination with ifosfamide, although other chemotherapeutic agents have also been used. Cisplatin and ifosfamide are the most widely studied systemic agents in the treatment of recurrent uterine MMMTs, with reported response rates of 18% to 44% for single-agent cisplatin and 39% for single-agent ifosfamide. Trials of combination therapy reveal higher response rates for cisplatin plus ifosfamide than for ifosfamide alone (57% vs 39%) but no significant improvement in survival for cisplatin plus ifosfamide over ifosfamide alone in patients with advanced, recurrent, or persistent disease.

Experience with paclitaxel in uterine MMMTs is limited. However, at M. D. Anderson, we recently completed a study of single-agent paclitaxel in uterine papillary serous carcinoma, 1 of the many subtypes of the carcinomatous component of uterine MMMTs. In this study, the overall response rate was 77%. Because of the significant influence of the carcinomatous component on survival, the use of paclitaxel in combination with carboplatin for advanced uterine MMMTs has become standard at our institution.

As mentioned in the preceding section, we are conducting a phase II trial of adjuvant pelvic radiation therapy concurrent with weekly cisplatin followed by 4 courses of carboplatin and paclitaxel in patients with uterine MMMTs. This trial is based on the evidence that postoperative radiation therapy may improve local control in patients with uterine MMMTs; the previously documented response rate of 18% to 44% for single-agent cisplatin in patients with uterine MMMTs; and moderate response rates with paclitaxel for uterine papillary serous carcinoma and ovarian MMMTs. The adjuvant radiation therapy with cisplatin as a radiosensitizer is designed to maintain local control, while the 4 additional courses of systemic therapy are designed to minimize any risk of distant recurrence. We believe that our new regimen may have better activity than the previous regimen of cisplatin and ifosfamide because of the addition of paclitaxel. In addition, eliminating ifosfamide and substituting carboplatin for cisplatin should improve tolerability and reduce the incidence and severity of neurotoxicity, nephrotoxicity, and gastrointestinal toxicity in these often elderly patients. This regimen will also allow patients with uterine MMMTs to be treated as outpatients, thus reducing the overall cost of treatment and potentially improving patients' quality of life.

Only patients with stage I, II, or IIIA uterine MMMTs with no gross residual disease after surgical treatment are eligible for this protocol. Treatment of patients with no gross residual disease can be justified by the poor outcomes observed in patients with small-volume extrauterine disease: recurrence rates of 40% to 60% have been observed in patients with disease that is apparently limited to the uterus. Patients will be evaluated for adverse reactions and progression-free survival.

Hormonal Therapy

Approximately 30% of uterine MMMTs express estrogen or progesterone receptors. At M. D. Anderson, we consider hormonal therapy for recurrent disease in patients with estrogen- or progesterone-receptor-positive tumors heavily pretreated with chemotherapy.

Treatment Summary

Ultimately, the ideal treatment for uterine MMMTs may be combined radiation therapy and chemotherapy or molecular targeted therapy after optimal surgical debulking. However, the best treatment has yet to be determined. Because current therapies are associated with poor response rates and high recurrence rates, it is critical to search for additional treatment options. Because of the rarity of uterine MMMTs, we believe patients with these tumors should be referred to major cancer treatment centers, where larger and more informative trials can be conducted to help answer these questions more efficiently and effectively.

LEIOMYOSARCOMA

Epidemiology and Tumor Features

Uterine LMS accounts for approximately 1% of all uterine malignancies but 40% of all uterine sarcomas. The average patient age at diagnosis of LMS is 53 years. Unfortunately, because of the tumor's stromal rather than endometrial origin, LMS is not often diagnosed preoperatively. Although some patients complain of pain or bleeding and undergo endometrial biopsy because of these symptoms, most women with LMS lack symptoms, although some present with a rapidly enlarging pelvic mass and thus do not undergo biopsy before surgery. Even with an endometrial biopsy, LMS is diagnosed preoperatively in only 15% of cases.

Uterine LMS presents as a solitary, poorly demarcated myometrial mass. This sarcoma arises from myometrial smooth muscle and smooth muscle from the myometrial vessels. Histologically, LMS usually consists of highly cellular, spindle-shaped smooth muscle cells with hyperchromatic nuclei and many mitoses (Figure 9–3). The nuclei are characterized by moderate to marked atypia, and mitotic counts of more than 10 mitoses per 10 high-power fields are common. Coagulative necrosis also may be present.

Smooth muscle tumors of uncertain malignant potential (STUMP) have atypical features that are not fully diagnostic of LMS. These tumors may have (1) more than 20 mitoses per 10 high-power fields and no necrosis or atypia, (2) fewer than 10 mitoses per 10 high-power fields and diffuse significant nuclear atypia but no coagulative necrosis, or (3) fewer than 10 mitoses per 10 high-power fields with coagulative necrosis but no atypia. These tumors are generally associated with a low risk of recurrence.

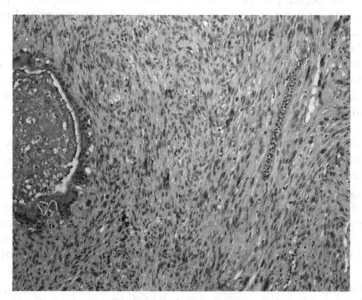

Figure 9–3. Leiomyosarcoma. This tumor involving the endocervix is characterized by fascicles of spindle cells with moderate to marked nuclear atypia and mitotic figures.

Another distinct subtype of LMS, myxoid LMS, is characterized by malignant behavior even when the mitotic count is fewer than 2 mitoses per 10 high-power fields. Histologically, myxoid LMS has an intercellular myxoid substance and infiltrates the myometrium. Myxoid LMS may be highly aggressive despite a low mitotic count and only mild to moderate nuclear atypia.

Sixty percent of women with LMS present with disease clinically limited to the uterus. Cure rates for these patients range from 20% to 60%, with rates depending on the success of primary resection. Recurrent disease is not curable unless it is resectable. Favorable prognostic features include premenopausal status, low mitotic count, pushing margins, hyalinization, absence of necrosis, origin in a uterine leiomyoma, and small tumor size. The recurrence rate is approximately 70% for stage I and II disease, and the site of recurrence is often distant. Recurrence risk is higher with higher stage or higher mitotic count. Unlike the case with uterine MMMTs, in patients with uterine LMS, pelvic and para-aortic lymph nodes are not typically involved at primary surgical evaluation.

Surgical Treatment

The M. D. Anderson approach to clinical evaluation and treatment of patients with uterine LMS is outlined in Figure 9–4. If the diagnosis is made or suspected preoperatively, we ordinarily recommend computed tomography or magnetic resonance imaging of the abdomen and pelvis prior to surgical exploration to evaluate for extrauterine spread. In addition, chest radiography and possibly chest computed tomography should be considered to rule out distant metastasis. The staging of uterine LMS has been adopted from a modified International Federation of Gynecology and Obstetrics system for uterine corpus cancer, and therefore surgery is required for staging (see the chapter "Treatment of Endometrial Cancer").

At M. D. Anderson, we consider total abdominal hysterectomy and bilateral salpingo-oophorectomy to be the minimum standard surgical treatment for uterine LMS. For patients with extrauterine disease detected at surgery, there are no clear guidelines regarding surgical debulking. After metastasis is proven by computed tomography–guided biopsy, patients are discussed in a multidisciplinary conference. Random biopsies of retroperitoneal lymph nodes rarely reveal metastatic spread; thus, we do not typically include lymph node sampling in our surgical treatment plan.

If the diagnosis of LMS is made after a myomectomy, we recommend a completion hysterectomy and surgical staging. We aim for optimal surgical cytoreduction because the literature suggests a survival benefit in patients with minimal residual disease.

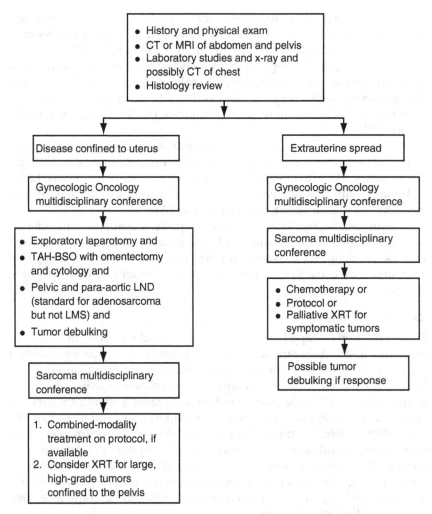

Figure 9–4. Algorithm for clinical evaluation and treatment of patients with leiomyosarcoma or adenosarcoma of the uterus. CT, computed tomography; MRI, magnetic resonance imaging; TAH-BSO, total abdominal hysterectomy and bilateral salpingo-oophorectomy; XRT, radiation therapy; LND, lymph node dissection; LMS, leiomyosarcoma.

Pathologic Evaluation

Important features that should be included in the gross and microscopic evaluation of uterine LMS are tumor size, presence or absence of coagulative tumor cell necrosis, degree of nuclear atypia, highest mitotic count per 10 high-power fields, presence or absence of vascular invasion, and status of the surgical margins. The 3 main criteria used to determine treatment and prognosis are necrosis, nuclear atypia, and mitotic count.

In tumors that lack necrosis and nuclear atypia, classification is as follows: 5 to 20 mitoses per 10 high-power fields, mitotically active leiomyoma; more than 20 mitoses per 10 high-power fields, STUMP.

In tumors that lack coagulative necrosis but have diffuse moderate to severe nuclear atypia, classification is as follows: fewer than 2 mitoses per 10 high-power fields, atypical leiomyoma; 2 to 10 mitoses per 10 high-power fields, STUMP; more than 10 mitoses per 10 high-power fields, uterine LMS.

In tumors with coagulative necrosis but without significant nuclear atypia, classification is as follows: fewer than 10 mitoses per 10 high-power fields, STUMP; at least 10 mitoses per 10 high-power fields, LMS.

Tumors with coagulative necrosis and significant nuclear atypia, regardless of mitotic count, are classified as LMS.

The prognostic significance of tumor grade in patients with uterine LMS is controversial. Past studies of the significance of grade have used various criteria for the diagnosis of LMS, have used different grading systems, and have come to different conclusions. Currently, we do not grade uterine LMS.

Radiation Therapy

Pelvic radiation therapy has historically been used for adjuvant treatment of uterine LMS. Adjuvant irradiation is considered for patients with a high risk of recurrence due to a high mitotic count or advanced stage. However, although radiation therapy has been shown to reduce the pelvic relapse rate by 50%, studies have not demonstrated a significant survival benefit with this approach. In patients with LMS, in contrast to patients with other uterine sarcomas, the dominant pattern of recurrence is outside the pelvis and abdominal cavity. At least two thirds of patients with uterine LMS have some component of distant disease at first recurrence. Thus, although the rate of recurrence in the pelvis is not insubstantial, little is potentially gained by delivering pelvic radiation therapy as a postoperative adjuvant treatment.

We reserve pelvic radiation therapy for patients with the highest risk of pelvic recurrence, such as patients with close surgical margins. Because lymph node metastasis is uncommon, when radiation therapy is necessary, irradiation of the operative bed (usually the lower pelvis) is usually sufficient for local control.

Chemotherapy

A randomized Gynecologic Oncology Group phase III trial evaluating adjuvant doxorubicin compared with no treatment in patients with stage I or II uterine sarcoma failed to find any significant survival advantage with chemotherapy (Omura et al, 1985). There are no established potentially curative therapies for unresectable LMS. First-line treatment for LMS is usually doxorubicin and/or ifosfamide. Single-agent ifosfamide has a response rate of 17% (Sutton et al, 1992). Doxorubicin has been associated with a response rate of 10% to 19% alone or in combination with ifosfamide (Hannigan et al, 1983; Berchuck et al, 1988). Although a response rate as high as 30% for the combination has been reported, it does not appear to offer a survival advantage (Sutton et al, 1996a). Median survival remains approximately 11 months. High-dose chemotherapy with doxorubicin and ifosfamide is associated with a 25% response rate in recurrent and advanced LMS. Gemcitabine is associated with a response rate of 20%, docetaxel has a response rate of approximately 15%, and liposomal doxorubicin has a response rate of 16% (Sutton et al, 2005). Other regimens include vincristine, doxorubicin, and cyclophosphamide; platinum, doxorubicin, and cyclophosphamide; paclitaxel and carboplatin; and dacarbazine. These regimens have shown no additional benefit and increased toxicity compared with doxorubicin alone. Regardless of the agent, 80% of patients with uterine LMS who are treated with chemotherapy eventually have progression of disease.

Treatment of Recurrent Disease

In contrast to uterine MMMTs, which tend to recur intra-abdominally, LMS frequently recurs outside the abdomen. There are no clear treatment guidelines for patients with recurrent LMS. Surgical treatment can be considered, especially in patients with a solitary liver or lung metastasis. Five-year survival rates can be as high as 33% to 55% in such patients. Levenback et al (1992) published a review of 45 patients who underwent resection of pulmonary metastases of uterine sarcoma (LMS in 84%; MMMT or ESS in 16%). Five- and 10-year survival rates after hysterectomy were 65% and 50%, respectively, with a mean follow-up time of 25 months. Patients with unilateral and small-volume metastases had a better prognosis than those with bilateral metastases. The only factor identified as a contraindication to resection of pulmonary metastases was extrathoracic tumor. We also consider surgical treatment for local recurrences if resection is feasible.

ENDOMETRIAL STROMAL SARCOMA

Epidemiology and Tumor Features

ESSs represent fewer than 5% of all uterine sarcomas. Historically, ESSs have been referred to as endolymphatic stromal myosis. These tumors are most commonly seen in premenopausal women, but age at presentation may range from 20 to 80 years. Patients typically present with bleeding and pain.

ESS may arise from uterine stroma, adenomyosis, or possibly endometriosis. ESS resembles cells from the endometrial stroma during the proliferative phase of the menstrual cycle. Histologically, ESS is composed of sheets of uniform cells with darkly staining small round or ovoid nuclei. Vascular invasion is common. Historically, ESS has been classified as low grade or high grade. Low-grade ESS is characterized by fewer than 10 mitoses per 10 high-power fields and lack of significant atypia and often expresses estrogen and progesterone receptors. We no longer include high-grade ESS in the category of ESS; rather, we now group high-grade ESS together with high-grade or undifferentiated uterine sarcomas. This is important because the low-grade and high-grade variants have vastly different prognostic factors and therapeutic options. Throughout the remainder of this section, "ESS" will refer to low-grade ESS.

As with uterine LMS, it is rare to make the diagnosis of uterine ESS preoperatively because of the tumor's stromal rather than endometrial origin. However, the finding on endometrial biopsy of hyperplastic stroma with few glands may suggest the presence of ESS. Grossly, ESS resembles pale yellow rubbery growths extending through the myometrium into lymphatic and venous channels (Figure 9–5). On evaluation of a hysterectomy specimen, close attention should be given to vessels in the broad ligament and adnexa.

Although low-grade ESSs tend to be less aggressive than other uterine sarcomas, one third have spread beyond the uterus at the time of diagnosis. As many as 30% to 50% of patients have recurrence, although recurrence may be delayed as long as 36 months to 10 years. Recurrences are

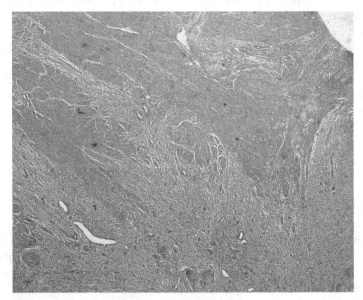

Figure 9–5. Endometrial stromal sarcoma. This sarcoma is characterized by tissue resembling proliferative endometrial stroma, diffusely invading the myometrium.

usually local, but late recurrences may involve the lung and abdomen. Stage at presentation is the best predictor of recurrence risk. Tumors are frequently estrogen receptor and progesterone receptor positive.

Surgical Treatment

The M. D. Anderson approach to clinical evaluation and treatment of patients with uterine ESS is outlined in Figure 9–6. Surgical treatment of ESS typically includes an exploratory laparotomy, total abdominal hysterectomy and bilateral salpingo-oophorectomy, omental biopsy, and aspiration of abdominal fluid for cytologic evaluation. There is little need for lymph node sampling. If tumor is palpable in the parametrium, a more extensive procedure, such as a radical hysterectomy, should be performed. Nodal involvement by low-grade ESS is rare. Bilateral oophorectomy is essential because of the high rate of expression of estrogen and progesterone receptors in ESS.

All recurrences should be evaluated for resectability. Occasionally with long-term remissions, surgery can be considered for recurrences. Prognosis, if excision is successful, is good; the 5-year survival rate is up to 90%.

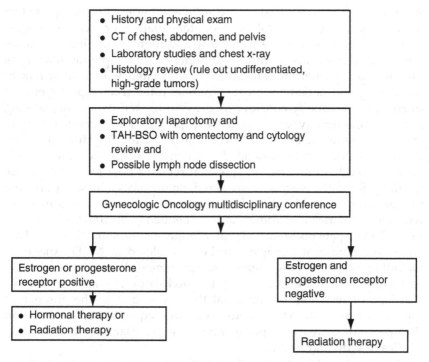

Figure 9–6. Algorithm for clinical evaluation and treatment of patients with endometrial stromal sarcomas. CT, computed tomography; TAH-BSO, total abdominal hysterectomy and bilateral salpingo-oophorectomy.

Radiation Therapy

The combination of adjuvant radiation therapy and high-dose progesterone has shown some benefit in patients with ESS. Although many
institutions recommend this combination for early-stage disease, at
M. D. Anderson we recommend hormonal therapy alone for early-stage
disease, and we reserve the combination of hormonal therapy and radiation therapy for recurrent or high-grade ESS. Adjuvant radiation therapy
clearly reduces the incidence of pelvic recurrence.

Chemotherapy

Doxorubicin, ifosfamide, paclitaxel, and carboplatin have been associated
with minimal response rates in patients with ESS. However, in patients
with estrogen or progesterone receptor expression, hormonal therapy is
the first choice for systemic therapy. Interpretation of ESS treatment
response rates in the literature is made difficult by the fact that many of
the earlier studies may have failed to differentiate between low-grade and
high-grade ESS.

Hormonal Therapy

At M. D. Anderson, the first-choice adjuvant therapy for low-grade ESS
has historically been leuprolide, depot formulation, or medroxyprogesterone acetate. Unfortunately, the dose and route of administration are
not standardized. Large tumors and tumors with lymph-vascular space
invasion or parametrial extension are associated with a high risk of
recurrence, and patients with such tumors often receive postoperative
treatment. We usually consider medroxyprogesterone acetate, 100 mg
per day indefinitely or until disease progression, versus radiation
therapy. Options include 1 month, 2 months, or for life. However, often
patients cannot tolerate extended hormonal therapy because of side
effects. In such situations, the question remains how long to continue
the drug. Recently, we have considered, on the basis of case reports, the
use of aromatase inhibitors for adjuvant therapy and treatment of
recurrent endometrial stromal tumors (Leunen et al, 2004). We also try
to enroll these patients in clinical trials of adjuvant hormonal therapy. Many
innovative hormonal therapies are being explored at M. D. Anderson,
including selective progesterone receptor modulators (mifepristone)
and newer selective estrogen receptor modulators. Because we believe
that lack of response to hormonal therapy is due to the absence of
estrogen or progesterone receptors and that sequential or combination
therapy may increase response rates, we are planning combination
studies in vitro and in vivo.

The presence of estrogen and progesterone receptors has been shown
to correlate directly with survival and response to hormonal therapy
and inversely with tumor grade. Fifty to 60% of primary endometrial

cancers and the majority of low-grade ESSs are both estrogen and progesterone receptor positive. Progesterones in the primary treatment of well-differentiated and recurrent endometrial cancers have been associated with response rates of 18% to 25% and stable disease rates of 20% to 50%. Progesterones in the treatment of low-grade ESS have been associated with response rates ranging from 33% to 45%.

The role of mifepristone, an antiprogesterone, in the treatment of endometrial cancer is currently being explored in a clinical trial at M. D. Anderson. Mifepristone acts on the endometrium and blocks the action of progesterone at the cellular level by binding the progesterone receptor. The affinity of mifepristone for the progesterone receptor is 5-fold greater than that of endogenous progesterone. As a result, mifepristone can produce a progesterone-like effect in the absence of progesterone. In our clinical trial, we are administering mifepristone to patients with progesterone-receptor-positive advanced or recurrent endometrial cancer or low-grade ESS.

UNDIFFERENTIATED SARCOMAS

Epidemiology and Tumor Features

Undifferentiated uterine sarcomas are high-grade epithelioid or spindle cell sarcomas that cannot be classified into 1 of the standard categories. These tumors usually present with abdominal or pelvic pain in postmenopausal women and represent less than 5% of all uterine sarcomas. Necrosis is a common finding. Recurrence often occurs within 2 years. The stage at diagnosis is the most significant predictor of prognosis.

Surgical Treatment

The treatment of choice for undifferentiated uterine sarcomas is surgery. Lymph node dissection is indicated after total abdominal hysterectomy and bilateral salpingo-oophorectomy to determine risk of recurrence. Extended surgical exploration is important to determine the appropriate type and extent of therapy.

Adjuvant Therapy

Radiation therapy is typically recommended for stage I and II undifferentiated sarcomas. However, concern about distant recurrences has led to consideration of combination treatment.

ADENOSARCOMA

Epidemiology and Tumor Features

Adenosarcomas consist of a benign epithelial component and a malignant mesenchymal component and make up about 25% of all uterine sarcomas

(Figure 9–7). The mean patient age at presentation is 58 years. Abnormal bleeding, pain, and tissue protruding from the cervical os are common. These tumors tend to form fleshy masses filling the uterine cavity, and deep invasion is rare. The mesenchymal component of adenosarcomas generally resembles ESS or fibrosarcoma. The stromal element is characterized by increased cellularity around the glands; generally, there is little nuclear atypia in the stromal cells, and usually there are at least 2 mitotic figures per 10 high-power fields. Adenosarcomas are typically low-grade malignancies that rarely metastasize, although up to 20% recur locally. Risk of recurrence is greater with greater depth of invasion as well as with pleomorphism or sarcomatous overgrowth.

A variant of the classic adenosarcoma is adenosarcoma with sarcomatous overgrowth, defined as either a sarcomatous component occupying 25% or more of the total tumor volume or the presence of an area of high-grade pure sarcoma. Sarcomatous overgrowth significantly worsens the patient's prognosis. The presence of sarcomatous overgrowth also increases the likelihood of lymphatic spread. Recurrences are much more likely with this variant and with adenosarcomas containing rhabdomyosarcoma or with lymph-vascular space invasion. Recurrences of adenosarcoma may consist of pure sarcoma, and resistance to chemotherapy is common.

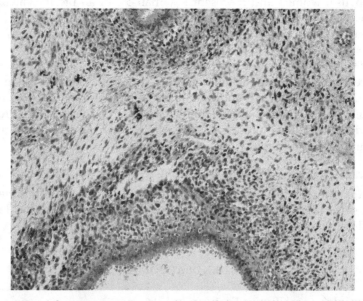

Figure 9–7. Adenosarcoma. Benign glands are surrounded by a cuff of hypercellular stroma. There is mild atypia, and mitotic figures are present.

Surgical Treatment

The M. D. Anderson approach to clinical evaluation and treatment of patients with uterine adenosarcoma is outlined in Figure 9–4. Complete surgical resection is the only treatment that has been successful for patients with adenosarcoma. We support full surgical therapy, including total abdominal hysterectomy and bilateral salpingo-oophorectomy, omentectomy, aspiration of abdominal fluid for cytologic evaluation, and lymph node dissection.

Radiation Therapy

Adenosarcoma is rare and is associated with a fairly good prognosis; therefore, it is difficult to assess the role of adjuvant radiation therapy. We use radiation therapy occasionally; the need for radiation therapy is decided on a case-by-case basis.

Chemotherapy

Cisplatin, doxorubicin, ifosfamide, cyclophosphamide, and vincristine have been used to treat uterine adenosarcoma and have produced various response rates. We especially consider adjuvant chemotherapy in cases with sarcomatous overgrowth.

Hormonal Therapy

Because of the low grade of the sarcoma component in most uterine adenosarcomas, hormonal therapy also remains an option.

SUMMARY

Surgical Approach for Uterine Sarcomas

In patients with uterine sarcomas, exploratory laparotomy, total abdominal hysterectomy, and bilateral salpingo-oophorectomy are recommended, even in patients with metastatic disease, for palliation of symptoms and possibly improved response to therapy. In patients with low-grade ESS, removal of the ovaries is recommended because of the hormonal responsiveness of this tumor. Cytoreductive surgery should be attempted in all patients with uterine sarcomas because of the lack of successful adjuvant and salvage therapies. Except in patients with LMS, extended staging with pelvic and para-aortic lymph node sampling is appropriate to facilitate the evaluation of new therapies.

Radiation Therapy Approach for Uterine Sarcomas

There are no controlled trials showing a survival benefit for adjuvant radiation therapy in patients with uterine sarcomas. The decision to use adjuvant radiation therapy is based on the hypothesis that decreasing the local recurrence rate will improve quality of life by reducing the risk of a pelvic recurrence. Thus, a careful discussion of the potential risks and possible benefits of radiation therapy in women with stage I/II sarcoma is required. There is very little evidence to support the use of adjuvant radiation therapy in women with higher-stage disease, but randomized trials currently in progress may provide important information on the use of radiation therapy in the future. At M. D. Anderson, we rely heavily on a multidisciplinary approach to treating uterine sarcomas.

KEY PRACTICE POINTS

- Patients with uterine sarcomas should be referred to large academic centers for participation in clinical trials.
- Multidisciplinary evaluation is important and should include specialists in radiation oncology, gynecologic oncology, and sarcoma.
- Optimal tumor debulking at presentation is ideal.
- Adjuvant radiation therapy improves local control and may delay recurrence but does not improve survival.
- Treatment of patients with extrauterine disease should be discussed in a multidisciplinary setting.

Suggested Readings

Arrastea CD, Fruchter RG, Clark M, et al. Uterine carcinosarcomas: incidence and trends in management and survival. *Gynecol Oncol* 1997;65:158–163.

Berchuck A, Rubin SC, Hoskins WJ, et al. Treatment of uterine leiomyosarcoma. *Obstet Gynecol* 1988;71:845–850.

Berchuck A, Rubin SC, Hoskins WJ, et al. Treatment of endometrial stromal tumors. *Gynecol Oncol* 1990;36:60–65.

Bitterman P, Chun B, Kurman RJ. The significance of epithelial differentiation in mixed mesodermal tumors of the uterus. *Am J Surg Pathol* 1990;14:317–328.

Callister M, Ramondetta LM, Jhingran A, et al. Malignant mixed mullerian tumors of the uterus: analysis of patterns of failure, prognostic factors, and treatment outcome. *Int J Radiat Oncol Biol Phys* 2004;58:786–796.

Curtin JP, McGuire WP, Brooker D. Evaluation of paclitaxel in the treatment of persistent or recurrent mixed mesodermal tumors of the uterus. GOG Statistical Report, 1998. GOG protocol #130B (July).

Dinh TA, Oliva EA, Fuller AF Jr., et al. The treatment of uterine leiomyosarcoma. Results from a 10-year experience (1990–1999) at the Massachusetts General Hospital. *Gynecol Oncol* 2004;92:648–652.

DiSaia PJ, Castro JR, Rutledge FN. Mixed mesodermal sarcoma of uterus. *Am J Roentgenol Radium Ther Nucl Med* 1973;117:632–636.

Echt G, Jepson J, Steel J, et al. Treatment of uterine sarcomas. *Cancer* 1990;66:35–39.

Eltabbakh GH, Yadav R. Good response of malignant mixed mullerian tumor of the ovary to paclitaxel and cisplatin chemotherapy. *Eur J Gynaecol Oncol* 1999;20:355–356.

Ferrer F, Sabater S, Farrus B, et al. Impact of radiotherapy on local control and survival in uterine sarcomas: a retrospective study from the Group Oncologic Catala-Occita. *Int J Radiat Oncol Biol Phys* 1999;44:47–52.

Fotiou S, Hatjieleftheriou G, Kyrousis G, et al. Long term tamoxifen treatment: a possible aetiological factor in the development of uterine carcinosarcoma: two case reports and review of the literature. *Anticancer Res* 2000;20:2015–2020.

Gershenson DM, Kavanagh JJ, Copeland LJ, et al. Cisplatin therapy for disseminated mixed mesodermal sarcoma of the uterus. *J Clin Oncol* 1987;5:618–621.

Hannigan EV, Freedman RS, Elder KW, et al. Treatment of advanced uterine sarcoma with adriamycin. *Gynecol Oncol* 1983;16:101–104.

Harlow BL, Weiss NS, Lofton S. The epidemiology of sarcomas of the uterus. *J Natl Cancer Inst* 1986;76:399–402.

Hoffmann W, Schmandt S, Kortmann RD, et al. Radiotherapy in the treatment of uterine sarcomas: a retrospective analysis of 54 cases. *Gynecol Obstet Invest* 1996;19:49–57.

Hornback NB, Omura G, Major FJ. Observations on the use of adjuvant radiation therapy in patients with stage I and II uterine sarcoma. *Int J Radiat Oncol Biol Phys* 1986;12:2127–2130.

Knocke TH, Kurcera H, Dörfler D, et al. Results of postoperative radiotherapy in the treatment of sarcoma of the corpus uteri. *Cancer* 1998;83:1972–1979.

Kushner DM, Webster KD, Belinson JL, et al. Safety and efficacy of adjuvant single-agent ifosfamide in uterine sarcomas. *Gynecol Oncol* 2000;78:221–227.

Leunen M, Breugelmans M, DeSutter P, et al. Low-grade endometrial stromal sarcoma treated with the aromatase inhibitor letrozole. *Gynecol Oncol* 2004;95:769–771.

Levenback C, Rubin SC, McCormack PM, et al. Resection of pulmonary metastases from uterine sarcomas. *Gynecol Oncol* 1992;45:202–205.

Levenback CF, Tortolero-Luna G, Pandey DK, et al. Uterine sarcoma. *Obstet Gynecol Clin North Am* 1996;23:457–473.

Look KY, Sandler A, Blessing JA, et al. Phase II trial of gemcitabine as second-line chemotherapy of uterine leiomyosarcoma: a Gynecologic Oncology Group (GOG) study. *Gynecol Oncol* 2004;92:644–647.

Major FJ, Blessing JA, Silverberg SG, et al. Prognostic factors in early-stage uterine sarcoma: a Gynecologic Oncology Group study. *Cancer* 1993;71:1702–1709.

Manolitsas TP, Wain GV, Williams KE, et al. Multimodality therapy for patients with clinical stage I and II malignant mixed müllerian tumors of the uterus. *Cancer* 2001;91:1937–1943.

Markman M, Kennedy A, Webster K, et al. Persistent chemosensitivity to platinum and/or paclitaxel in metastatic endometrial cancer. *Gynecol Oncol* 1999;73:422–423.

Muss HB, Bundy B, DiSaia PJ, et al. Treatment of recurrent or advanced uterine sarcoma. A randomized trial of doxorubicin versus doxorubicin and cyclophosphamide (a phase III trial of the Gynecologic Oncology Group). *Cancer* 1985;55:1648–1653.

Nasu K, Kawano Y, Hirota Y, et al. Immunohistochemical study of c-erb B-2 expression on MMMT of the female genital tract. *J Obstet Gynaecol Res* 1996;22:347–351.

Omura GA, Blessing JA, Major F, et al. A randomized clinical trial of adjuvant adriamycin in uterine sarcomas: a Gynecologic Oncology Group Study. *J Clin Oncol* 1985;3:1240–1245.

Omura GA, Major FJ, Blessing JA, et al. A randomized study of adriamycin with and without dimethyl triazenoimidazole carboxamide in advanced uterine sarcomas. *Cancer* 1983;52:626–632.

Ramondetta LM, Burke TW, Levenback C, et al. Treatment of uterine papillary serous carcinoma with paclitaxel. *Gynecol Oncol* 2001;82:156–161.

Resnick E, Chambers SK, Carcangiu ML, et al. A phase II study of etoposide, cisplatin, and doxorubicin chemotherapy in mixed mullerian tumors (MMT) of the uterus. *Gynecol Oncol* 1995;56:370–375.

Rose PG, Boutselis JG, Sachs L. Adjuvant therapy for stage I uterine sarcoma. *Am J Obstet Gynecol* 1987;156:660–662.

Schwartz SM, Weiss NL, Saling JR, et al. Exogenous sex hormone use, correlates of endogenous hormone levels and the incidence of histologic types of sarcoma of the uterus. *Cancer* 1996;4:717–724.

Silverberg SG, Major FJ, Blessing JA, et al. Carcinosarcoma (malignant mixed mesodermal tumor) of the uterus: a GOG pathologic study. *Int J Gynecol Pathol* 1990;9:1–19.

Sit AS, Price FV, Kelley JL, et al. Chemotherapy for malignant mixed mullerian tumors of the ovary. *Gynecol Oncol* 2000;79:196–200.

Spanos WJ, Peters LJ, Oswald MJ. Patterns of recurrence in malignant mixed mullerian tumor of the uterus. *Cancer* 1986;57:155–159.

Sutton G, Blessing J, Hanjana P, et al. Phase II evaluation of liposomal doxorubicin (Doxil) in recurrent or advanced leiomyosarcoma of the uterus: a Gynecologic Oncology Group study. *Gynecol Oncol* 2005;96:749–752.

Sutton G, Blessing JA, Park R, et al. Ifosfamide treatment of recurrent or metastatic endometrial stromal sarcomas previously unexposed to chemotherapy: a study of the Gynecologic Oncology Group. *Obstet Gynecol* 1996a;87:747–750.

Sutton GP, Ashbury R, Silverberg S. Adjuvant ifosfamide, mesna, and cisplatin in patients with completely resected stage I or II carcinosarcoma of the uterus: a study of the Gynecologic Oncology Group. *Proceedings of the American Society of Clinical Oncology* 1997;15:A1288.

Sutton GP, Blessing JA, Barnhill DL. Phase II trial of ifosfamide and mesna in patients with recurrent or advanced endometrial stromal sarcoma of the uterus—preliminary report [abstract]. *Proceedings of the American Society of Clinical Oncology* 1991.

Sutton GP, Blessing JA, Barrett RJ, et al. Phase II trial of ifosfamide and mesna in leiomyosarcoma of the uterus: a Gynecologic Oncology Group study. *Am J Obstet Gynecol* 1992;166:556–559.

Sutton GP, Blessing JA, Malfetano JH. Ifosfamide and doxorubicin in the treatment of advanced leiomyosarcomas of the uterus: a Gynecologic Oncology Group Study. *Gynecol Oncol* 1996b;62:226–229.

Sutton GP, Blessing JA, Rosenshein N, Photopulos G, DiSaia PJ. Phase II trial of ifosfamide and mesna in mixed mesodermal tumors of the uterus (a Gynecologic Oncology Group study). *Am J Obstet Gynecol* 1989;191:309–312.

Sutton GP, Williams SD, Hsiu JG. Ifosfamide and the uroprotector mesna with or without cisplatin in patients with advanced, persistent or recurrent mixed mesodermal tumors of the uterus [abstract]. *Proceedings of the Society of Gynecologic Oncologists* 1998.

Swisher EM, Gown AM, Skelly M, et al. The expression of epidermal growth factor receptor, Her-2/Neu, p53, and Ki-67 antigen in uterine malignant mixed mesodermal tumors and adenosarcoma. *Gynecol Oncol* 1996;60:81–88.

Szlosarek PW, Lofts FJ, Pettengell R, et al. Effective treatment of a patient with a high-grade endometrial stromal sarcoma with an accelerated regimen of carboplatin and paclitaxel. *Anticancer Drugs* 2000;11:275–278.

Thigpen JT, Blessing JA, Beecham J, et al. Phase II trial of cisplatin as first line chemotherapy in patients with advanced or recurrent uterine sarcomas: a Gynecologic Oncology Group study. *J Clin Oncol* 1991;9:1962–1966.

Thigpen JT, Blessing JA, Orr JW, et al. Phase II trial of cisplatin in the treatment of patients with advanced or recurrent mixed mesodermal sarcomas of the uterus: a Gynecologic Oncology Group study. *Cancer Treatment Reports* 1986;70:271–274.

10 TREATMENT OF ENDOMETRIAL CANCER

Lois M. Ramondetta, Thomas W. Burke,
Russell Broaddus, and Anuja Jhingran

CHAPTER OUTLINE

CHAPTER OVERVIEW

The treatment of endometrial cancer continues to evolve as we begin to understand issues related to nodal spread, peritoneal disease, risk of recurrence, and combination therapy. Advances in treatment for recurrent disease have been slow, however, owing to the minimal number of recurrences in patients with early-stage disease and the poor prognosis of those with advanced disease. For patients with disease confined to the uterus, surgical staging remains the mainstay of therapy. Surgical evaluation of nodal spread is considered important in all stages beyond those characterized by superficial endometrial involvement. For patients with advanced disease, tumor debulking also appears to improve progression-free survival but not overall survival. In patients with intermediate-risk disease confined to the uterus, radiation therapy increases local control rates but does not improve survival. For patients with high-risk factors such as deeply invasive grade 3 or stage IIB or higher disease, radiation therapy probably improves survival as well as local control. The role of chemotherapy in the treatment of endometrial cancer is evolving and is beginning to include the treatment of patients with advanced disease.

INTRODUCTION

The treatment of endometrial cancer is in a state of flux. Most endometrial cancers have clear risk factors and early warning signs. However, at present, little is known about why some patients have recurrent disease and which patients should receive adjuvant radiation therapy. Data are beginning to mature that will define the true impact of radiation therapy and cytotoxic therapy, and recent data suggest a benefit for aggressive lymphadenectomy. As more is learned about the molecular components of endometrial cancer, the risks of recurrence may be more clearly identified, and more effective modalities of treatment and schedules of surveillance may be found. Molecular profiling is expected to provide clinicians with the ability to employ targeted agents.

In this chapter, we present an overview of the way we at M. D. Anderson Cancer Center approach endometrial cancer treatment, and we point out areas where new knowledge may change our current care practices.

EPIDEMIOLOGY

Endometrial cancer is the most common gynecologic cancer in the United States. The American Cancer Society estimates that about 7,310 women in the United States will die of uterine cancer and 40,880 women will develop uterine cancer in 2005. The survival rate across all stages is approximately 84%. Fortunately, most endometrial cancers are discovered at an early stage because of warning signs such as irregular or postmenopausal bleeding. Therefore, it is incumbent upon physicians and all women to be aware of the significance of these signs. Although the majority of endometrial cancers occur in postmenopausal women, up to 25% may occur before menopause, so awareness is important throughout a woman's life.

There are many clearly identifiable risk factors for endometrial cancer that can raise suspicion and possibly provide indications for early screening. These risk factors include obesity, hypertension, nulliparity, hypothyroidism, and diabetes as well as a history of breast or colon cancer. The degree of obesity has a proportional effect on a woman's risk of endometrial cancer. If a woman is 30 pounds overweight, her risk of endometrial cancer may be up to 3 times that of the general population, and if she is 50 pounds or more overweight, her risk rises to greater than 5 times that of the general population. There is controversy regarding the actual independent risk associated with diabetes mellitus and hypertension, but most investigators factor in these comorbidities as independent but less significant risk factors. After controlling for weight, however, many investigators have found no independent risk related to these comorbidities.

Prolonged endogenous or exogenous exposure to estrogen, due to early menarche or late menopause, also increases a woman's risk of endometrial cancer. Women with late menopause, defined as occurring at or after 52 years of age, have a 2- to 3-fold increase in the risk of endometrial cancer. Prolonged estrogen replacement therapy, without the concomitant use of progesterone, increases the risk of endometrial cancer compared with the risk in women not using estrogens at all. This is a timely concern, as a recent Women's Health Initiative study reported an increase in breast cancer in women using the Premarin and Provera hormone replacement therapy combination (Rossouw et al, 2002). Therefore, practitioners need to be diligent in recognizing the risks of unopposed, as well as opposed, estrogen when prescribing hormone replacement therapy.

Women taking tamoxifen represent another high-risk group that occasionally may require early screening. A National Surgical Adjuvant Breast and Bowel Project (NSABP) trial revealed that endometrial cancer occurred at a 2- to 7.5-fold higher rate in tamoxifen-treated women. However, the majority of the endometrial cancers diagnosed in that study were stage I and low grade (78% and 88%, respectively). Because of the beneficial effects of tamoxifen in preventing recurrent breast cancer, the use of tamoxifen has continued despite the risk of endometrial cancer. Fortunately, a 5-year maximum on the use of tamoxifen has been established, and newer selective estrogen receptor (ER) modulators with protective uterine effects are now being used to prevent recurrences.

PRETREATMENT EVALUATION

Surgery is the standard treatment for endometrial cancer. Although most women present with early-stage disease, aggressive histology and comorbidities may alter even the best-prepared surgical plans. Routine preoperative evaluation should include hematologic, renal, and hepatologic evaluation, electrocardiography, and chest radiography. If extrauterine pelvic disease is suspected, computed tomography (CT) and magnetic resonance imaging (MRI) may offer additional information that can help with treatment planning as well as clarify patient expectations for the surgery. At M. D. Anderson, we prefer MRI to CT for evaluating suspected invasion of the rectum, bladder, or cervix. If primary colon cancer or colon involvement is suspected and not detected on CT or MRI, a colonoscopy as well as a determination of the preoperative carcinoembryonic antigen level is recommended for surgical planning.

Positron emission tomography may be a reasonable alternative in the future for evaluation of lymph node metastasis; however, at present, we rely primarily on CT or MRI for evaluation of retroperitoneal nodes. For most patients, the value of intravenous pyelography, sigmoidoscopy, or cystoscopy has been minimized because more comprehensive information is often obtained from CT or MRI. However, although both CT and MRI can detect retroperitoneal disease with 40% to 69% sensitivity, these results only rarely alter the surgical treatment plan. At present, there is no steadfast rule for surgical staging of retroperitoneal lymph nodes at M. D. Anderson, although we do consider patients for enrollment in lymphatic mapping protocols. Surgical management of retroperitoneal nodes varies among our many gynecologic oncologists. Some recommend lymphadenectomy for "at risk" cases only, while others perform lymphadenectomy on all patients. However, recent data suggesting that all patients benefit from surgical staging of retroperitoneal lymph nodes have been considered (Ben-Shachar et al, 2005).

The value of serum CA-125 measurement in determining the preoperative spread of endometrial cancer is still unclear. Patients with lymph node metastasis have an 8.7-fold higher risk than those without metastasis of having a CA-125 level greater than 40 U/mL. A CA-125 value greater than 20 U/mL and a grade 3 histologic classification can correctly identify 75% to 87% of patients with nodal disease. A serum CA-125 level greater than 20 U/mL alone correctly predicted the need for lymphadenectomy in 70% of patients (Sood et al, 1997).

Although the usefulness of preoperative evaluation with imaging and serum CA-125 measurement in patients with endometrial cancer remains to be determined, we believe that such evaluation may be beneficial in women whose medical conditions suggest increased surgical risk. Nearly 30% of women with stage I endometrial cancer diagnosed by preoperative biopsy will need surgical staging at the time of hysterectomy. Furthermore, 25% to 30% of histologic grade 1 cancers will be upgraded or will have unexpected deep invasion at the time of surgery. The ability to preoperatively identify patients who do or do not need surgical staging would be advantageous because it could rule out the need for extended lymphadenectomy in some patients. This is particularly beneficial in a population with so many comorbidities. Preoperative findings suggesting a need for surgical staging would also allow a general obstetrician and gynecologist to consider arranging for oncologic backup or simply to refer the patient to a gynecologic oncologist. If preoperative histologic evaluation suggests a low risk for lymph node spread and thus no need for surgical staging, the results of additional preoperative radiologic evaluation might permit surgery to proceed transvaginally laparoscopically or via a Pfannenstiel incision. MRI evaluation of the abdomen and pelvis might also decrease the number of unnecessary lymph node dissections if used in combination with CA-125 measurement and histologic evaluation. Such information could assist a clinician in planning surgery in patients with contraindications to surgical staging.

SURGICAL TREATMENT

Surgery is always the treatment of choice for endometrial cancer that is clinically confined to the uterus. The goal of surgery is to provide definitive treatment of patients whose tumors are limited to the uterus, to obtain specimens that provide prognostic information, and to identify patients with extrauterine spread. However, in patients who are poor surgical candidates and who have at least a 20% mortality risk, treatment with either brachytherapy or empiric pelvic radiation therapy can be considered. Alternatively, younger women with low-grade tumors who wish to preserve their fertility could be offered treatment with progestins, although data are limited, other than from case series, to support this plan of treatment. First and foremost, we advise these young patients that progestin therapy is not the standard of care and that we do not consider it the safest option. Our experience has been that most women will opt to discontinue these medications and have surgery because of the significant side effects of progestins, which include weight gain, mood swings, and bloating. Before such a conservative treatment is considered, we recommend that the patient undergo dilatation and curettage as well as MRI to determine the extent, grade, and depth of invasion of the tumor.

Standard surgery for endometrial cancer is a hysterectomy and bilateral salpingo-oophorectomy done either via a vertical midline incision or laparoscopically to allow adequate access for retroperitoneal staging of aortic lymph nodes. In well-chosen patients, we plan a laparoscopic lymph node dissection and vaginal hysterectomy, with no increased surgical risk and the potential benefits of early hospital discharge and decreased risk of wound infection.

At M. D. Anderson, a lymph node dissection is now performed in most endometrial cancer patients, although the ratio of dissection to sampling is based almost entirely on physician preference. Other factors determining the degree of surgical dissection may include the grade, depth, and size of the lesion and the age and comorbidities of the patient.

Patients with endometrial cancer who are poor surgical candidates present difficult situations. At M. D. Anderson, these patients are always discussed in a multidisciplinary conference. Radiation therapy as primary therapy, without surgery, is reserved for very rare cases in which the operative risk is considered to be extraordinarily high. Disease-specific survival rates of 75% to 85% and local recurrence rates of 10% to 20% have been reported for patients with clinical stage I or II endometrial carcinoma treated with radiation therapy alone. At M. D. Anderson, we weigh the risk of surgical mortality against the risk of recurrence with radiation therapy alone. In cases in which the surgical mortality risk is greater than 20%, we consider primary treatment with radiation.

SURGICAL STAGING

The current International Federation of Gynecology and Obstetrics (FIGO) staging system for carcinoma of the endometrium is surgical (Gal et al, 1992) (Table 10–1). The staging procedure, although not defined by FIGO, typically includes hysterectomy, bilateral salpingo-oophorectomy, washings for cytologic evaluation, pelvic nodal sampling, para-aortic nodal sampling, and biopsy of any suspicious areas. Through a midline vertical abdominal incision or laparoscopically, the peritoneal cavity is entered and saline washings of the cavity, particularly the pelvic peritoneum, are collected and forwarded for cytologic examination. Extrafascial hysterectomy with bilateral salpingo-oophorectomy is then performed. The uterine specimen is sent directly to the pathology laboratory, where it is grossly and microscopically evaluated. Next, the endometrial cavity is inspected to assess the extent of tumor involvement. Full-thickness frozen sections are then obtained, and the depth of myometrial invasion is determined by light microscopy.

At the time of frozen section analysis, a preliminary determination of tumor histologic type is communicated to the surgeon. At M. D. Anderson, we have an excellent gynecologic pathology division and rely on their assessment of the specimen when considering the need for surgical staging. The surgical procedure is terminated at that point for patients with grade 1 tumors with superficial myometrial invasion. In addition to tumor histologic type and depth of invasion, microscopic evaluation of the cervix is also important. Tumor invasion of the cervix raises the tumor stage and increases the chance of pelvic nodal spread; thus, complete staging is considered more valuable in these cases.

Our approach after the initial collection of pelvic washings and hysterectomy with bilateral salpingo-oophorectomy is to perform lymph node dissection in all patients with grade 2 disease and more than one-third invasion and all grade 3 endometrioid adenocarcinoma, uterine papillary serous carcinoma (UPSC), or clear cell carcinoma regardless of invasion. In all other patients, many of our surgeons wait for intraoperative pathologic analysis of frozen sections before sampling nonsuspicious lymph nodes. If the tumor is minimally invasive and grade 1 endometrioid adenocarcinoma, we typically do not perform lymph node dissection.

Table 10-1. International Federation of Gynecology and Obstetrics Staging of
Endometrial Cancer

Stage I
IA
Tumor limited to endometrium
IB
Invasion to < 1/2 the myometrium
IC
Invasion to > 1/2 the myometrium

Stage II
IIA
Endocervical glandular involvement
IIB
Cervical stromal invasion

Stage III
IIIA
Tumor invades serosa and/or adnexa and/or positive peritoneal cytology
IIIB
Vaginal involvement
IIIC
Metastases to pelvic and/or para-aortic lymph nodes

Stage IV
IVA
Tumor invasion of bladder and/or bowel mucosa
IVB
Distant metastases including intra-abdominal and/or inguinal lymph nodes

Modified from Benedet et al (2000).

If grade 2 or grade 3 endometrioid adenocarcinoma is present with even
minimal invasion, we tend to perform lymph node dissection to clearly
define the need for adjuvant therapy and to avoid overtreatment.

Tumor Features

Endometrial cancer is histopathologically diverse. Approximately 80% of
endometrial cancers are of the endometrioid histotype, while papillary
serous carcinoma, clear cell carcinoma, malignant mixed müllerian tumors,
and other rare types make up the other 20% (Sherman, 2000). On the basis
of histologic characteristics, molecular profiling, and clinical behavior,
endometrial cancer can be divided into 2 broad categories (Matias-Guiu
et al, 2001). Type 1 cancers are typically low-grade (grade 1 or grade 2)
endometrioid adenocarcinoma. These tumors are related to excess estrogen
and are frequently preceded or accompanied by the premalignant change

complex atypical hyperplasia. Mutations of K-*ras*, *PTEN*, and *β-catenin* and microsatellite instability are common in type 1 cancers (Mutter et al, 1999; Matias-Guiu et al, 2001). Usually, type 1 cancers are diagnosed at an early stage and have a favorable prognosis. In contrast, type 2 cancers are composed of papillary serous carcinoma, clear cell carcinoma, malignant mixed müllerian tumors, or high-grade (grade 3) endometrioid adenocarcinoma. Type 2 cancers usually arise in older women, are not related to estrogen exposure, and are not associated with endometrial hyperplasia. Typically, type 2 cancers have *P53* mutations and loss of heterozygosity at several chromosomal loci (Matias-Guiu et al, 2001). Type 2 cancers are typically associated with advanced-stage disease at diagnosis and poor prognosis.

Although these categories are applicable to many endometrial cancers, there are numerous exceptions. A small percentage of low-grade endometrioid adenocarcinomas are either advanced stage at diagnosis or recur years after hysterectomy. Papillary serous carcinoma and endometrioid adenocarcinoma can coexist in the same tumor. Some type 2 cancers have the molecular alterations associated with type 1 tumors (mutations of K-*ras*, *PTEN*, or *β-catenin* or microsatellite instability), suggesting that type 2 tumors can arise through dedifferentiation of a preexisting type 1 cancer (Matias-Guiu et al, 2001). It is often difficult to predict how high-grade endometrioid adenocarcinomas will behave clinically, as these tumors can be associated with early-stage disease at diagnosis with no evidence of lymphatic spread at the time of hysterectomy. Of note, transitioning into this type 2 category are uterine mixed müllerian carcinomas, which until recently have been grouped with uterine sarcomas. (Details regarding the treatment of uterine mixed müllerian carcinomas are included in the chapter "Uterine Sarcomas.") At M. D. Anderson, we treat tumors with even a small percentage of papillary serous carcinoma or clear cell histology as we would a tumor with 100% aggressive histology. We approach papillary serous carcinoma and clear cell tumors aggressively and systemically because of their associated early and distant lymphatic spread. Thus, we routinely perform lymph node dissection in these tumors regardless of the degree of invasion.

The FIGO staging system does not define a specific method of lymph node assessment for surgical staging operations. We believe that accurate staging information should be obtained in all but the lowest-risk subset of patients. Caution should be exercised, however, because lymphatic dissection is associated with the following risks: vessel injury and infection, lymphedema of the lower extremities, and small bowel injuries in patients who undergo radiation therapy. We currently are attempting to evaluate techniques for retroperitoneal sentinel lymph node identification. The benefits of sentinel node biopsy include a lower risk of surgical morbidity, the reduction of side effects of surgical dissection followed by radiation therapy, and the avoidance of over- or undertreatment due to limited information obtained from incomplete dissections. Furthermore, retroperitoneal dissection can be difficult in obese patients, physicians may lack the necessary surgical skills to perform it, or physicians may believe that lymphadenectomy is not required in early-stage disease.

Retrospective reviews suggest that para-aortic lymph nodes are positive in less than 2% of patients if the pelvic nodes are negative. Previously, we employed a selective approach to lymph node sampling, but some of us now prefer a full nodal dissection to the level of the renal vessels on the basis of retrospective data indicating a survival advantage for such cases and our own sentinel node data. At M. D. Anderson, we have adopted a staging approach similar to that used in staging ovarian carcinomas, an approach designed to provide the greatest chance of detecting extrauterine spread. Lymph nodes from the major pelvic node chains are dissected or sampled bilaterally between the bifurcation of the iliac arteries and the circumflex iliac vein and superior to the obturator nerve. Additional lymph node samples are obtained from the para-aortic nodes to the level of the renal vessels. A careful exploration is then performed, and peritoneal, diaphragmatic, or serosal surfaces that look or feel abnormal are biopsied. No additional benefit has been found from random peritoneal biopsies during the staging of endometrial cancer. After a generous portion of the infracolic omentum is removed as a biopsy specimen, the procedure is completed.

PATHOLOGIC EVALUATION OF THE HYSTERECTOMY SPECIMEN

The pathologic evaluation of hysterectomy specimens for endometrial cancer must take into account tumor characteristics that influence the clinical management of the disease both intraoperatively and postsurgically. Such characteristics include the histologic type of tumor, depth of myometrial invasion, presence or absence of vascular/lymphatic invasion, and involvement of the cervix, serosa, or adnexa. All hysterectomy specimens for cases of endometrial cancer are submitted to the Department of Pathology at M. D. Anderson for frozen section intraoperative evaluation. The pathologist performs a longitudinal bivalve incision of the uterus to expose the tumor in the endometrial cavity. The entire endometrium is then carefully sectioned at 2-mm intervals. Areas of suspected gross myometrial invasion are evaluated by frozen section analysis for depth of myometrial invasion. If no gross myometrial invasion is detected, 2 to 3 random sections of tumor with underlying myometrium are analyzed. If the tumor is grossly adjacent to the cervix, the cervix is also sampled. Additionally, the ovaries are carefully inspected, and if any suspicious lesions are detected grossly, they are sampled for frozen section analysis. Information conveyed to the surgeon after frozen section analysis includes the histologic type of tumor, tumor grade, if applicable, depth of myometrial invasion, presence of vascular/lymphatic invasion, and involvement of the cervix or ovaries.

Following frozen section evaluation, sections of the hysterectomy specimen are submitted for routine histopathologic evaluation. If frozen section analysis revealed endometrial hyperplasia or a low-grade tumor, the entire endometrium is examined microscopically to rule out the presence of a higher-grade component. Full-thickness sections of endometrial tumor and underlying myometrium are microscopically analyzed to obtain an accurate measurement of the depth of myometrial invasion. If the cervix is grossly normal, 2 representative sections of the ectocervix and endocervix are analyzed. If the ovaries and fallopian tubes are grossly normal, representative sections are evaluated microscopically. However, if the endometrial tumor is a serous carcinoma, the entire fallopian tubes and ovaries are examined microscopically.

ADJUVANT TREATMENT

We routinely discuss the need for adjuvant therapy in a multidisciplinary setting, taking into account not only the depth of myometrial invasion, histologic type, and lymph node involvement but also comorbidities and individual patient wishes. We categorize endometrial cancer, using the information obtained from surgical staging, into 3 groups based on the risk of recurrence. Low-risk tumors are defined as stage IA/B, grade 1, or stage IA, grade 2 (Table 10–2). Intermediate-risk tumors are defined as stage IA, grade 3; stage IB, grade 2–3; stage IC, grade 1–2; or stage IIA. Deeply invasive grade 3 tumors or stage IIB tumors are considered high risk. Recurrence rates for low-risk, intermediate-risk, and high-risk tumors are 5%, 10%, and 14% to 42%, respectively. We recommend adjuvant brachytherapy for intermediate-risk tumors to reduce the rate of vaginal apex recurrence. We believe that lymph node status is the most important prognosticator in endometrial cancer, and we support the use of surgical staging for additional determination of the best treatment for all patients.

Adjuvant Radiation Therapy

Controversy surrounds the efficacy of and indications for adjuvant radiation therapy following surgery. Postoperative pelvic irradiation clearly reduces the risk of pelvic recurrence but has not been shown to improve survival rates when disease is confined to the uterus. Three randomized studies have examined postoperative radiation therapy in intermediate-risk patients. In the first of these studies, done by Aalders and colleagues (1980), patients with endometrial cancer clinically confined to the uterus were randomized prospectively to undergo primary surgery and vaginal brachytherapy, with or without additional external-beam irradiation. A significant reduction in the rate of vaginal and pelvic recurrences was observed in the group that received adjuvant radiation therapy (1.9% vs 6.9%), but there was no difference in overall survival. In the second

Table 10–2. M. D. Anderson Cancer Center Adjuvant Treatment Guidelines for
Endometrial Cancer after Full Surgical Staging*

Risk	Surgical Stage	Adjuvant Therapy
Low	Stage IA, Grade 1 or 2 Stage IB, Grade 1	None
Low Intermediate	Stage IB, Grade 2 Stage IA, Grade 3	Vaginal cuff irradiation or none
High Intermediate	Stage IC, Grade 1 or 2 Stage IB, Grade 3 Stage IIA, Grade 1, 2, or 3	Vaginal cuff irradiation +/– pelvic irradiation
High	Stage IC, Grade 3 Stage IIB, Grade 1, 2, or 3	Pelvic irradiation + vaginal cuff irradiation
High	Stage III, Grade 1, 2, or 3	Chemotherapy or radiation therapy or both (Treatment for stage IIIA disease with positive cytology is controversial.)
High	Stage IV, Grade 1, 2, or 3	Chemotherapy with or without palliative radiation therapy

*Excluding uterine papillary serous carcinoma and clear cell carcinoma.

prospective randomized trial, Gynecologic Oncology Group Study 99 (Keys et al, 2004), patients with endometrial adenocarcinoma underwent complete surgical staging with pelvic and para-aortic lymph node dissection. Patients were randomized to receive no further therapy or pelvic radiation therapy, and the incidence of recurrence was significantly lower in the pelvic radiation therapy arm (12% vs 3%, $P = .007$). There was again no significant difference in the 4-year overall survival rate (86% vs 92%, $P = .557$). In this study, a subgroup analysis found that one third (132) of the patients fell into a "high-risk group" that actually had improvement in overall survival with radiation therapy compared with surgery alone. This high intermediate–risk group consisted of patients older than 70 years with moderate to poorly differentiated tumors, lymphovascular invasion, and outer-third myometrial invasion.

The last of the 3 randomized trials was conducted in the Netherlands (Creutzberg, 2004). In this trial, 715 patients with intermediate-risk endometrial carcinoma were randomly assigned after surgery to radiation therapy with 46 Gy or no radiation therapy. The overall survival rates at 5 years were the same in the radiation and no radiation groups (81% vs 85%); however, 5-year local-regional recurrence rates were 4% in the irradiated group and 14% in the control group. Pathologic review revealed that 90% of the patients in this trial had grade 1 or 2 endometrioid adenocarcinoma, with the majority having less than 50% myometrial invasion. Of note, because their risk of recurrence is considered low, the majority of these patients would not have been treated with postoperative radiation therapy at M. D. Anderson.

Several studies have documented survival rates of 80% to 90% for patients with high-risk disease (high-grade, deeply invasive, or cervical involvement) disease treated with postoperative radiation therapy. In our opinion, patients with cervical stromal involvement or positive pelvic or para-aortic nodes benefit from postoperative radiation therapy, although a role for chemotherapy in these patients is being explored.

At M. D. Anderson, patients with fully staged intermediate-risk disease are treated with high-dose-rate vaginal cuff radiation therapy that consists of treatment with 5 fractions of 6 Gy each using a vaginal cylinder. This treatment is prescribed to the vaginal surface, and only the length of the dome is treated. The size of the dome is determined by patient comfort level. Treatment is given every other day, except in special circumstances. In general, patients tolerate this treatment well.

Patients with high-risk disease (i.e., deeply invasive disease, high-grade histologic type, or cervix involvement [stage II]) or high intermediate–risk disease are treated with external-beam radiation therapy to the pelvis followed by a vaginal cuff boost. The pelvic irradiation is delivered using a 4-field technique. Pelvic treatment fields typically extend from the L4 or L5 lumbar vertebra to the mid or lower pubic ramus. The lateral field's anterior border is usually in front of the symphysis pubis, and the posterior border is treated to the S1 or S2 level. Sacral nodes are not commonly involved with metastatic endometrial carcinoma unless the cervix is involved and therefore do not need to be covered by external-beam fields. In the lateral field, we try to block out as much of the small bowel as possible while still treating the nodal beds. We usually recommend that our patients have their bladders full, which pushes the bowel up and out of the pelvis, decreasing the amount of bowel in the treatment field. We treat the pelvis to 45 Gy in 25 fractions, followed by 5 Gy to the vaginal cuff in 3 fractions. Recently, we have begun treating some of our patients with high-risk endometrial cancer on a protocol of intensity-modulated radiation therapy to the pelvis (Figure 10–1). In this protocol, we are evaluating the feasibility of this individualized treatment and are comparing its acute and late toxicity to that of the standard 4-field technique. It is our thought that intensity-modulated radiation therapy may decrease the area of the small bowel that is exposed to radiation and therefore reduce both acute and late bowel toxic effects without sacrificing effectiveness.

Adjuvant Hormonal Therapy

The Norwegian Radium Hospital studied more than 1,100 patients with endometrial cancer and failed to identify a benefit for adjuvant hormonal therapy with progestins (Vergote et al, 1989). In fact, no trial has demonstrated a benefit for adjuvant progestins in this disease. Also, cardiac and

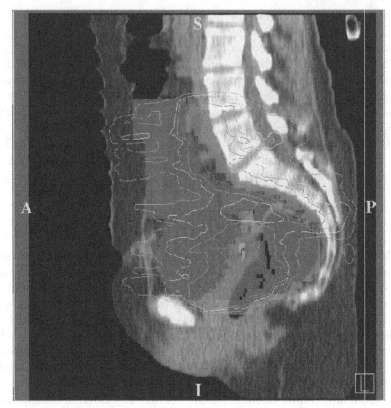

Figure 10–1. Intensity-modulated radiation therapy treatment plan for a patient being treated for endometrial cancer postoperatively.

coagulopathic events are more frequent in progestin-treated women. Therefore, we do not recommend this type of adjuvant treatment.

Adjuvant Chemotherapy

Multiple studies have shown no advantage for adjuvant chemotherapy, whereas others have suggested that in high-risk patients there may be a slight survival advantage. Other than for protocol-based exploration of its use as a radiation sensitizer in the setting of endometrioid endometrial cancer, we at M. D. Anderson do not routinely administer chemotherapy for adjuvant therapy in endometrial cancer patients. We do, however, use adjuvant chemotherapy to treat patients with UPSC or clear cell carcinoma. We approach the treatment of these patients as we would that of those with a similar stage of ovarian cancer. The rationale for this treatment approach is that the high risk for peritoneal spread with these histologic types as well as their predilection for distant metastasis warrants systemic treatment. If possible, we treat these patients on protocols that combine regional and systemic treatment.

The treatment of high-risk tumors, including clear cell and UPSC histologic subtypes, is still controversial. Because of the rarity of clear cell carcinoma, it is still usually grouped with endometrioid cancers in treatment protocols, even though the response to chemotherapy has been very poor. However, consenting patients with surgically staged stage I–IIIA UPSC are treated on protocol using a combination of chemotherapy and radiation therapy. Our current protocol involves pelvic irradiation with weekly radiosensitizer followed by chemotherapy with paclitaxel. The basis for this protocol is a 77% response rate treating UPSC recurrences with paclitaxel (Ramondetta et al, 2001). Because of the early risk of distant spread with this histology, we envision always using a combined chemotherapy and radiation therapy approach.

TREATMENT OF RESIDUAL DISEASE

Treatment decisions at diagnosis are highly individualized for patients with advanced endometrial cancer. Long-term survival is uncommon, and a multimodality treatment approach is often indicated. The primary goals of treatment should be control of the pelvic tumor and relief of symptoms caused by metastatic disease.

Stage III Disease

Tumors outside the uterus but confined to the pelvis may be approached with curative intent. We often treat these patients using a multimodality approach of surgery and radiation therapy for local control and chemotherapy to sensitize tissue to radiation and to also treat distant metastatic cells. Although others have advocated treating advanced disease with preoperative radiation, it is standard at M. D. Anderson to proceed initially with surgery, attempt debulking, and then administer radiation, with or without chemotherapy, on protocol 3 to 6 weeks after surgery if indicated for residual disease or high-risk status. However, if tumor extension to the cervix is palpated during a preoperative physical examination, we typically treat the patient with 45 Gy of preoperative pelvic radiation and 72-hour ALTO (afterloading tandem ovoid), followed by an extrafascial hysterectomy 4 to 6 weeks later.

Stage IIIA disease is defined as endometrial cancer with invasion of the uterine serosa or adnexa or positive peritoneal cytologic findings. The grouping of this latter finding with uterine serosal or adnexal involvement always leads to a difficult treatment decision for the physicians at M. D. Anderson. In 1981, Creasman et al reported on 167 patients with stage I endometrial cancer. Fifteen percent of the patients were found to have positive cytologic findings, and these patients had poorer survival than did the patients with negative cytologic findings. In another study, 10% of 93 patients were found to have positive cytologic findings, but survival did not differ among patients with and without carcinoma cells in the abdominal cavity (Piver et al, 1993). In a third study of 278 women with clinical stage I compared with 53 women with stage IIIA endometrial cancer who underwent surgical staging, no difference was seen in survival for these patients when cytologic results alone were compared (Tebeu et al, 2004). At M. D. Anderson, aggressive histologic subtypes such as clear cell carcinoma or UPSC with isolated positive cytologic findings are treated with systemic therapy, whereas with endometrioid tumors with positive cytologic findings, in the absence of other metastasis, surgery alone is considered a reasonable option.

The current trend in the treatment of patients with advanced disease (greater than stage II) is tumor-reductive surgery followed by combination chemotherapy and radiation therapy. A recent report suggested that patients with stage IIIB to IIIC disease, in the absence of positive peritoneal cytology and adnexal disease, have survival rates in the 40% to 65% range (Ayhan et al, 2002). Our standard adjuvant treatment for patients with stage IIIC disease is radiation therapy, although consideration is given to chemotherapy delivered as part of a protocol. In patients with positive pelvic nodes and negative para-aortic nodes, we treat the pelvis using a 4-field technique, as described above, to a total dose of 45 Gy, followed by a vaginal cuff boost of 5 Gy in 3 fractions prescribed to the vaginal surface using high-dose-rate brachytherapy. A recent Gynecologic Oncology Group study reported a 70% 5-year survival rate in 63 patients with positive pelvic nodes and negative para-aortic nodes who were treated with pelvic external-beam radiation therapy (Morrow et al, 1991).

We treat patients with positive para-aortic nodes or positive pelvic nodes and para-aortic nodes of unknown status with extended-field radiation therapy using a 4-field technique from T12 at the top of the field to the pelvis at the bottom. The entire field is treated with 45 Gy in 25 fractions, and a boost is given to a smaller area if there is extranodal extension or residual disease. Patients will usually also receive a vaginal cuff boost as previously described. Several retrospective studies have reported 5-year survival rates of 40% to 70% in patients with positive para-aortic nodes treated with this technique. Our clinical treatment guidelines for endometrial cancer can be found in the appendix to chapter 1, and order sets for patients undergoing total abdominal hysterectomy can be seen in Figure 10–2 (see the next 3 pages).

Stage IV Disease

The management of stage IV endometrial cancer is based on the individual presentation and includes assessments of the extent of disease, the risks of surgical removal of the tumor, and the patient's comorbidities. Initial tumor debulking, performed on the basis of "ovarian criteria," remains the mainstay of treatment. In patients with significant comorbidities, chemotherapy

M. D. Anderson Cancer Center & Physician's Network Post-Op Orders

MD's signature indicates all orders are activated.
To delete an order, draw one line through the item, write "delete", and initial your entry.

Site/Sub-site: Gyn/Endometrial
Pathway: GynS2 Total Abdominal Hysterectomy
Continued on next page—Page 1 of 2

Attending Physician: _____

Date: _____ **Height:** _____ **Weight:** _____ **Diagnosis:** _____

Allergies: _____
Diagnostic Tests CBC in am POD #1 at 0400.

Vital Signs
1. Every 4 hours for 48 hours; then every shift. Call House Officer (H.O.) if:
SBP greater than _____ less than _____ **HR** greater than _____ less than _____
DBP greater than _____ less than _____ **RR** greater than _____less than _____
Urine Output less than 30 ml/hr **Temp** greater than 38.3°C
2. Respiratory rate every 2 hours for 8 hours, then every 4 hours while on PCA.
If respiratory rate less than 10, hold IV PCA infusion and notify team managing PCA.
If respiratory rate less than or equal to 6, hold IV infusion, and give Naloxone as indicated below, and call primary team, resident of staff on call (or pain service, if consulted).

Interventions
1. While on PCA, if unarousable and/or respiratory rate less than or equal to 6 give Naloxone STAT as indicated under medications below.
2. Compression Boots at all times when in bed. Discontinue when ambulating four times a day.
3. Incentive Spirometer every hour while awake on day of surgery; then every 2 hours.
4. Turn, Cough, Deep Breathe every 2 hours.
5. Remove OR dressing on POD #1.
6. Incision care with soap and water, starting POD #1.
7. Foley to bedside. Discontinue Foley at noon POD #1. If no void in 6 hours after Foley discontinued notify H.O.

IV Fluids
1. D5NS at 100 ml/hr for 24 hours; then decrease IVFs to 75 ml/hr for 24 hours; then Heparin Lock on POD #2; flush with 100 units Heparin every day and prn.

Activity
1. Bedrest; dangle on side of bed, to chair if tolerated in P.M. day of surgery.
2. Ambulate POD #1 with assistance 4 times daily.
3. Increase ambulation with assistance 5-6 times daily POD #2-3.

Diet
1. NPO; may have 30 ml ice chips (not to exceed 60 ml every 4 hours).
2. Clear Liquid Diet POD #1 for dinner. POD #2 for breakfast and luch.
3. Soft/Bland Diet: No bacon or milk products on POD #2, starting at dinner.
4. Continue soft/bland diet POD #3 through discharge, advance as tolerated.
Medications and Other Orders Continued on Next Page

Physician's Signature/ID Code: _____
Pager: _____ **Date:** _____ **Time:** _____

M. D. Anderson Cancer Center & Physician's Network Post-Op Orders

MD's signature indicates all orders are activated.
To delete an order, draw one line through the item, write "delete", and initial your entry.

Site/Sub-site: Gyn/Endometrial
Pathway: GynS2 Total Abdominal Hysterectomy
—*Page 2 of 2*

Medication
Scheduled Medications
1. Analgesia—*administer regimen indicated below:*
    Ketorolac Tromethamine 30 mg IV every 6 hours after intraoperative dose for
    6 doses IF age less than or equal to 60 years.
    Ketorolac Tromethamine 15 mg IV every 6 hours after intraoperative dose for
    6 doses IF age more than 60 years.
2. Start PCA pump: Morphine Sulfate 5 mg/ml (note concentration)
    PCA should not be used in mentally compromised patients or those with sleep apnea. For
    changes or renewals after 72 hours, use the PCA IV Medications order set in the On-line
    Order Set Repository.

Loading Dose (optional)	Basal Dose (optional)	PRN Dose	Lockout Time	Hourly Max (optional)
____ mg (0-3 mg) every 5 m in for a max of ____ mg (less than 8 mg)	____ mg/hr (0-0.5-1 mg/hr)	____ mg (1-3 mg)	____ min (5-15 min)	____ mg/hr

Discontinue PCA Basal in AM on POD #1. Discontinue PCA pump in AM on POD #2 at 6AM.
3. Routine Meds: _____

Medication as needed (prn)
1. Prochlorperazine 10 mg IVPB every 6 hours prn N/V.
2. Naloxone 0.4 mg IV STAT, if unarousable and/or respiratory rate less than or equal to 6
    while on PCA. May repeat Naloxone 0.4 mg IV in 2 minutes if respiratory rate remains
    less than or equal to 6.
3. Start Hydrocodone 7.5 mg/Acetaminophen 500 mg 1 or 2 po every 4 hours prn pain on
    POD #2.
4. Diphenhydramine 12.5 mg or 25 mg IV/PO every 6 hours prn for pruritis.

Instruction/Education
1. Reinforce Pre-op teaching and Care Path with patient and significant other.
2. Review Needs Assessment.
3. Begin Discharge Instructions POD #2.
4. Anticipated Discharge POD #3.
5. Special Discharge Needs: _____

Physician's Signature/ID Code: _____
Pager: _____ Date: _____ Time: _____

M. D. Anderson Cancer Center & Physician's Network

Pathway: GynS2 Total Abdominal Hysterectomy

This path is a general guideline: Care is revised to meet the individual patient's needs based on medical necessity.

Date Category of Care Consult	Pre-Operative Visit Surgery Scheduling Additional consults as indicated per multidisiplinary screening criteria	Same Day Admit Surgery	Post-Op Day #1	Post-Op Day #2	Post-Op Day #3 Discharge Day
Diagnostic Test	CBC (within 14 days) Glucose, BUN, Creat within 30 days Type & Screen CXR (if over 60 years old) ECG (if over 40 years old)	CBC if blood loss greater than 1,000 ml or Hgb pre-op less than 11 gm	CBC at 0400	Incentive Spirometer continued Inspect incision line/staples Observe for excessive bleeding	Incentive Spirometer continued Inspect incision line/staples Observe for excessive bleeding
Treatment	Fleets enema	Incentive Spirometer Turn/Cough/ Deep Breath every 2 hours Observe for excessive bleeding Foley to bedside Compression boots	Incentive Spirometer continued Inspect incision line/staples Observe for excessive bleeding Discontinue Foley at Noon Remove O.R. Dressing		
Medication	Meds as per anesthesia Magnesium Citrate 1 bottle po 48 hrs. before surgery	IV Fluids at 100 ml/hr Ketorolac Tromethamine 30mg IV if over 60 yrs or 60 mg if less than or equal to 60 yrs PCA pump basal	IV Fluids at 75ml/hr Ketorolac Tromethamine 30mg IV every 6 hrs if less than or equal to 60 yrs or 15 mg every 6 hrs if over 60 yrs Discontinue PCA basal, continue demand	Discontinue PCA at 6AM Cap IV line Oral pain meds (Hydrocodone 7.5/Acetamino- phen 500mg)	Oral pain meds (Hydrocodone 7.5/Acetamino- phen 500mg)
Performance Status/Activity	Activities of daily living	Bedrest dangle at the bedside this pm, stand up to chair as tolerated	Ambulate in halls four times daily	Increase ambulation in halls	Increase ambulation in halls
Nutrition	NPO after midnight prior to surgery	Ice Chips 30 ml prn, not to exceed 60 ml every 4 hours	Ice Chips 30 ml prn, not to exceed 60 ml every 4 hours Clear liquids for supper	Soft/bland diet (no bacon or milk products) Diet changes as ordered	Soft/bland diet
Teaching/ Psychosoc	Assess patient for barriers to learning Provide educational materials Pre-op educational materials per standard Instructions on use of incentive spirometer Clarify any concerns	Reinforce pre-op teaching with pt/significant other	Review care path and length of stay with pt/significant other	Start discharge teaching with pt/significant other	Reinforce discharge teaching with pt/significant other
Discharge Planning	Needs assessment		Needs assessment reviewed	Discharge plan agreed upon	Discharge orders and meds written for Lortab & Senkot if needed

Figure 10–2. M. D. Anderson Cancer Center order set for patients with endometrial cancer undergoing a total abdominal hysterectomy.

might be considered initially. However, for all other patients, debulking seems to be associated with decreased morbidity (Goff et al, 1994; Lambrou et al, 2004). Following debulking, treatment usually includes chemotherapy on protocols such as Gynecologic Oncology Group trial 209 (randomization to paclitaxel and carboplatin vs paclitaxel, doxorubicin, and cisplatin).

TREATMENT OF RECURRENT DISEASE

Recurrent endometrial cancer can be much more difficult to treat than primary disease and requires assessment of the presence of hormonal receptors in the recurrent tumor; assessment of the location of the recurrence, including its proximity to the rectum and bladder; and an emphasis on achieving the best quality of life possible for the patient.

Disease usually recurs within the first 3 years after treatment, making early surveillance very important. We suggest a surveillance schedule that includes pelvic examination, vaginal cytologic evaluation, and serum CA-125 measurement at 6- to 12-month intervals for women with grade 2–3 adenocarcinomas. Patients with higher-risk disease should be seen at 3- to 6-month intervals. Obviously, prompt attention to symptomatic women is also recommended. Using these guidelines, one could expect to identify 95% of recurrences (Reddoch et al, 1995). Furthermore, because patients with endometrial cancer have an increased risk of cancers of the breast, ovary, and colon, our surveillance schedule includes screening for new primary tumors at these sites. We also do breast and rectal examinations and schedule mammography and colonoscopies per the American Cancer Society guidelines. When an abnormality is detected by surveillance, a biopsy is performed to confirm the presence of a recurrence or new primary tumor. This is either a direct biopsy of the mass or a CT-guided deep biopsy performed by the Section of Interventional Radiology at M. D. Anderson.

Surgical treatment of endometrial cancer recurrences is considered only in certain situations. If the recurrence is isolated and solitary, for instance a lung metastasis, or if the recurrent cancer is causing a bowel obstruction, surgery may be considered. This is especially so in situations where patients have not been treated for their recurrences and thus have not been shown to be resistant to chemotherapy options. Surgical approaches to recurrent endometrial cancer may also be considered to improve quality of life, as in the case of enterocutaneous fistulas, and to debulk nodal recurrences before using directed radiation therapy in cases of isolated nodal recurrence. Finally, pelvic exenteration is considered in the case of an isolated central recurrence.

Radiation Therapy

Radiation therapy is our initial choice for patients with recurrences at a single site, e.g., the vaginal apex or urethra. We also can give external-beam radiation therapy to the region surrounding the recurrence to reduce tumor bulk. The most common site of recurrence in patients with endometrial carcinoma is in the apical vagina in the region of the hysterectomy scar. Patients with isolated vaginal recurrence who were previously treated with surgery alone can be treated with definitive radiation therapy, which has a 5-year local control rate of 40% to 80% and a 5-year survival rate of 30% to 80%. The treatment consists of a combination of external-beam radiation therapy and brachytherapy. We usually treat the pelvis with external-beam radiation to a total dose of 45 to 50 Gy. As with vaginal cancer, the thickness of the residual disease after external-beam radiation therapy is the most important factor in determining the type of brachytherapy. If the residual disease is thicker than 3 to 5 mm, we use interstitial brachytherapy. For apical tumors, we place the needles using a vaginal template under laparoscopic guidance. A total dose of between 75 and 85 Gy (including the external-beam radiation dose) is given after careful evaluation of the clinical situation, balancing the risks of tumor recurrence and normal tissue complications. For tumors in other parts of the vagina, except the posterior vagina, the lesion is usually boosted with a combination of intracavitary and interstitial brachytherapy. If the lesion involves the posterior vagina and is thicker than 3 mm after external-beam radiation therapy, we continue to deliver external-beam radiation therapy in smaller fields to a total dose of 60 to 66 Gy.

Hormonal Therapy

Hormonal treatment of recurrent endometrial cancer primarily refers to progestational agents but may also refer to gonadotropin-releasing hormone agonists and newer selective ER or PR modulators. The response rates for these agents have been approximately 30%. Response is more likely in ER- and PR-positive and low-grade tumors. Tamoxifen has a response rate similar to that of progesterone in endometrial cancers. We suspect that tamoxifen works by binding to the cell's ER and preventing activation. The Gynecologic Oncology Group showed a response rate of 15% for endometrial cancers treated with leuprolide (Lupron) (Covens et al, 1997), and this response rate is similar to that for tamoxifen. The mechanism of action for gonadotropin-releasing hormone agonists, however, remains unclear.

At M. D. Anderson, we believe hormonal therapy is often the best treatment option for selected patients because of the ease of oral administration and the low risk of side effects, including thrombosis, weight gain, and fluid retention. The question remains how long to continue treatment with progestational agents in the face of remission or any response. We typically recommend that if the toxic effects are tolerable, hormonal therapy should be continued indefinitely or at least 2 to 5 years.

Many innovative hormonal therapies are being explored at our institution, including the use of selective PR modulators (such as mifepristone [RU-486]) and newer selective ER modulators. Because we believe that lack of response to hormonal therapy is due to the absence of PR or ER expression and that sequential or combination therapy may increase response rates, we are planning to look at combination studies in vitro and in vivo. The presence of ER and PR has been shown to correlate with improved survival and response to hormonal therapy and with lower tumor grade. Fifty percent to 60% of primary endometrial cancers and the majority of low-grade endometrial stromal sarcomas are both ER and PR positive. The treatment of well-differentiated primary and recurrent endometrial cancer with progesterones has been associated with a response rate of 18% to 25% and a stable disease rate of 20% to 50%. Used in the treatment of low-grade endometrial stromal sarcomas, progesterone was associated with response rates of 33% to 45%.

We presently offer a trial in which we administer mifepristone to patients with PR-positive advanced recurrent endometrial cancer or low-grade endometrial stromal sarcoma.

Chemotherapy

At M. D. Anderson, we administer chemotherapy for recurrent endometrial cancer only in the context of treatment protocols. Because recurrent endometrial cancer is rare, these trials are often phase II, and they allow for the evaluation of the type of response, its duration, and any toxic effects. Historically, chemotherapy trials in patients with recurrent endometrial cancer show response rates in the 25% to 30% range (not much better than that of hormonal agents). Higher response rates are seen with agents given in combination, but the duration of response typically remains short (7 to 8 months). Owing to the short duration of response, balancing the toxicity of new chemotherapeutic agents with the effects of treatment on quality of life becomes all the more important. Because we feel strongly about these issues at M. D. Anderson, we include a quality-of-life evaluation in all therapeutic trials.

In regards to the actual agents in use, we tend to focus on platinum-based agents or combinations. Studies have indicated that cisplatin and doxorubicin are the most active drugs in recurrent endometrial cancer. Unfortunately, response rates even for these agents remain at about 30%. Thigpin et al (2004) reviewed the use of carboplatin alone for endometrial recurrence and found a response rate of 33% but a duration of response of only 2 to 5 months. Although higher response rates have been seen for combinations of cisplatin, doxorubicin, and cyclophosphamide, the duration of response still remains short (Pustilnik and Burke, 2000). Therefore, the benefit of available chemotherapy for patients with recurrent endometrial cancer is unclear, and we are continually studying in protocols new agents to treat this population.

Patients with recurrent disease of the UPSC histologic subtype are treated on innovative research protocols. We do not include them in endometrioid endometrial cancer protocols unless they have already been included in a national consortium such as the Gynecologic Oncology Group. Presently, we are exploring in a protocol the treatment of patients with recurrent UPSC with imatinib and paclitaxel. Patients not on this protocol are treated primarily with paclitaxel or carboplatin.

HORMONE REPLACEMENT THERAPY

Because estrogen has been implicated as a cause of endometrial cancer, many investigators have recommended no treatment with estrogen replacement therapy after hysterectomy for endometrial cancer. However, it seems likely that estrogen replacement therapy improves the quality of life for patients with hot flashes and those at risk for osteoporosis. On the basis of the literature, it appears that estrogen replacement therapy does not significantly increase the risk of recurrence in endometrial cancer patients at low risk. At M. D. Anderson, we have historically believed that patients with low-risk tumors and no extrauterine disease who have been treated with hysterectomy can be safely offered replacement therapy without a high risk of recurrence. We have not routinely used combined estrogen-progestogen or cycled estrogen-progestogen and have instead prescribed estrogen alone. However, the recent Women's Health Initiative results have altered the practice of many of the gynecologic oncologists at M. D. Anderson. At present, we consider estrogen replacement therapy only for patients with unbearable hot flashes. In patients who do not have hot flashes but who are at increased risk for osteoporosis, a bone density test is usually performed, and bisphosphonate is given, if appropriate.

KEY PRACTICE POINTS

- Recognizing the risk factors for and symptoms of endometrial cancer is key to obtaining a good prognosis.

- Careful preoperative planning and thorough intraoperative staging can help prevent over- and undertreatment.

- In almost all endometrial cancer surgeries, lymph node dissections require sampling to the level of the renal vessels.

- Adjuvant radiation therapy does improve local control, but in intermediate-risk patients its effect on survival remains to be determined. In high-risk groups and in patients with stage IIB disease there is evidence that adjuvant radiation therapy improves both local control and overall survival.

- Treatment for recurrent disease may include radiation therapy, chemotherapy, or hormonal therapy. In patients with isolated vaginal recurrence, radiation therapy is associated with a 5-year local control rate of 40% to 80% and a 5-year survival rate of 30% to 80%. With chemotherapy or hormonal therapy, the response rates are generally between 15% and 30%.

- Estrogen replacement therapy should be offered to patients who have been treated for endometrial cancer only in the case of unbearable hot flashes, and extended counseling regarding the unknown effects on recurrence rates is recommended.

SUGGESTED READINGS

Aalders J, Abeler V, Kolstad P, Onsrud M. Postoperative external irradiation and prognostic parameters in stage I endometrial carcinoma: clinical and histopathologic study of 540 patients. *Obstet Gynecol* 1980;56:419–427.

Ayhan A, Taskiran C, Celik C, Aksu T, Yuce K. Surgical stage III endometrial cancer: analysis of treatment outcomes, prognostic factors and failure patterns. *Eur J Gynaecol Oncol* 2002;23:553–556.

Ball HG, Blessing JA, Lentz SS, Mutch DG. A phase II trial of paclitaxel in patients with advanced or recurrent adenocarcinoma of the endometrium: a Gynecologic Oncology Group study. *Gynecol Oncol* 1996;62:278–281.

Bancher-Todesca D, Neunteufel W, Williams KE, et al. Influence of postoperative treatment on survival in patients with uterine papillary serous carcinoma. *Gynecol Oncol* 1998;71:344–347.

Benedet JL, Bender H, Jones H 3rd, Ngan HY, Pecorelli S. FIGO staging classifications and clinical practice guidelines in the management of gynecologic cancers. FIGO Committee on Gynecologic Oncology. *Int J Gynaecol Obstet* 2000;70:209–262.

Ben-Shachar I, Pavelka J, Cohn DE, et al. Surgical staging for patients presenting with grade 1 endometrial carcinoma. *Obstet Gynecol* 2005;105:487–493.

Brown JJ, Thurnher S, Hricak H. MR imaging of the uterus: low-signal-intensity abnormalities of the endometrium and endometrial cavity. *Magn Reson Imaging* 1990;8:309–313.

Burke TW, Gershenson DM, Morris M, et al. Postoperative adjuvant cisplatin, doxorubicin, and cyclophosphamide (PAC) chemotherapy in women with high-risk endometrial carcinoma. *Gynecol Oncol* 1994;55:47–50.

Corn BW, Lanciano RM, Greven KM, et al. Impact of improved irradiation technique, age, and lymph node sampling on the severe complication rate of surgically staged endometrial cancer patients: a multivariate analysis. *J Clin Oncol* 1994;12:510–515.

Covens A, Thomas G, Shaw P, et al. A phase II study of leuprolide in advanced/recurrent endometrial cancer. *Gynecol Oncol* 1997;64:126–129.

Creasman WT, DiSaia PJ, Blessing J, Wilkinson RH Jr, Johnston W, Weed JC Jr. Prognostic significance of peritoneal cytology in patients with endometrial cancer and preliminary data concerning therapy with intraperitoneal radiopharmaceuticals. *Am J Obstet Gynecol* 1981;141:921–929.

Creasman WT, Henderson D, Hinshaw W, Clarke-Pearson DL. Estrogen replacement therapy in the patient treated for endometrial cancer. *Obstet Gynecol* 1986;67:326–330.

Creutzberg CL. GOG-99: ending the controversy regarding pelvic radiotherapy for endometrial carcinoma? [comment]. *Gynecol Oncol* 2004;92:740–743.

Creutzberg CL, van Putten WL, Koper PC, et al. Surgery and postoperative radiotherapy versus surgery alone for patients with stage-1 endometrial carcinoma: multicentre randomised trial. PORTEC Study Group. Post operative radiation therapy in endometrial carcinoma. *Lancet* 2000;355:1404–1411.

Faquin WC, Fitzgerald JT, Lin MC, Boynton KA, Muto MG, Mutter GL. Sporadic MSI is specific to neoplastic and preneoplastic endometrial tissues. *Am J Clin Pathol* 2000;113:576–582.

Fukuchi T, Sakamoto M, Tsuda H, Maruyama K, Nozawa S, Hirohashi S. β-catenin mutation in carcinoma of the uterine endometrium. *Cancer Res* 1998;58:3526–3528.

Gal D, Recio FO, Zamurovic D. The new International Federation of Gynecology and Obstetrics surgical staging and survival rates in early endometrial carcinoma. *Cancer* 1992;69:200–202.

Goff BA, Goodman A, Muntz HG, et al. Surgical stage IV endometrial carcinoma: a study of 47 cases. *Gynecol Oncol* 1994;52:237–240.

Goff BA, Kato D, Schmidt RA, et al. Uterine papillary serous carcinoma: patterns of metastatic spread. *Gynecol Oncol* 1994;54:264–268.

Greven KM, Lanciano RM, Corn B, Case D, Randall ME. Pathologic stage III endometrial carcinoma. Prognostic factors and patterns of recurrence. *Cancer* 1993;71:3697–3702.

Gurin CC, Federici MG, Kang L, Boyd J. Causes and consequences of MSI in endometrial carcinoma. *Cancer Res* 1999;59:462–468.

Hendrickson M, Ross J, Eifel P, Martinez A, Kempson R. Uterine papillary serous carcinoma: a highly malignant form of endometrial adenocarcinoma. *Am J Surg Pathol* 1982;6:93–108.

Ichikawa Y, Lemon SJ, Wang S, et al. MSI and expression of MLH1 and MSH2 in normal and malignant endometrial and ovarian epithelium in HNPCC family members. *Cancer Genet Cytogenet* 1999;112:2–8.

Ikeda T, Yoshinaga K, Semba S, Kondo E, Ohmori H, Horii A. Mutational analysis of the CTNNB1 (β-catenin) gene in human endometrial cancer: frequent mutations at codon 34 that cause nuclear accumulation. *Oncology Reports* 2000;7:323–326.

Inoue M. Current molecular aspects of the carcinogenesis of the uterine endometrium. *Int J Gynecol Cancer* 2001;11:339–348.

International Federation of Gynecology and Obstetrics: classification and staging of malignant tumors in the female pelvis. *Int J Gynaecol Obstet* 1971;9:172.

Ito K, Watanabe K, Nasim S, Sasano H, Saito S, Yajima A. Prognostic significance of p53 overexpression in endometrial cancer. *Cancer Res* 1994;54:4667–4670.

Jovanovic AS, Boynton KA, Mutter GL. Uteri of women with endometrial carcinoma contain a histopathologic spectrum of monoclonal putative precancers, some with MSI. *Cancer Res* 1996;56:1917–1921.

Kadar N, Homesley HD, Malfetano JH. Positive peritoneal cytology is an adverse factor in endometrial carcinoma only if there is other evidence of extrauterine disease. *Gynecol Oncol* 1992;46:145–149.

Kato DT, Ferry J, Goodman A, et al. Uterine papillary serous carcinoma (UPSC): a clinicopathologic study of 30 cases. *Gynecol Oncol* 1995;59:384–389.

Keys HM, Roberts JA, Brunetto VL, et al. A phase III trial of surgery with or without adjunctive external pelvic radiation therapy in intermediate risk endometrial adenocarcinoma: a Gynecologic Oncology Group study. *Gynecol Oncol* 2004;92:744–751.

Kong D, Suzuki A, Zou TT, et al. PTEN1 is frequently mutated in primary endometrial carcinomas. *Nat Genet* 1997;17:143–144.

Kucera H, Vavra N, Weghaupt K. Benefit of external irradiation in pathologic stage I endometrial carcinoma: a prospective clinical trial of 605 patients who received postoperative vaginal irradiation and additional pelvic irradiation in the presence of unfavorable prognostic factors. *Gynecol Oncol* 1990;38:99–104.

Lambrou NC, Gomez-Marin O, Mirhashemi R, et al. Optimal surgical cytoreduction in patients with stage III and stage IV endometrial carcinoma: a study of morbidity and survival. *Gynecol Oncol* 2004;93:653–658.

Lanciano RM, Greven KM. Adjuvant treatment for endometrial cancer: who needs it? *Gynecol Oncol* 1995;57:135–137.

Lee RB, Burke TW, Park RC. Estrogen replacement therapy following treatment for stage I endometrial carcinoma. *Gynecol Oncol* 1990;36:189–191.

Levenback C, Burke TW, Silva E, et al. Uterine papillary serous carcinoma (UPSC) treated with cisplatin, doxorubicin, and cyclophosphamide (PAC). *Gynecol Oncol* 1992;46:317–321.

Levine RL, Cargile CB, Blazes MS, van Rees B, Kurman RJ, Ellenson LH. PTEN mutations and microsatellite instability in complex atypical hyperplasia, a precursor lesion to uterine endometrioid carcinoma. *Cancer Res* 1998;58:3254–3258.

Mallipeddi P, Kapp DS, Teng N. Long-term survival with adjuvant whole abdominopelvic irradiation for uterine papillary serous carcinoma. *Cancer* 1993;71:3076–3081.

Matias-Guiu X, Catasus L, Bussaglia E, et al. Molecular pathology of endometrial hyperplasia and carcinoma. *Hum Pathol* 2001;32:569–577.

Mirabelli-Primdahl L, Gryfe R, Kim H, et al. Beta-catenin mutations are specific for colorectal carcinomas with microsatellite instability but occur in endometrial carcinomas irrespective of mutator pathway. *Cancer Res* 1999; 59:3346–3351.

Moore DH, Fowler WC Jr, Walton LA, Droegemueller W. Morbidity of lymph node sampling in cancers of the uterine corpus and cervix. *Obstet Gynecol* 1989;74:180–184.

Morrow C, Bundy B, Kurman RJ, et al. Relationship between surgical-pathological risk factors and outcome in clinical stage I and II carcinoma of the endometrium: a Gynecologic Oncology Group study. *Gynecol Oncol* 1991;40:55–65.

Murphy AA, Morales AJ, Kettel LM, Yen SS. Regression of uterine leiomyomata to the antiprogesterone RU486: dose-response effect. *Fertil Steril* 1995;64:187–190.

Mutter GL, Boynton KA, Faquin WC, et al. Allelotype mapping of unstable microsatellites establishes direct lineage continuity between endometrial precancers and cancer. *Cancer Res* 1996;56:4483–4486.

Mutter GL, Wada H, Faquin WC, Enomoto T. K-ras mutations appear in the premalignant phase of both microsatellite stable and unstable endometrial carcinogenesis. *Mol Pathol* 1999;52:257–262.

Nei H, Saito T, Yamasaki H, Mizumoto H, Ito E, Kudo R. Nuclear localization of β-catenin in normal and carcinogenic endometrium. *Mol Carcinog* 1999;25:207–218.

Piver MS, Recio FO, Baker TR, Hempling RE. A prospective trial of progesterone therapy for malignant peritoneal cytology in patients with endometrial carcinoma. *Gynecol Oncol* 1993;47:373–376.

Podratz KC, O'Brien PC, Malkasian GD Jr, Decker DG, Jefferies JA, Edmonson JH. Effects of progestational agents in treatment of endometrial carcinoma. *Obstet Gynecol* 1985;66:106–110.

Pustilnik T, Burke TW. Adjuvant chemotherapy for high-risk endometrial cancer. *Semin Radiat Oncol* 2000;10:23-28.

Ramondetta L, Burke TW, Levenback C, Bevers M, Bodurka-Bevers D, Gershenson DM. Treatment of uterine papillary serous carcinoma with paclitaxel. *Gynecol Oncol* 2001;82:156–161.

Reddoch JM, Burke TW, Morris M, et al. Surveillance for recurrent endometrial carcinoma: development of a follow-up scheme. *Gynecol Oncol* 1995;59:221–225.

Risinger JI, Hayes AK, Berchuck A, Barrett JC. PTEN/MMAC1 mutations in endometrial cancers. *Cancer Res* 1997;57:4736–4738.

Risinger JI, Hayes K, Maxwell GL, et al. PTEN mutation in endometrial cancers is associated with favorable clinical and pathologic characteristics. *Clin Cancer Res* 1998;4:3005–3010.

Rossouw JE, Anderson GL, Prentice RL, et al. Risks and benefits of estrogen plus progestin in healthy postmenopausal women: principal results from the Women's Health Initiative randomized controlled trial. *JAMA* 2002; 288:321–333.

Schneider CC, Gibb RK, Taylor DD, Wan T, Gercel-Taylor C. Inhibition of endometrial cancer cell lines by mifepristone (RU 486). *J Soc Gynecol Investig* 1998;5:334–338.

Sherman ME. Theories of endometrial carcinogenesis: a multidisciplinary approach. *Mod Pathol* 2000;13:295–308.

Sherman ME, Bur ME, Kurman RJ. p53 in endometrial cancer and its putative precursors: evidence for diverse pathways of tumorigenesis. *Hum Pathol* 1995;26:1268–1274.

Silva EG, Jenkins R. Serous carcinoma in endometrial polyps. *Mod Pathol* 1990;3:120–128.

Sood AK, Buller RE, Burger RA, Dawson JD, Sorosky JI, Berman M. Value of preoperative CA 125 level in the management of uterine cancer and prediction of clinical outcome. *Obstet Gynecol* 1997;90:441–447.

Staebler A, Lax SF, Ellenson LH. Altered expression of hMLH1 and hMSH2 protein in endometrial carcinomas with MSI. *Hum Pathol* 2000;31:354–358.

Stringer CA, Gershenson DM, Burke TW, Edwards CL, Gordon AN, Wharton JT. Adjuvant chemotherapy with cisplatin, doxorubicin, and cyclophosphamide (PAC) for early-stage high-risk endometrial cancer: a preliminary analysis. *Gynecol Oncol* 1990;38:305–308.

Sun M, Zhu G, Zhou L. Effect of mifepristone on the expression of progesterone receptor messenger RNA and protein in uterine leiomyomata [in Chinese]. *Zhonghua Fu Chan Ke Za Zhi* 1998;33:227–231.

Sutton GP, Blessing JA, DeMars LR, Moore D, Burke TW, Grendys EC. A phase II Gynecologic Oncology Group trial of ifosfamide and mesna in advanced or recurrent adenocarcinoma of the endometrium. *Gynecol Oncol* 1996;63:25–27.

Tashiro H, Blazes MS, Wu R, et al. Mutations in PTEN are frequent in endometrial carcinoma but rare in other common gynecological malignancies. *Cancer Res* 1997;57:3935–3940.

Tashiro H, Isacson C, Levine R, Kurman RJ, Cho KR, Hedrick L. p53 gene mutations are common in uterine carcinoma and occur early in their pathogenesis. *Am J Pathol* 1997;150:177–185.

Tebeu PM, Popowski Y, Verkooijen HM, et al. Positive peritoneal cytology in early-stage endometrial cancer does not influence prognosis. *Br J Cancer* 2004;91:720–724.

Thigpen JT, Blessing JA, DiSaia PJ, Yordan E, Carson LF, Evers C. A randomized comparison of doxorubicin alone versus doxorubicin plus cyclophosphamide in the management of advanced or recurrent endometrial carcinoma: a Gynecologic Oncology Group study. *J Clin Oncol* 1994;12:1408–1414.

Thigpen JT, Blessing JA, Hatch KD, et al. A randomized trial of medroxyprogesterone acetate (MPA) 200 mg versus 1000 mg daily in advanced or recurrent endometrial carcinoma: a Gynecologic Oncology Group study [abstract]. *Proc ASCO* 1991;10:185.

Thigpen JT, Blessing JA, Homesley H, Creasman WT, Sutton G. Phase II trial of cisplatin as first-line chemotherapy in patients with advanced or recurrent endometrial carcinoma: a Gynecologic Oncology Group study. *Gynecol Oncol* 1989;33:68–70.

Thigpen JT, Brady MF, Homesley HD, et al. Phase III trial of doxorubicin with or without cisplatin in advanced endometrial carcinoma: a Gynecologic Oncology Group study. *J Clin Oncol* 2004;22:3902–3908.

Thigpen JT, Buchsbaum HJ, Mangan C, Blessing JA. Phase II trial of adriamycin in the treatment of advanced or recurrent endometrial carcinoma: a Gynecologic Oncology Group study. *Cancer Treat Rep* 1979;63:21–27.

Tritz D, Pieretti M, Turner S, Powell D. Loss of heterozygosity in usual and special variant carcinomas of the endometrium. *Hum Pathol* 1997;28:607–612.

Vergote I, Kjorstad K, Abeler V, Kolstad P. A randomized trial of adjuvant progestagen in early endometrial cancer. *Cancer* 1989;64:1011–1016.

Watson P, Vasen HF, Mecklin JP, Jarvinen H, Lynch HT. The risk of endometrial cancer in hereditary nonpolyposis colorectal cancer. *Am J Med* 1994;96:516–520.

Zanotti KM, Belinson JL, Kennedy AW, Webster KD, Markman M. The use of paclitaxel and platinum-based chemotherapy in uterine papillary serous carcinoma. *Gynecol Oncol* 1999;74:272–277.

Zeng C, Gu M, Huang H. A clinical control study of the treatment of uterine leiomyoma with gonadotrophin releasing hormone agonist or mifepristone [in Chinese]. *Zhonghua Fu Chan Ke Za Zhi* 1998;33:490–492.

11 SURGERY FOR OVARIAN CANCER

Judith K. Wolf and J. Taylor Wharton

CHAPTER OUTLINE

CHAPTER OVERVIEW

At M. D. Anderson Cancer Center, exploratory laparotomy is the standard of care for patients with presumed ovarian cancer, and total abdominal hysterectomy, bilateral salpingo-oophorectomy, and tumor-reductive surgery are the standard of care for patients with confirmed ovarian cancer. Optimal tumor-debulking surgery—i.e., surgery resulting in no residual tumor nodules larger than 1 cm—is known to be associated with improved survival; therefore, the goal of surgery is optimal tumor debulking whenever feasible. Only patients who are unable to tolerate surgery or who have cancer that is known preoperatively to preclude optimal tumor reduction are considered for neoadjuvant chemotherapy. If neoadjuvant chemotherapy is administered, patients are reassessed after 3 or 6 cycles to see if they have become candidates for surgical debulking. Surgical debulking performed in this situation is referred to as interval debulking surgery or interval cytoreductive surgery.

We do not routinely perform second-look surgery outside the context of clinical trials because this procedure is of no known benefit to patients. Patients who have a complete clinical response to primary tumor debulking and adjuvant chemotherapy are offered a second-look procedure only if they are candidates for and are interested in protocol therapy. If patients opt for second-look surgery, it is generally performed as a laparoscopic procedure, if technically possible.

Secondary tumor debulking can be considered for patients with residual disease detected on second-look surgery and for patients with isolated late recurrence. Palliative surgery can be used to relieve bowel obstruction and symptoms. Tumor debulking is not recommended in patients who will not receive postoperative chemotherapy.

Introduction

Most patients with suspected ovarian cancer have either an isolated pelvic mass or masses or suspected abdominal carcinomatosis. These can be found on clinical examination or on imaging studies, most commonly computed tomography (CT), ultrasonography, or both. Magnetic resonance imaging is not routinely used, as it is no more accurate than CT in the detection of abnormalities and generally costs more. Staging of ovarian cancer is surgical; therefore, surgery is important not only to establish the diagnosis but also to establish the extent of disease. Because of the potential for spread of early ovarian cancer, biopsy of sites of suspected malignancy alone is not recommended. Thus, when a patient presents with findings suggestive of ovarian cancer, evaluation for possible exploratory laparotomy is indicated.

Patients with ovarian cancer who wish to maintain fertility should be carefully evaluated, and several prognostic factors should be considered (see the chapter "Fertility-Sparing Options for Treatment of Women with Gynecologic Cancers"). In patients diagnosed with ovarian germ cell tumors and sex cord-stromal tumors, fertility conservation is the standard practice.

Exploratory Laparotomy
and Primary Tumor Debulking

Exploratory laparotomy is used for diagnosis and staging, and in patients with confirmed ovarian cancer, primary tumor debulking, if feasible, is performed during the exploration.

Preoperative Assessment

For patients with suspected ovarian cancer, the preoperative assessment should include a careful personal and family history, a review of systems, and an assessment of surgical risk. Important points to cover in the history include gynecologic and obstetric history, gynecologic surgeries, infections, endometriosis, oral contraceptive use, and personal and family history of cancer. A personal history of breast cancer or family history of ovarian cancer can increase the risk of ovarian cancer. Another consideration in patients with a personal history of breast cancer is metastatic breast cancer presenting as a pelvic mass or abdominal carcinomatosis. In breast cancer survivors with findings suggestive of ovarian cancer, a search for other sites of breast cancer recurrence—specifically, with mammography, clinical breast examination, and bone scan—may be indicated.

Careful review of any changes in bowel habits, such as constipation, diarrhea, early satiety, bloating, nausea, vomiting, blood in the stool, or change in the caliber of the stool, can help identify patients who may have a primary tumor of the colon or may need bowel surgery as part of tumor debulking. Change in bladder function is common in patients with ovarian cancer; however, routine preoperative cystoscopy is not indicated.

On physical examination, the clinician should look for signs of distant spread of disease—specifically, groin, supraclavicular, or, less commonly, axillary lymphadenopathy. The lungs should be carefully auscultated for signs of pleural effusion. The abdomen should be palpated for evidence of ascites, hepatomegaly or splenomegaly, or masses. The pelvic examination should include both vaginal and rectovaginal examinations to evaluate for pelvic masses and rectal compression or extension. A Papanicolaou test should be performed if results from a test performed within the previous 12 months are not available.

Preoperative laboratory work should include a complete blood cell count, evaluation of kidney and liver function, and a type and screen procedure or cross-matching to determine blood type. Tumor markers measured should include CA-125; carcinoembryonic antigen if a primary tumor of the bowel is suspected; and alpha fetoprotein, beta human chorionic gonadotropin, and lactate dehydrogenase if a germ cell tumor is suspected. Germ cell tumors are more common in young patients.

Preoperative imaging studies should include chest radiography and a CT scan of the abdomen and pelvis. Most patients referred to a gynecologic oncologist have already had these tests performed. Patients who have not had a mammogram within the previous 12 months and patients with abnormal findings on mammography within the previous 12 months should undergo further evaluation. Decisions regarding other radiographic testing should be tailored to the individual patient's signs and symptoms. Routine use of magnetic resonance imaging or positron emission tomography is not indicated.

If findings on the history, physical examination, or CT suggest the possibility of large bowel involvement, a barium enema may help to determine if a large bowel resection or colostomy might be needed at the time of ovarian tumor debulking. If the need for a colostomy is anticipated, we refer the patient for a consultation with an enterostomal therapy nurse before surgery so that the abdomen can be marked for appropriate colostomy placement to ensure that ostomy bags fit well and the ostomy site does not interfere with normal function or clothing. The consultation with the enterostomal therapy nurse also provides an opportunity to teach the patient about proper ostomy care. We do not routinely perform colonoscopy, but this would be another way to evaluate the large bowel.

Patients with significant medical problems should be evaluated by the appropriate medical specialist to determine the risks associated with surgery and to provide recommendations regarding preoperative management (e.g., the use of beta blockers).

On the day before surgery, patients follow an outpatient bowel preparation regimen consisting of a polyethylene glycol electrolyte mechanical cleansing. Patients also take oral antibiotics, most commonly erythromycin and neomycin base, 1 g each, at 1 pm, 2 pm, and 10 pm. Patients are instructed to eat or drink nothing after midnight. Almost all patients are able to tolerate this preparation on an outpatient basis and are admitted to the hospital the day of surgery. Perioperatively, we also give an intravenous dose of a cephalosporin, such as cefoxitin. We use intermittent pneumatic compression stockings for prophylaxis against deep venous thrombosis.

Surgical Technique

After general anesthesia induction, the patient is placed in a modified lithotomy position in Allen stirrups, and a pelvic and abdominal examination is performed to try to further delineate the disease. This position is particularly helpful when a low rectal anastomosis is created, and it also gives excellent access to the para-aortic region for nodal dissection.

After the abdomen and vagina are prepared, a vertical midline incision is made. Peritoneal washings are obtained or ascites fluid is removed, if present (Figure 11–1). The entire abdomen and pelvis are then explored, and the bowel is examined in its entirety. Masses apparently confined to the ovary are removed intact (Figure 11–2). Once the amount and distribution of disease is delineated, a decision is made regarding the feasibility of optimal tumor debulking, defined as surgery resulting in no residual tumor nodules larger than 1 cm. This is one of the most important decisions made during exploratory laparotomy and can be made only with complete information about the extent of disease and the patient's overall medical status. If the patient is relatively healthy and can tolerate a lengthy and possibly bloody procedure, the surgeon may decide to take the time to try to remove disease from critical structures such as the diaphragm. However, if there is significant disease in an area that cannot be resected, such as the small bowel mesentery, tumor debulking would not be prudent, as it would result in additional surgical risk with no gain for the patient. In the rare patient in whom all or most of the disease involves the bowel or other vital organs, any debulking is risky. In such cases, although it is difficult to admit that one cannot remove the

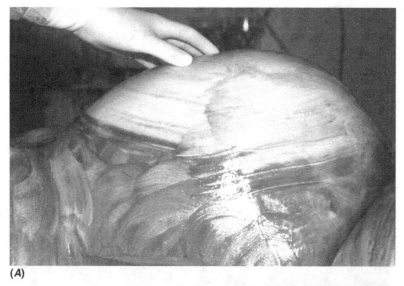

(A)

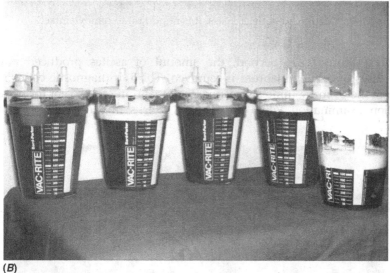

(B)

Figure 11–1. Preoperative (A) and intraoperative (B) findings of ascites in a patient with ovarian cancer.

tumor, the surgeon must remember the Hippocratic oath and "first do no harm." The proper approach in such situations is to obtain a tumor biopsy specimen and close the abdomen.

Once the decision is made to proceed with tumor debulking, omentectomy is often a good choice for the initial approach, for several reasons. First, removal of the omentum facilitates packing the bowel out of the

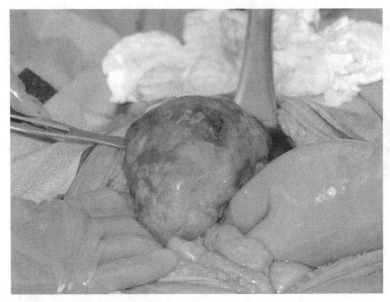

Figure 11–2. Malignant adnexal mass. It is important to remove intact.

pelvis (Figure 11–3). Second, the amount of ascites produced often decreases once the omentum is removed. Third, if diagnostic confirmation of the primary tumor is needed, the omentum can be sent for frozen section examination while the surgeon works in the pelvis. A good

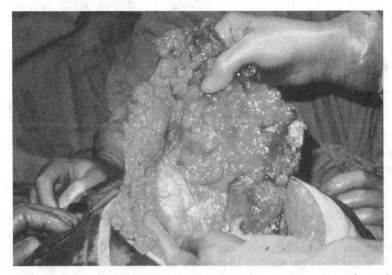

Figure 11–3. Omentum with tumor. Resection can be started on the undersurface, at the edge of the transverse colon.

approach to removing the omentum is from the posterior inferior attachment to the transverse colon. This allows access to the lesser sac and careful dissection from the colon without significant blood loss. Once the omentum is freed from the colon, the blood supply from the stomach can be ligated. On the left side, omental disease may extend to the spleen or near the spleen. Atraumatic dissection here is imperative. Occasionally, to achieve optimal debulking, splenectomy is also done.

After the bowel is packed out of the pelvis, opening of the retroperitoneum on the pelvic sidewalls from the round ligament superiorly allows for identification of the infundibulopelvic ligaments, ureters, and pelvic spaces. Ligation of the infundibulopelvic ligaments can decrease the amount of bleeding to adnexal structures, including masses. Opening the pelvic spaces allows inspection of the extent of disease and determination of the extent of pelvic dissection required for tumor removal. Hysterectomy, bilateral salpingo-oophorectomy, and colon resection, if required, can be done in an en bloc dissection.

After removal of the omentum and pelvic disease, with or without colon resection, attention can be turned to other residual disease, including disease of the small bowel, lymph nodes, and peritoneal surfaces. If bowel resection is required, we use stapling devices to decrease operative time. When lymph nodes must be removed, the retroperitoneal spaces can be opened further to facilitate access to pelvic and para-aortic nodes. Large areas of disease on the peritoneal surfaces or diaphragm can be removed using either a cavitron ultrasonic surgical aspirator or an argon-beam coagulator. However, removal of disease on the peritoneal surface or diaphragm rarely results in a difference between optimal and suboptimal outcome; therefore, it is imperative to weigh the risks and benefits of such procedures.

If a bowel resection or splenectomy is performed, a drain may be left in the area. If a large amount of ascites continues to be produced throughout the surgery, a peritoneal drain for ascites fluid may be left in place. After surgery is completed, hemostasis is assured, and the peritoneal cavity is irrigated, we usually close the abdomen with a running mass closure using a single-filament suture such as a polydioxanone suture. Skin staples are used for the skin closure. If the patient has had significant blood loss or ascites fluid production or has serious comorbid conditions, she may recover in the intensive care unit. Otherwise, standard postanesthesia recovery and postoperative care is used.

INTERVAL DEBULKING SURGERY

Interval debulking surgery, also known as interval cytoreductive surgery, is performed after a few courses of neoadjuvant chemotherapy or in the middle of adjuvant chemotherapy administered after less-than-optimal primary tumor debulking. Two prospective trials of the effect of interval debulking found different results. A European trial of patients who underwent suboptimal debulking surgery followed by 3 cycles of cisplatin and cyclophosphamide and were randomly assigned to interval surgery or none, followed by 3 more cycles of chemotherapy, found a survival benefit in patients who underwent interval debulking surgery (Van der Burg et al, 1995). However, a Gynecologic Oncology Group trial that used the same general approach in a similar population, but with cisplatin and paclitaxel, found no survival benefit of interval debulking (Rose et al, 2002).

Given these conflicting results and the more recent United States trial showing no benefit of interval debulking (Rose et al, 2004), we generally reserve interval debulking for 2 types of patients. The first are patients who at the time of presentation at our institution are not good candidates for surgery (e.g., those with poor performance status due to cancer burden or comorbid conditions, poor nutritional status [serum albumin level less than 2.0 g/dL], or bilateral pleural effusions) and thus are treated with neoadjuvant chemotherapy. Only patients who are unable to tolerate surgery or who have cancer that is known preoperatively to preclude optimal tumor reduction are considered for neoadjuvant chemotherapy. If neoadjuvant chemotherapy is administered, patients are reassessed after 3 or 6 cycles to see if they have become candidates for surgical debulking. The second group of patients in whom interval debulking is considered are patients who have undergone a suboptimal surgical procedure elsewhere. Sometimes patients are referred to us after an exploratory laparotomy with only a biopsy or a minimal attempt at tumor debulking. These patients may be considered individually for repeat exploratory laparotomy before chemotherapy or interval debulking.

SECOND-LOOK SURGERY

After a patient has completed primary therapy—most commonly primary tumor debulking followed by 6 to 8 courses of chemotherapy—a second surgery may be considered. This is traditionally called a second-look surgery when it is done in a patient in complete clinical remission. Today, that would be a patient with normal findings on physical examination, serum CA-125 analysis, and imaging. Imaging may include radiography, CT, magnetic resonance imaging, and even positron emission tomography. A second-look surgery has traditionally been offered to patients in clinical remission to further define their disease status. However, this surgery has no proven clinical benefit.

Of patients in clinical remission, approximately 30% to 40% are found to have gross disease on second-look surgery, another 20% to 30% are found to have microscopic disease, and 30% to 50% have no gross or microscopic cancer identified. The problem is that for patients with residual disease, either gross or microscopic, there is no known treatment that is proven to increase survival. Even for patients with no cancer identified on second-look surgery, the recurrence rate is 50%. There is no proven treatment to prevent recurrence, and it is impossible to determine which 50% of patients will have recurrence.

Because of all these issues, we do not routinely perform second-look surgery. That being said, we are always looking for new and better treatments for patients with ovarian cancer, and we have clinical trials designed to deliver additional therapy depending on patients' disease status after primary tumor debulking. Patients with a complete clinical response to primary tumor debulking followed by 6 to 8 courses of chemotherapy are offered a second-look procedure if they are candidates for and are interested in protocol therapy.

When we perform a second-look surgery, we often use a laparoscopic approach. Laparoscopy allows adequate visualization and access for biopsies in most patients. This approach can often save the patient the morbidity of a second major abdominal procedure. Since most patients have had a vertical midline incision, a 5-mm laparoscope is often first placed in the left upper quadrant to avoid adhesions from previous surgery. This first view allows inspection and facilitates safe placement of a larger scope and other trocars for peritoneal access. The patient has to undergo a laparotomy only if the laparoscopic approach does not provide sufficient access, if a complication occurs, or if there is a large area of disease that will be secondarily debulked (see the next section).

During second-look surgery, biopsies of any abnormal areas, adhesions, and sites of previous known disease are routinely performed. Depending on whether lymph nodes have been evaluated before, pelvic and para-aortic lymph nodes may be removed.

If the surgery is performed laparoscopically, it can be done on an outpatient basis with minimal recovery time.

SECONDARY TUMOR DEBULKING

For patients with gross disease found at the time of second-look surgery, a few small studies show a survival benefit from further tumor debulking to remove all but microscopic disease. Such a benefit has not been proven in a large prospective randomized trial, but there may be a benefit for a few patients who have had a response to the initial adjuvant therapy and can receive further active therapy after the secondary surgery.

The other situation in which we consider secondary tumor debulking is for patients with a long disease-free interval, usually at least 12 months after completion of chemotherapy, who present with recurrent disease that appears on preoperative imaging to be localized and resectable. Such patients are presumed to have chemotherapy-responsive cancer, and it is theorized that a second "optimal" debulking may have a benefit similar to that of the primary tumor debulking. There is some information from retrospective studies suggesting that this may in fact be true, but the benefit of secondary tumor debulking in this group of patients has not been proven in prospective studies. The Gynecologic Oncology Group is currently performing a clinical trial to try to answer this question. The study randomizes patients who might be candidates for secondary surgery to surgery or chemotherapy and is designed to determine whether surgery provides a survival benefit.

While we await answers from clinical trials, we limit secondary tumor debulking to patients who have a long disease-free interval (at least 12 months); are presumed to have a good chance to respond again to chemotherapy; have disease that appears preoperatively to be resectable; and are physically able to tolerate surgery. Patients whose cancer recurs quickly (less than 6 months after primary tumor debulking followed by 6 to 8 courses of chemotherapy) are unlikely to respond well to further treatment, and we do not recommend secondary debulking in this situation.

Some patients have disease that appears on preoperative imaging to be localized and resectable but at the time of surgery is found to be widespread or unresectable. Unfortunately, there is no good way to predict this before surgery.

Surgical principles for secondary debulking are the same as those outlined earlier in this chapter in the section Exploratory Laparotomy and Primary Tumor Debulking. The surgeon must always keep in mind that most patients with recurrent disease, even those with a long disease-free interval, are not ultimately cured of their cancer. Thus, special caution should be exercised when deciding whether to pursue extensive, risky resections in such patients.

SURGERY FOR PALLIATION

In patients with recurrent ovarian cancer, palliative surgery can be considered for relief of bowel obstruction or symptoms. In patients with recurrence, surgery for tumor reduction is not recommended unless postoperative chemotherapy is planned.

Patients with recurrent ovarian cancer and bowel obstruction are usually quite debilitated and malnourished and have a limited life expectancy. Usually, these patients have chemorefractory disease. Even if the disease is chemoresponsive, it must be kept in mind that in patients with a bowel obstruction, giving further chemotherapy can be dangerous.

Stagnant bowel contents can breed bacteria, and if a patient becomes neutropenic, this can lead to life-threatening infection.

Patients with recurrent ovarian cancer who develop bowel obstruction can have a small or large bowel obstruction or both. Obstruction can be partial or complete and can occur at multiple sites. Many of these patients have a so-called "tumor ileus," with cancer encasing much of the bowel from the outside, narrowing multiple areas and slowing peristalsis to the point that the patient cannot tolerate oral intake. When we consider operating on a patient with this problem, we try to obtain a preoperative assessment of the extent of disease and bowel involvement. Although there is no test that gives all the information needed, a CT scan, barium enema, or small bowel series may help determine if the obstruction can be relieved. There have been no prospective trials showing what is best for these patients, but several small case series give some information about surgery to try to resolve obstruction. In general, the bowel obstruction is relieved in about two thirds of patients who undergo surgery, and about two thirds of patients in whom surgery is successful are able to tolerate a regular diet after surgery. In one third of patients who undergo surgery, the obstruction cannot be relieved. In such cases, life expectancy is usually 1 to 2 months. In patients whose obstruction is relieved, the average life expectancy is about 6 months.

Surgery for obstruction may include colostomy, bowel resection, bowel bypass, ileostomy, or a combination of these procedures. If the obstruction cannot be relieved because of the extent of bowel involvement, an attempt is always made to place a gastrostomy tube, as this may be the only relief the patient can get from gastric distention, nausea, and vomiting. Surgery to relieve bowel obstruction should be limited to that goal; tumor debulking should not be attempted.

Patients facing surgery for bowel obstruction should be informed of the data available regarding the possibility of relieving the obstruction and the average life expectancy. Those who choose not to have surgery or who are too debilitated to tolerate surgery can usually be offered placement of a gastrostomy tube, via either an endoscopic or an interventional radiologic procedure.

Occasionally a patient presents with a recurrent ovarian cancer mass that does not cause a bowel obstruction but does cause pain or some other symptom that can best be relieved by surgical removal. When surgery is considered for such a patient, it is important to think about life expectancy, the morbidity of surgery, and other possible palliative measures that could be undertaken. For example, in a patient with a painful pelvic mass or symptomatic supraclavicular lymphadenopathy, palliative radiotherapy may be safer than palliative surgery, although a few patients may best be treated with surgery.

SUMMARY

Surgery has several roles in the treatment of ovarian cancer. Today, diagnosis, staging, and primary tumor debulking are probably the most established and important roles for surgery. However, surgery for patients with recurrent disease should be considered in certain circumstances after careful consideration of the risks and benefits.

KEY PRACTICE POINTS

- Complete surgical staging is important for all ovarian cancers.
- On exploratory laparotomy, the surgeon must be prepared to stage any ovarian mass.
- Optimal primary tumor debulking should be attempted whenever feasible in patients with advanced ovarian cancer.
- Interval debulking surgery may be appropriate for patients who have poor performance status at presentation and thus are not eligible for primary tumor debulking.
- Routine second-look surgery offers no survival benefit.
- Secondary tumor debulking may be considered in patients with chemosensitive recurrent ovarian cancer and potentially resectable disease.
- Surgery to relieve bowel obstruction can prolong survival in patients with recurrent ovarian cancer.

SUGGESTED READINGS

Eisenkop SM, Friedman RL, Spirtos NM. The role of secondary cytoreductive surgery in the treatment of patients with recurrent epithelial ovarian carcinoma. *Cancer* 2000;88:144–153.

Greer BE, Bundy BN, Ozols RF, et al. Implications of second-look laparotomy (SLL) in the context of Gynecologic Oncology Group (GOG) protocol 158: a non-randomized comparison using an explanatory analysis [abstract]. *Gynecol Oncol* 2003;88:156–157.

Hoskins WJ, Bundy BN, Thigpen JT, et al. The influence of cytoreductive surgery on recurrence-free interval and survival in small-volume stage III epithelial ovarian cancer: a Gynecologic Oncology Group study. *Gynecol Oncol* 1992;47:159–166.

Hoskins WJ, McGuire WP, Brady MF, et al. The effect of diameter of largest residual disease on survival after primary cytoreductive surgery in patients with suboptimal residual epithelial ovarian carcinoma. *Am J Obstet Gynecol* 1994;170:974–979.

Morris M, Gershenson DM, Wharton JT, et al. Secondary cytoreductive surgery for recurrent epithelial ovarian cancer. *Gynecol Oncol* 1988;34:334–338.

Pothuri B, Vaidya A, Aghajanian C, Venkatraman E, Barakat RR, Chi DS. Palliative surgery for bowel obstruction in recurrent ovarian cancer: an updated series. *Gynecol Oncol* 2004;89:306–313.

Rose PG, Nerenstone S, Brady M. A phase III randomized study of interval secondary cytoreduction in patients with advanced stage ovarian carcinoma with suboptimal residual disease: a Gynecologic Oncology Group study [abstract]. *Proc Am Soc Clin Oncol* 2002;21:201a (abstract 802).

Rose PG, Nerenstone S, Brady MF, et al; Gynecologic Oncology Group. Secondary surgical cytoreduction for advanced ovarian carcinoma. *N Engl J Med* 2004;351:2489–2497.

Rubin SC, Hoskins WJ, Benjamin I, Lewis JL. Palliative surgery for intestinal obstruction in advanced ovarian cancer. *Gynecol Oncol* 1989;34:16–19.

Tuxen MK, Strauss G, Lund B, Hansen M. The role of second-look laparotomy in the long-term survival in ovarian cancer. *Ann Oncol* 1997;8:643–648.

Van der Burg MEL, Van Lent M, Buyse M, et al. The effect of debulking surgery after induction chemotherapy in the prognosis in advanced epithelial ovarian cancer. *N Engl J Med* 1995;332:629–634.

Venesmaa P, Ylikorkala O. Morbidity and mortality associated with primary and repeat operations for ovarian cancer. *Obstet Gynecol* 1992;79:168–172.

12 CHEMOTHERAPY FOR EPITHELIAL OVARIAN CANCER

Michele L. Donato, Xipeng Wang, John J. Kavanagh, and David M. Gershenson

CHAPTER OUTLINE

CHAPTER OVERVIEW

Chemotherapy has been an integral part of the treatment of epithelial ovarian cancer at M. D. Anderson Cancer Center since the 1950s. Since the introduction of paclitaxel in the early 1990s, the combination of a taxane and a platinum drug has been the standard. Concomitantly, a growing menu of chemotherapeutic agents has been discovered, tested in phase I and II trials, and used to treat recurrent ovarian cancer at M. D. Anderson. For over 2 decades, our standard treatment for early-stage epithelial ovarian cancer at M. D. Anderson, based on experience and clinical trials in advanced-stage disease, has included 6 cycles of platinum-based combination chemotherapy. Since the mid-1990s, we have recommended the combination of paclitaxel plus carboplatin every 3 weeks for 6 cycles because of its superior therapeutic index. For patients with advanced-stage disease, indications for neoadjuvant chemotherapy and interval debulking include the following: (1) unresectable disease on the basis of computed tomographic characteristics, (2) 1 or more comorbidities that increase the patient's risk of major perioperative complications, (3) massive effusions, or (4) stage IV disease. An ongoing randomized clinical trial should further elucidate the role of neoadjuvant chemotherapy. Recent reports of a survival benefit associated with intraperitoneal chemotherapy for patients with optimal advanced-stage disease have resulted in a re-examination of this approach. However, unresolved issues include determining the optimal regimen, number of cycles, and method of administration. A single randomized study from the Southwest Oncology Group and Gynecologic Oncology Group has demonstrated a progression-free survival benefit associated with 12 cycles of monthly paclitaxel following completion of primary chemotherapy; future studies will further clarify the role of consolidation therapy. Finally, the role of both autologous and allogeneic stem cell transplantation remains under study.

INTRODUCTION

Ovarian cancer is the most common cause of cancer death among women with gynecologic cancer and the fourth leading cause of cancer death in women in the United States; estimates for 2004 included 25,580 new cases and 16,090 deaths (Jemal et al, 2004). Most types of ovarian cancer (about 90%) are derived from celomic epithelium. The current standard for treatment of ovarian cancer consists of primary cytoreductive surgery followed by paclitaxel and platinum-based chemotherapy (McGuire et al, 1996). The past 30 years has seen some improvement in the diagnosis and management of ovarian cancer; 5-year survival rates for all stages in the United States have increased from 37% for patients diagnosed from 1974 to 1976 to 41% for those diagnosed from 1983 to 1985 to 53% for those diagnosed from 1992 to 1999 (Greenlee et al, 2000; Jemal et al, 2004). However, the tendency for ovarian cancer to progress and recur has led to its being considered a long-term or chronic disease, one that is best managed with a combination of surveillance, surgery, chemotherapy, and palliative care (Armstrong, 2002).

Chemotherapy has been an integral part of the treatment of epithelial ovarian cancer at M. D. Anderson Cancer Center since the 1950s. For primary postoperative treatment, single-agent regimens of alkylating agents dominated from the late 1950s through the mid-1970s. Beginning in the mid-1970s, the introduction of new agents—cisplatin, doxorubicin, and hexamethylmelamine—expanded our armamentarium and subsequently led to the development of combination chemotherapy regimens. From the late 1970s until the early 1990s, the combination of cisplatin and cyclophosphamide was the most popular regimen, on the basis of literature support of it as the standard postoperative treatment. With the introduction of paclitaxel in the early 1990s, however, the standard changed; since that time, the combination of a taxane and a platinum drug has become the standard. Concomitantly, a growing menu of chemotherapeutic agents has been discovered, tested in phase I and II trials, and used to treat recurrent ovarian cancer at M. D. Anderson.

This chapter will describe the contemporary M. D. Anderson approach to the use of chemotherapy for primary treatment, consolidation or maintenance therapy, and treatment of recurrence in patients with ovarian cancer. In addition, our experience with high-dose chemotherapy over the past decade will be discussed. Although the focus of this chapter will be on standard therapy, it should be emphasized that clinical trials have played a dominant role in the treatment of our patient population during this era.

PRIMARY CHEMOTHERAPY

Early-Stage Disease

Approximately 30% of women with epithelial ovarian cancer present with stage I or II disease. The keys to optimal clinical management of patients with apparent early-stage ovarian cancer include comprehensive surgical staging and subsequent risk assessment. Comprehensive surgical staging leading to a diagnosis of early-stage disease allows patients the opportunity to participate in clinical trials. For patients referred with apparent stage I or II disease but with incomplete staging, reoperation, possibly using a minimally invasive approach, is an option.

Risk assessment separates patients into low-risk and high-risk cohorts. Low-risk epithelial ovarian cancer is defined by the following 2 characteristics: (1) stage IA or IB disease (intact capsule, no tumor excrescences, and no malignant ascites or negative peritoneal cytology) and (2) grade 1 or 2 disease. The standard treatment for this group of patients is surgery alone, and the 5-year survival rate is at least 95% (Young et al, 1990). A controversy regarding whether grade 2 disease belongs in the low-risk or high-risk category remains unresolved and is compounded by the lack of uniformity in grading systems. At M. D. Anderson, we recommend a 2-tier grading system—low grade and high grade—based on nuclear atypia and, secondarily, mitotic count (Malpica et al, 2004), which would obviate the confusion surrounding grade 2 disease.

Patients with high-risk early-stage epithelial ovarian cancer have 1 or more of the following characteristics: (1) stage IC (ruptured capsule, tumor excrescences, positive peritoneal cytology, or malignant ascites) to II (involvement of 1 or both ovaries with pelvic extension) disease;

(2) grade 3 disease; or (3) clear cell histology. In some classification systems, dense adherence is also considered an indication of high-risk disease; however, in the view of many experts, dense adherence is simply another term for stage II disease. Patients with high-risk disease are thought to have a relapse rate in the range of 40% to 50% and are the focus of adjuvant therapy trials.

For over 2 decades, our standard treatment for early-stage epithelial ovarian cancer at M. D. Anderson, based on experience and clinical trials in advanced-stage disease, has included 6 cycles of platinum-based combination chemotherapy. Until the early 1990s, this meant 6 cycles of the cisplatin plus cyclophosphamide regimen. However, following the report of Gynecologic Oncology Group (GOG) Study 111 (McGuire et al, 1996) and the extrapolation of their results to patients with early-stage disease, we began to recommend 6 cycles of paclitaxel plus cisplatin. Since the mid-1990s, we have recommended the combination of paclitaxel plus carboplatin every 3 weeks for 6 cycles on the basis of its superior therapeutic index. Although the dose of carboplatin in various clinical trials has ranged from area under the curve (AUC) = 4 to AUC = 7.5, our standard dose has been AUC = 5 because of the lack of data to support a dose-intensity relationship with carboplatin.

Recently, randomized trials have reported that platinum-based chemotherapy is associated with a survival benefit in early-stage epithelial ovarian cancer. In a report of 2 parallel randomized phase III trials—International Collaborative Ovarian Neoplasm 1 and Adjuvant Chemotherapy in Ovarian Neoplasm—platinum-based chemotherapy improved recurrence-free and overall survival at 5 years in the combined group (Trimbos et al, 2003). In GOG trial 157 (Bell et al, 2003), patients with high-risk early-stage ovarian cancer were randomized to receive 3 or 6 cycles of paclitaxel plus carboplatin. Preliminary results of this trial indicate no definite statistically significant advantage in terms of relapse-free survival for 6 cycles, but there is a trend toward better outcomes. The interpretation of this trial remains controversial; however, our conclusion is that the trend toward superior outcomes associated with 6 cycles of paclitaxel plus carboplatin cannot be ignored.

Advanced-Stage Disease

With the publication of the results of GOG trial 111 (McGuire et al, 1996), the standard therapy for patients with advanced-stage epithelial ovarian cancer at M. D. Anderson changed from cisplatin plus cyclophosphamide to the combination of paclitaxel and a platinum drug. Initially, this regimen included paclitaxel administered over 24 hours at a dose of 135 mg/m^2 in combination with cisplatin at 75 mg/m^2. Although this study was conducted in patients with residual disease, this new combination became standard for all patients with advanced-stage disease, regardless of residual disease status. Subsequently, the GOG conducted a phase III randomized trial (GOG trial 158) comparing cisplatin to carboplatin, both in combination with paclitaxel (Ozols et al, 2003). Once the preliminary findings of this study became known, the standard postoperative therapy at M. D. Anderson for patients with advanced-stage ovarian cancer became paclitaxel 175 mg/m^2 over 3 hours plus carboplatin AUC = 5. Although the carboplatin dose in GOG trial 158 was AUC = 7.5, the lack of support for increased platinum dose intensity between the range of AUC = 4 and AUC = 8 has informed our decision regarding the carboplatin dosing.

The combination of paclitaxel plus carboplatin has remained our standard regimen despite several phase I, II, and III studies of novel combinations. We currently recommend 6 cycles of therapy administered every 3 weeks. Strategies that have been pursued recently by several groups, including our own, as well as by cooperative groups in the phase III setting, include the following: (1) the addition of a third agent—either a chemotherapy or biologic agent—to the paclitaxel plus carboplatin regimen (Gershenson et al, 1999) or (2) the comparison of the paclitaxel plus platinum regimen with single agents such as cisplatin, carboplatin, or paclitaxel (Muggia et al, 2000; International Collaborative Ovarian Neoplasm Group, 2002). To date, no regimen that includes a third agent has demonstrated survival superiority over the standard of paclitaxel plus carboplatin. In addition, a phase III trial comparing the combination of paclitaxel plus carboplatin to the combination of docetaxel plus carboplatin has recently been published (Vasey et al, 2004). The results of this trial indicate equivalent efficacy for the 2 regimens. However, the docetaxel arm was associated with less neurotoxicity but significantly more grade 3 to 4 neutropenia. On the basis of the results of this study, the docetaxel plus carboplatin regimen appears to be a reasonable alternative to the standard, particularly for patients who are experiencing neurotoxicity or who have conditions that would warrant avoidance of paclitaxel.

Neoadjuvant Chemotherapy

Since the late 1970s, we have employed neoadjuvant chemotherapy followed by interval debulking surgery in selected patients with advanced-stage epithelial ovarian cancer. This approach continues to the present. One of the possible benefits of neoadjuvant chemotherapy and interval debulking surgery compared with the standard approach is reduced perioperative morbidity. However, several years ago, we recognized that only a prospective randomized trial would determine how the efficacy and complication rate associated with this approach compared with those associated with the standard treatment of primary cytoreductive surgery followed by chemotherapy. Two trials—GOG trial 152 and a European

Organization for Research and Treatment of Cancer (EORTC) study—have tested the concept of interval debulking surgery in patients with advanced ovarian cancer (van der Burg et al, 1995; Rose et al, 2004). However, neither of these trials addressed the use of true neoadjuvant chemotherapy because all patients in both studies underwent an attempt, albeit suboptimal, at primary cytoreductive surgery. Also, there is considerable confusion surrounding these trials; both tested the concept of interval debulking surgery as secondary cytoreductive surgery rather than primary cytoreductive surgery. Despite receiving submissions of protocol concepts, the GOG's Protocol Committee has chosen not to pursue this strategy in a phase III setting. However, the EORTC is currently conducting such a trial—EORTC trial 5597.

In the interim, we are left with clinical experience and data from retrospective studies to place neoadjuvant chemotherapy into context when making treatment decisions at the initial diagnosis of women with advanced-stage epithelial ovarian cancer. In the experience of our group over almost 3 decades, potential candidates for neoadjuvant chemotherapy and interval debulking surgery have 1 or more of the following characteristics: (1) unresectable disease on the basis of interpretation of computed tomography (CT) scans; (2) 1 or more comorbidities that place the patient at high risk of complications from primary surgery; (3) massive effusions, particularly pleural effusion, potentially compromising the postoperative recovery; or (4) stage IV disease. In fact, without randomized controlled trial data, the decision to recommend neoadjuvant chemotherapy rather than the standard approach is often based on subjective information. Although computed tomographic criteria to predict resectability have been studied, it remains unproven whether this approach has sufficient accuracy.

If neoadjuvant chemotherapy is considered for 1 of the reasons above, we believe that it is important to establish the diagnosis as accurately as possible prior to initiation of therapy. Diagnostic options include fine-needle biopsy or core biopsy performed by an interventional radiologist or laparoscopy and biopsy to establish a diagnosis and to determine resectability. The latter approach, although more costly, has its merits. Typically, we administer 3 cycles of neoadjuvant chemotherapy; if the patient is responding on the basis of serum marker analysis and computed tomography, then interval debulking surgery is performed.

Our retrospective review of the M. D. Anderson experience with neoadjuvant chemotherapy and interval debulking surgery was one of the first publications on this topic (Jacob et al, 1991). Although not adequately powered to answer the question of which approach is the best, this study revealed equivalent survival for neoadjuvant chemotherapy and interval debulking compared with the standard approach in 18 matched controls. In addition, the perioperative complication rate was lower in the neoadjuvant chemotherapy group. Other retrospective reports have demonstrated similar findings.

INTRAPERITONEAL CHEMOTHERAPY

The concept of intraperitoneal chemotherapy to treat ovarian cancer is not new, having been studied since the 1950s. In the 1980s and 1990s, several phase II studies of intraperitoneal chemotherapy for recurrent or persistent ovarian cancer were reported. Although our group has studied the intraperitoneal approach for both gene therapy and biologic agents over the past several years, like many other groups, we have not embraced the concept of intraperitoneal chemotherapy for a variety of reasons. The principal reason has been the lack of definitive data in randomized trials proving the superiority of the intraperitoneal approach over the intravenous approach. In addition, it has been our belief that the complications and morbidity associated with intraperitoneal chemotherapy, particularly catheter-related complications, have been underreported.

Nevertheless, 3 American phase III trials over the past decade or so have suggested a potential role for intraperitoneal chemotherapy, although each trial has had design flaws or significant associated toxicities. A Southwest Oncology Group and GOG trial compared intravenous cisplatin plus cyclophosphamide with intraperitoneal cisplatin plus intravenous cyclophosphamide in patients with optimal advanced ovarian cancer (Alberts et al, 1996). This trial revealed a survival advantage for patients in the intraperitoneal chemotherapy arm (median survival duration, 49 vs 41 months). However, criticisms leveled against this trial include the almost complete lack of reporting of catheter-related complications and the fact that the subgroup with the most minimal residual disease was expanded during the trial. In addition, by the time the trial was reported, paclitaxel had already replaced cyclophosphamide in standard ovarian cancer therapy.

In a second trial of the GOG—GOG trial 114—patients were randomized to receive standard chemotherapy with intravenous cisplatin plus paclitaxel for 6 cycles or 2 cycles of moderate-dose carboplatin followed by 6 cycles of intraperitoneal cisplatin plus intravenous paclitaxel (Markman et al, 2001). Patients in the intraperitoneal chemotherapy arm experienced superior progression-free survival (PFS) (28 vs 22 months) as well as improved overall survival (63 vs 52 months; $P = .05$). However, design flaws associated with this trial included the following: (1) 8 cycles of chemotherapy in the experimental arm versus 6 cycles in the standard arm; (2) the 2 cycles of carboplatin in the experimental arm led to significant myelosuppression, particularly thrombocytopenia, and were responsible for 18% of patients in the experimental arm receiving 2 or fewer cycles of intraperitoneal therapy; and (3) the experimental arm was, strictly speaking, not intraperitoneal chemotherapy since patients received intravenous carboplatin for the initial 2 cycles.

The most recent GOG trial—GOG trial 172—was reported preliminarily at the 2002 annual meeting of the American Society of Clinical Oncology (Armstrong, 2002). This trial compared standard intravenous cisplatin plus paclitaxel with intraperitoneal cisplatin and intravenous paclitaxel on day 1 followed by intraperitoneal paclitaxel on day 8. Preliminary results demonstrated an improvement in PFS and overall survival but significantly greater toxicity associated with the experimental arm. In addition, once again, a significant proportion of patients in the intraperitoneal arm did not complete 6 cycles of chemotherapy.

The preliminary GOG trial 172 report showing that intraperitoneal chemotherapy was associated with a significant improvement in overall survival will most certainly cause the gynecologic oncology community to reexamine its attitudes and clinical management related to intraperitoneal chemotherapy. However, even with such survival data, unresolved issues will remain, including the optimal intraperitoneal chemotherapy regimen, the optimal number of cycles, and the best method of administration.

CONSOLIDATION THERAPY

For patients who are clinically disease free (normal serum CA-125 level and negative computed tomography scan of abdomen and pelvis) at the completion of primary chemotherapy, 3 options are typically discussed with them and their families: (1) discontinuation of therapy (observation only), (2) second-look surgery, and (3) consolidation therapy. Second-look surgery outside a clinical trial is increasingly uncommon in our practice. The most popular choice of patients is observation only, largely because neither of the other 2 options is associated with a survival advantage.

Consolidation therapy, however, has been given increasing consideration owing to recent information. The optimal number of cycles of primary chemotherapy for patients with advanced-stage epithelial ovarian cancer remains unknown. Once combination chemotherapy became standard for such patients, 6 cycles emerged as the most popular number, but this decision was arbitrary and not evidence based. Two early randomized trials found no difference in survival based on the number of primary chemotherapy cycles, but these studies were almost certainly underpowered to answer the question (Hakes et al, 1992; Bertelsen et al, 1993). At about the same time, our group published the findings of a retrospective study focused on prolonged chemotherapy (12 vs 6 cycles of chemotherapy with cisplatin plus cyclophosphamide) and demonstrated a PFS benefit for those patients receiving 12 cycles of chemotherapy

(Gershenson et al, 1992). On the basis of these provocative findings, we recommended a prospective randomized trial.

The Southwest Oncology Group and GOG recently reported a randomized trial comparing 3 monthly cycles versus 12 monthly cycles of paclitaxel following completion of primary chemotherapy (Markman et al, 2003). This trial was discontinued early by the data monitoring committee, so overall survival data will not be available. The median PFS durations were 21 and 28 months in the 3-cycle and 12-cycle arms, respectively. Therefore, this trial and the resulting data are part of our discussions with all patients who are disease free at the completion of primary therapy. Well-designed second-generation consolidation trials will hopefully provide further PFS data as well as overall survival data associated with novel maintenance strategies.

THERAPEUTIC STRATEGIES
FOR RECURRENT OVARIAN CANCER

Current management strategies for relapsed ovarian cancer rely mainly on salvage chemotherapy, although surgery and hormonal therapy can be useful in some carefully selected patients. The choice of systemic salvage therapy for relapsed ovarian cancer should include consideration of the treatment-free interval as well as the bulk of disease, symptoms, and performance status. Patients with platinum-sensitive disease may benefit from reinduction with paclitaxel, a platinum-based compound, or both. For patients with platinum-refractory or platinum-resistant disease, consideration should be given to the sequential use of single-agent therapies such as topotecan, liposomal doxorubicin, or gemcitabine, with care taken to avoid the potential for cumulative toxicity. Experimental therapies may be appropriate for patients whose disease progresses during conventional therapy. Hormonal therapies may also be helpful in some patients. Other approaches being explored, such as immunotherapy and gene therapy, are as yet too new to allow definitive conclusions to be drawn. This section reviews the current status of treatment strategies for recurrent ovarian cancer.

Definitions

More than half of patients with newly diagnosed ovarian cancer will have a clinical complete response to primary paclitaxel plus platinum-based chemotherapy, and 50% of those women will have a pathologic complete response (typically verified by second-look surgery). During long-term follow-up, however, about half of all patients who have a complete response will have disease recurrence, and ultimately, only 10% to 12% of all patients given primary therapy will experience long-term remission or cure (Rubin et al, 1988). The choice of salvage treatment for recurrent disease depends on the interval between completion of the initial chemotherapy and the date of progression or recurrence; this so-called "treatment-free interval" is used to predict whether the disease is sensitive or resistant to platinum-based chemotherapy. Patients who experience disease progression during first-line therapy or relapse within 3 months after completing the initial treatment are considered to have platinum-refractory disease. Patients who show some evidence of response to primary treatment and experience relapse within 6 months after completing treatment are considered to have platinum-resistant disease, whereas those who experience relapse more than 6 months after the primary treatment are considered to have platinum-sensitive disease (Spriggs, 2004).

The most commonly used agents for salvage chemotherapy in patients with recurrent ovarian cancer are topotecan, liposomal doxorubicin, gemcitabine, oral etoposide, paclitaxel, docetaxel, and platinum-based compounds such as cisplatin or carboplatin. Results from many randomized trials suggest that the longer the treatment-free interval after first-line therapy, the more likely that the disease will respond to salvage therapy.

Salvage Chemotherapy for Platinum-Sensitive Disease

The M. D. Anderson approach to salvage chemotherapy for patients with platinum-sensitive disease includes carboplatin reinduction, occasionally with carboplatin combined with paclitaxel or docetaxel. Some patients with platinum-sensitive disease may benefit from reinduction therapy with single-agent paclitaxel, a platinum agent, or a combination of the 2. In a large multicenter study (Parmar et al, 2003), use of paclitaxel plus platinum-based chemotherapy in patients with relapsed platinum-sensitive ovarian cancer was compared with conventional single-agent platinum-based chemotherapy. Comparison of survival curves at 2 years showed a 7% improvement in survival in the combination chemotherapy group (57%) over that in the single-agent treatment group (50%) ($P = .02$). At the 1-year analysis, the median PFS time (the period between completion of second-line chemotherapy and next progression) was 9 months in the single-agent group and 12 months in the combination chemotherapy group ($P = .0004$). These results were interpreted to mean that the combination of paclitaxel with platinum-based chemotherapy was beneficial in terms of overall survival and PFS in platinum-sensitive ovarian cancer. However, analysis of patient characteristics in both groups in that study reveals that 43% of patients in the paclitaxel-plus-platinum group were treated with a taxane (41% paclitaxel and 2% docetaxel) in their previous chemotherapy regimen and 42% of patients in the platinum-only group received previous taxane treatment. Although the percentages of patients in the 2 groups previously treated with taxane therapy were virtually the same, the role of paclitaxel combined with platinum as salvage therapy cannot be excluded, and previous taxane treatment might be the reason why patients in the paclitaxel-plus-platinum group demonstrated improved PFS and 2-year survival. In another study (Dizon et al, 2002), a retrospective analysis showed favorable outcomes with the combination of carboplatin and paclitaxel for patients with relapsed platinum-sensitive disease who had shown complete responses to first-line platinum-based chemotherapy.

Currently, single-agent paclitaxel or platinum-based chemotherapy is an accepted salvage therapy for platinum-sensitive disease at some institutions. In a retrospective analysis of the experience at Memorial Sloan-Kettering Cancer Center, Dizon et al (2003) reported that single-agent carboplatin is effective as salvage chemotherapy for patients with recurrent platinum-sensitive disease. However, they also found in a secondary analysis of 29 patients that paclitaxel plus carboplatin produced a higher overall response rate and longer overall survival time.

Weekly doses of paclitaxel are another common form of salvage therapy for relapsed disease. In an M. D. Anderson working group study, Kavanagh and colleagues (1995) suggested that extending the platinum-free treatment interval may improve outcome by increasing the sensitivity of tumors to subsequent reintroduction of platinum. This analysis suggests that retreatment with platinum compounds can induce a clinical response in patients who respond to intervening therapy and extend the platinum-free interval (more than 12 months) between primary and reinduction platinum therapy. Since all patients who responded to carboplatin were initially sensitive to a taxane, it can be presumed that previous prolonged taxane exposure may have eliminated the platinum-resistant clone or permitted the loss of resistance to platinum. This research proposed the new idea that extending the treatment-free interval by avoiding cross-resistance to platinum or the intervening therapy could improve patient sensitivity to the reinduction of platinum.

The topoisomerase I inhibitor topotecan is active in platinum-resistant or platinum-refractory recurrent ovarian cancer and has been proposed for use as first-line salvage therapy for platinum-sensitive recurrent ovarian cancer. Topotecan is typically given in 5-day or 3-day protocols and can be given intravenously or orally. In 1 GOG study (McGuire et al, 2000), patients with recurrent platinum-sensitive ovarian cancer were given 1.5 mg/m^2 of topotecan as a 30-minute intravenous infusion for 5 days of every 21-day cycle. This protocol produced significant neutropenia. In a different 3-day strategy for recurrent platinum-sensitive disease (Miller et al, 2003), topotecan was given at 2.0 mg/m^2 per day for 3 days in a 21-day cycle. The results were clinical outcomes and myelosuppression similar to those in the 5-day treatment; therefore, this 3-day topotecan treatment was thought to be no better than the 5-day treatment. Both strategies were associated with significant myelosuppression. In another study (Clarke-Pearson et al, 2001), oral topotecan (2.3 mg/m^2 daily for 5 days every 21 days) used to treat recurrent ovarian cancer led to a toxicity profile similar to those in previous reports, although the incidence of grade 4 neutropenia was lower. Because topotecan is associated with high rates of myelosuppression, the toxicity seems to be noncumulative and can be managed with supportive therapy for extended dosing periods.

As noted previously, the treatment-free interval is the best predictor of response to subsequent salvage treatment; prolonging that interval, by whatever means, may improve the likelihood of response to future therapy. Another study (Topuz et al, 2004) found that intraperitoneal cisplatin, given as consolidation treatment, could prolong the progression-free period for patients with a complete pathologic response.

In summary, current findings regarding salvage chemotherapy for platinum-sensitive recurrent disease favor reinduction with platinum-based chemotherapy, with or without paclitaxel. The best cutoff schedule for platinum reinduction—12 to 18 months, 18 to 24 months, or more than 24 months after tumor recurrence—remains to be found. However, some evidence suggests that the use of non-cross-resistant agents may enhance tumor response owing to their dissimilar mechanisms of action. Use of nonplatinum agents at first relapse might reduce the possibility that tumors will become increasingly resistant to platinum retreatment, but there are no scientific data to support this. Clinical trials are ongoing to identify more effective salvage chemotherapy regimens for recurrent platinum-sensitive ovarian cancer.

Salvage Chemotherapy for Platinum-Refractory or Platinum-Resistant Disease

The M. D. Anderson approach to salvage chemotherapy for platinum-refractory or platinum-resistant disease includes liposomal doxorubicin, topotecan, gemcitabine, and hormonal therapy. Oral etoposide is also used occasionally. Platinum-resistant disease is associated with poor outcomes and a decreased response to both platinum compounds and other agents. The mechanism underlying chemoresistance in ovarian cancer is not well understood. The response rates to salvage treatments are low, and the best choice of treatment is controversial. Therapeutic agents currently in clinical use as salvage therapy for platinum-refractory or platinum-resistant ovarian cancer include paclitaxel, platinum-based compounds, docetaxel, topotecan, doxorubicin, gemcitabine, and etoposide.

For platinum-refractory or -resistant disease in patients who have not received paclitaxel-based chemotherapy, paclitaxel is the main choice for salvage therapy. An overall response rate of 25% can be anticipated (Trimble et al, 1993). For patients with platinum-resistant disease who were given paclitaxel-plus-platinum-based combination therapy as primary therapy, reinduction with paclitaxel or platinum-based therapy is still an option. The optimal dose and schedule for paclitaxel have not been identified; 3 common protocols—175 mg/m^2 given over 3 hours,

135 mg/m² given over 24 hours, and low-dose (60 to 80 mg/m²) paclitaxel given weekly—produce similar response rates and PFS times (Boruta et al, 2003).

Topotecan has produced overall response rates of 14% to 23% in patients with platinum-resistant disease (Hoskins et al, 1998), compared with 33% in those with platinum-sensitive disease (McGuire et al, 2000). Several phase III clinical trials have been conducted comparing topotecan with paclitaxel and doxorubicin for treatment of relapsed ovarian cancer. In 1 such study (ten Bokkel Huinink et al, 1997), the response and disease-stabilization rates were similar for patients given topotecan and paclitaxel; however, the median duration of response was longer for the topotecan group (32 weeks) than for those given paclitaxel (20 weeks). A Kaplan-Meier analysis of the data from that study showed that topotecan was associated with longer PFS than paclitaxel (ten Bokkel Huinink et al, 2002). Another phase III clinical trial of topotecan in comparison with liposomal doxorubicin (Gordon et al, 2001) showed that these 2 treatments produced similar overall response rates, times to progression, and survival times but that topotecan was associated with significant myelosuppression.

Some authors have proposed that the best use of topotecan is as first-line therapy at first relapse (Armstrong, 2002). First, topotecan is a highly noncumulative myelosuppressive agent. Platinum-based chemotherapy in particular can have long-term effects on bone marrow function and recovery; therefore, use of topotecan late in the course of therapy is likely to cause severe hematologic toxicity. However, use of topotecan as salvage therapy for a first relapse should not diminish subsequent opportunities for the use of other chemotherapeutic agents. Second, patients given topotecan for a first relapse could benefit from the extension of the platinum-free interval by experiencing an enhanced tumor response rate (and, presumably, better PFS and overall survival times) after further platinum treatment.

Clinical trials of single-agent docetaxel therapy in recurrent ovarian cancer with platinum resistance show that it is a promising new regimen (Kaye et al, 1997). The general dose is from 75 to 100 mg/m², and the overall response rate to docetaxel varies from 17% to 40%. One phase II study performed at M. D. Anderson involved 55 patients with platinum-resistant disease (Kavanagh et al, 1996); the dose was 100 mg/m² over 1-hour intravenous infusion in a 21-day cycle. The overall response rate was 40%, and 38% of patients demonstrated stable disease. The median response duration was 4.5 months, and the median survival duration was 10 months.

Liposomal doxorubicin has also been used in single-agent or combination therapy for relapsed ovarian cancer. The standard dosage is 40 to 50 mg/m² given as a 1-hour infusion every 28 days. As single-agent salvage therapy, liposomal doxorubicin has been shown in some phase II studies to produce response rates of 6% to 30%, with a median time to progression of 2.4 to 5.7 months (Stebbing and Gaya, 2002). Two phase III studies of liposomal doxorubicin in comparison with paclitaxel and topotecan suggest that liposomal doxorubicin is active in salvage therapy for relapsed ovarian cancer (Gordon et al, 2001).

Gemcitabine has also been used as single-agent and combination therapy for relapsed ovarian cancer. The regimen is 800 mg/m^2 intravenously on days 1, 8, and 15, followed by 1 week of rest. Study findings (Lund et al, 1995) indicate that gemcitabine was well tolerated in patients with platinum-resistant disease, but no phase III trials have been performed to compare its performance with that of other chemotherapeutic agents.

Two other agents that can be given orally and have some activity in recurrent ovarian cancer are altretamine and etoposide. Altretamine, an alkylating agent, has produced response rates of 10% to 15% in platinum-resistant or platinum-refractory disease; a higher response rate and longer survival are possible for platinum-sensitive disease. Etoposide, a topoisomerase II inhibitor, has been used to treat relapsed ovarian cancer. The typical protocol involves low doses (e.g., 50 to 100 mg/day) given over long periods (e.g., for 10 to 14 days in 21-day cycles). A phase II trial by the GOG showed that oral etoposide was active in both platinum-sensitive and platinum-resistant disease, with an overall response rate of 27% (7% complete response rate) and a median survival time of 10.8 months in patients with platinum-resistant disease (Rose et al, 1998).

Hormonal Therapy

The significant toxicity associated with salvage chemotherapy for ovarian cancer has led to the investigation of alternative therapies. The most frequently used hormonal agents are gonadotrophin-releasing hormone (GnRH) agonists, tamoxifen, antiandrogens, and aromatase inhibitors such as letrozole.

One meta-analysis of tamoxifen for relapsed ovarian cancer (Williams, 2000), which included 11 nonrandomized series, 1 nonrandomized phase II study, and 1 randomized trial, showed that only 11% of women treated with tamoxifen (59 of 568) had an objective response to treatment, and 31% had stable disease (109 of 356 in 8 trials).

GnRH analogue has been proposed as a new hormonal therapy for ovarian cancer. Two classes of GnRH analogue—GnRH agonist and GnRH antagonist—with distinct mechanisms of antitumor effect have been studied in clinical trials for the treatment of relapsed platinum-refractory ovarian cancer. Many clinical trials of GnRH analogue have been performed in patients with relapsed platinum-resistant disease. In a study of 245 patients, 23 (9%) responded to treatment with GnRH analogue and 64 (26%) had stable disease (Emons et al, 2000). For patients who cannot receive chemotherapy because of its substantial toxicity or their poor condition, GnRH analogues may be their best choice for salvage therapy, especially compared with palliative chemotherapy.

High-Dose Chemotherapy

High-dose chemotherapy with autologous stem cell transplantation was developed on the basis of the in vitro observation that there is a dose-response correlation in certain tumors. Most current models suggest that the optimal use of high-dose chemotherapy is for the eradication of minimal residual disease.

The European Blood and Marrow Transplant Registry reported on 254 patients with ovarian carcinoma treated with hematopoietic transplantation (Ledermann, 2001). Patients with stage III disease who underwent transplantation during the first complete or partial remission had a median survival duration of 59 months. We recently reported on 96 patients with advanced-stage ovarian cancer treated at M. D. Anderson with autologous stem cell transplantation (Donato et al, 2004). It was again demonstrated that patients with low-volume disease are more likely to benefit from high-dose treatment. Concerns about high-dose chemotherapy have been the mortality risk and quality-of-life issues; however, current high-dose chemotherapy treatments have very low mortality risks. Quality-of-life trials will be necessary to compare patients undergoing high-dose chemotherapy and transplantation with those receiving other therapies. At the same time, a large and well-designed randomized trial is needed to further elucidate the role of high-dose therapy.

KEY PRACTICE POINTS

- Standard primary chemotherapy for patients at M. D. Anderson with high-risk early-stage or advanced-stage epithelial ovarian cancer consists of a combination of a taxane and carboplatin.

- Until information from randomized clinical trials becomes available, neoadjuvant chemotherapy followed by interval debulking surgery is considered for patients with apparent unresectable advanced-stage ovarian cancer, massive effusions, significant comorbidities, or stage IV disease.

- Evolving information from a series of cooperative group clinical trials suggests that intraperitoneal chemotherapy should be considered for patients with optimal advanced ovarian cancer; however, several questions remain unanswered, including the optimal regimen, the optimal number of cycles, and the best method of administration.

- On the basis of the evidence to date, consolidation therapy should be considered as 1 of 3 options for patients with advanced-stage ovarian cancer who are clinically disease free at the completion of primary chemotherapy.

- For patients with platinum-sensitive recurrent ovarian cancer, platinum-based chemotherapy is generally recommended; unanswered questions include the optimal regimen and the precise influence of the so-called "platinum-free interval."

- For patients with platinum-resistant recurrent ovarian cancer, a growing list of active agents is available for treatment, including paclitaxel, topotecan, liposomal doxorubicin, gemcitabine, docetaxel, altretamine, and oral etoposide.

- A variety of hormonal agents have demonstrated modest antitumor activity in patients with recurrent ovarian cancer.

- Although high-dose chemotherapy studies in subsets of patients with ovarian cancer have yielded provocative findings, large, well-designed randomized trials are required to definitively elucidate the role of this treatment strategy.

SUGGESTED READINGS

Alberts DS, Liu PY, Hannigan EV, et al. Intraperitoneal cisplatin plus intravenous cyclophosphamide versus intravenous cisplatin plus intravenous cyclophosphamide for stage III ovarian cancer. *N Engl J Med* 1996;335:1950–1955.

Armstrong DK. Relapsed ovarian cancer: challenges and management strategies for a chronic disease. *Oncologist* 2002;7(suppl 5):20–28.

Bell J, Brady M, Lage J, et al. A randomized phase III trial of three versus six cycles of carboplatin and paclitaxel as adjuvant treatment in early stage ovarian epithelial carcinoma: a Gynecologic Oncology Group Study. *Gynecol Oncol* 2003;88:156.

Bertelsen K, Jakobsen A, Stroyer I, et al. A prospective randomized comparison of 6 and 12 courses of cyclophosphamide, Adriamycin, and cisplatin in advanced epithelial ovarian cancer: a Danish Ovarian Study Group trial (DACOVA). *Gynecol Oncol* 1993;49:30–36.

Boruta DM, Fowler WC, Gehrig PA, et al. Weekly paclitaxel infusion as salvage therapy in ovarian cancer. *Cancer Invest* 2003;21:675–681.

Clarke-Pearson DL, Van Le L, Iveson T, et al. Oral topotecan as single-agent second-line chemotherapy in patients with advanced ovarian cancer. *J Clin Oncol* 2001;19:3967–3975.

Dizon DS, Dupont J, Anderson S, et al. Treatment of recurrent ovarian cancer: a retrospective analysis of women treated with single-agent carboplatin originally treated with carboplatin and paclitaxel. The Memorial Sloan-Kettering Cancer Center experience. *Gynecol Oncol* 2003;91:584–590.

Dizon DS, Hensley ML, Poynor EA, et al. Retrospective analysis of carboplatin and paclitaxel as initial second-line therapy for recurrent epithelial ovarian carcinoma: application toward a dynamic disease state model of ovarian cancer. *J Clin Oncol* 2002;20:1238–1247.

Donato ML, Aleman A, Champlin RE, et al. Analysis of 96 patients with advanced ovarian carcinoma treated with high-dose chemotherapy and autologous stem cell transplantation. *Bone Marrow Transplant* 2004;33:1219–1224.

Emons G, Weiss S, Ortmann O, et al. LHRH might act as a negative autocrine regulator of proliferation of human ovarian cancer. *Eur J Endocrinol* 2000;142: 665–670.

Gershenson DM, Mitchell M, Atkinson N. The effect of prolonged cisplatin-based chemotherapy on progression free survival in patients with optimal epithelial ovarian cancer. "Maintenance" therapy reconsidered. *Gynecol Oncol* 1992;47:7–13.

Gershenson DM, Morris M, Burke T, et al. A phase I trial of intravenous melphalan, paclitaxel, and cisplatin plus granulocyte colony-stimulating factor in patients with suboptimal advanced epithelial ovarian cancer or peritoneal cancer. *Cancer* 1999;86:2291–2300.

Gordon AN, Fleagle JT, Guthrie D, et al. Recurrent epithelial ovarian carcinoma: a randomized phase III study of pegylated liposomal doxorubicin versus topotecan. *J Clin Oncol* 2001;19:3312–3322.

Greenlee RT, Murray T, Bolden S, Wingo PA. Cancer statistics, 2000. *CA Cancer J Clin* 2000;50:7–33.

Hakes TB, Hoskins CE, Hoskins WJ, et al. Randomized prospective trial of 5 versus 10 cycles of cyclophosphamide, doxorubicin, and cisplatin in advanced ovarian carcinoma. *Gynecol Oncol* 1992;45:284–289.

Hoskins P, Eisenhauer E, Beare S, et al. Randomized phase II study of two schedules of topotecan in previously treated patients with ovarian cancer: a National Cancer Institute of Canada Clinical Trials Group study. *J Clin Oncol* 1998;16:2233–2237.

International Collaborative Ovarian Neoplasm Group. Paclitaxel plus carboplatin versus standard chemotherapy with either single-agent carboplatin or cyclophosphamide, doxorubicin, and cisplatin in women with ovarian cancer: the ICON3 randomized trial. *Lancet* 2002;360:505–515.

Jacob JN, Gershenson DM, Morris M, et al. Neoadjuvant chemotherapy and interval debulking surgery for advanced ovarian cancer. *Gynecol Oncol* 1991;42:146–150.

Jemal A, Tiwari RC, Murray T, et al. Cancer statistics. *CA Cancer J Clin* 2004;54:8–29.

Kavanagh JJ, Kudelka AP, de Leon CG, et al. Phase II study of docetaxel in patients with epithelial ovarian carcinoma refractory to platinum. *Clin Cancer Res* 1996;2:837–842.

Kavanagh J, Tresukosol D, Edwards C, et al. Carboplatin reinduction after taxane in patients with platinum-refractory epithelial ovarian cancer. *J Clin Oncol* 1995;13:1584–1588.

Kaye SB, Piccart M, Aapro M, et al. Phase II trials of docetaxel (Taxotere) in advanced ovarian cancer—an updated overview. *Eur J Cancer* 1997;33: 2167–2170.

Ledermann JA. High-dose chemotherapy with peripheral blood stem cell transplantation (PBSCT) in ovarian cancer. *Int J Gynecol Cancer* 2001;10 (suppl 1):53–56.

Lund B, Hansen OP, Neijt JP, et al. Phase II study of gemcitabine in previously platinum-treated ovarian cancer patients. *Anticancer Drugs* 1995;6:61–62.

Malpica A, Deavers M, Lu K, et al. Grading ovarian serous carcinoma using a two-tier system. *Am J Surg Pathol* 2004;28:496–504.

Markman M, Bundy BN, Alberts DS, et al. Phase III trial of standard-dose intravenous cisplatin plus paclitaxel versus moderately high-dose carboplatin followed by intravenous paclitaxel and intraperitoneal cisplatin in small-volume stage III ovarian carcinoma: an intergroup study of the Gynecologic Oncology Group, Southwestern Oncology Group, and Eastern Cooperative Oncology Group. *J Clin Oncol* 2001;19:1001–1007.

Markman M, Liu FY, Zilczynski S, et al. Phase III trial of 12 versus 3 months of maintenance paclitaxel in patients with advanced ovarian cancer after complete response to platinum and paclitaxel-based chemotherapy: a Southwest Oncology Group and Gynecologic Oncology Group trial. *J Clin Oncol* 2003;13:2460–2465.

McGuire WP, Blessing JA, Bookman MA, et al. Topotecan has substantial antitumor activity as first-line salvage therapy in platinum-sensitive epithelial ovarian carcinoma: a Gynecologic Oncology Group Study. *J Clin Oncol* 2000;18:1062–1067.

McGuire WP, Hoskins WJ, Brady MF, et al. Cyclophosphamide and cisplatin compared with paclitaxel and cisplatin in patients with stage III and stage IV ovarian cancer. *N Engl J Med* 1996;334:1–6.

Miller DS, Blessing JA, Lentz SS, et al. Phase II evaluation of three-day topotecan in recurrent platinum-sensitive ovarian carcinoma: a Gynecologic Oncology Group study. *Cancer* 2003;98:1664–1669.

Muggia FM, Braly PS, Brady MF, et al. Phase III randomized study of cisplatin versus paclitaxel versus cisplatin and paclitaxel in patients with suboptimal stage III or IV ovarian cancer: a Gynecologic Oncology Group study. *J Clin Oncol* 2000;18:106–115.

Ozols RF, Bundy BN, Greer BE, et al. Phase III trial of carboplatin and paclitaxel compared with cisplatin and paclitaxel in patients with optimally resected stage III ovarian cancer: a Gynecologic Oncology Group study. *J Clin Oncol* 2003;21:3194–3200.

Parmar MK, Ledermann JA, Colombo N, et al. Paclitaxel plus platinum-based chemotherapy versus conventional platinum-based chemotherapy in women with relapsed ovarian cancer: the ICON4/AGO-OVAR-2.2 trial. *Lancet* 2003;361:2099–2106.

Rose PG, Blessing JA, Mayer AR, et al. Prolonged oral etoposide as second-line therapy for platinum-resistant and platinum-sensitive ovarian carcinoma: a Gynecologic Oncology Group study. *J Clin Oncol* 1998;16:405-410.

Rose PG, Nerenstone S, Brady MF, et al. Secondary surgical cytoreduction for advanced ovarian carcinoma. *N Engl J Med* 2004;351:2489–2497.

Rubin SC, Hoskins WJ, Hakes TB, et al. Recurrence after negative second-look laparotomy for ovarian cancer: analysis of risk factors. *Am J Obstet Gynecol* 1988;159:1094–1098.

Spriggs D. Optimal sequencing in the treatment of recurrent ovarian cancer. *Gynecol Oncol* 2004;90:S39–S44.

Stebbing J, Gaya A. Pegylated liposomal doxorubicin (Caelyx) in recurrent ovarian cancer. *Cancer Treat Rev* 2002;28:121–125.

ten Bokkel Huinink W, Gore M, Carmichael J, et al. Topotecan versus paclitaxel for the treatment of recurrent epithelial ovarian cancer. *J Clin Oncol* 1997;15:2183–2193.

ten Bokkel Huinink W, Gore M, Carmichael J, et al. Topotecan versus paclitaxel for the treatment of recurrent epithelial ovarian cancer. *Classic Papers Curr Comments* 2002;7:133–143.

Topuz E, Eralp Y, Saglam S, et al. Efficacy of intraperitoneal cisplatin as consolidation therapy in patients with pathologic complete remission following frontline therapy for epithelial ovarian cancer. Consolidative intraperitoneal cisplatin in ovarian cancer. *Gynecol Oncol* 2004;92:147–151.

Trimble EL, Adams JD, Vena D, et al. Paclitaxel for platinum-refractory ovarian cancer: results from the first 1,000 patients registered to National Cancer Institute Treatment Referral Center 9103. *J Clin Oncol* 1993;11:2405–2410.

Trimbos JB, Parmar M, Vergote I, et al. International Collaborative Ovarian Neoplasm trial 1 and Adjuvant Chemotherapy in Ovarian Neoplasm trial: two parallel randomized phase III trials of adjuvant chemotherapy in patients with early-stage ovarian carcinoma. *J Natl Cancer Inst* 2003;95:105–112.

van der Burg MEL, van Lent M, Buyse M, et al. The effect of debulking surgery after induction chemotherapy on the prognosis in advanced epithelial ovarian cancer. *N Engl J Med* 1995;332:629–634.

Vasey PA, Jayson GC, Gordon A, et al. Phase III randomized trial of docetaxel-carboplatin versus paclitaxel-carboplatin as first-line chemotherapy for ovarian carcinomas. *J Natl Cancer Inst* 2004;96:1682–1691.

Vergote I, De Wever I, Tjalma W, et al. Neoadjuvant chemotherapy or primary debulking surgery in advanced ovarian carcinoma: a retrospective analysis of 285 patients. *Gynecol Oncol* 1998;71:431–436.

Williams CJ. Tamoxifen for relapse of ovarian cancer. *Cochrane Database Syst Rev* 2000;(2):CD001034.

Young RC, Walton LA, Ellenberg SS, et al. Adjuvant therapy in stage I and stage II epithelial ovarian cancer. Results of two prospective randomized trials. *N Engl J Med* 1990;322:1021–1027.

13 TREATMENT OF RARE OVARIAN MALIGNANCIES

Jubilee Brown and David M. Gershenson

CHAPTER OUTLINE

CHAPTER OVERVIEW

Although the vast majority of ovarian cancers are epithelial in origin, 10% of ovarian malignancies are nonepithelial. Most of these are sex cord–stromal tumors and germ cell tumors. Surgery, chemotherapy, radiation therapy, and hormonal therapy are all components of treatment for these rare ovarian tumors, but specific treatment recommendations are based on many factors, including histologic type, extent of disease, and patient-related factors such as age and karyotype. Conservative surgery to maintain reproductive potential is an important consideration in many of these patients, as germ cell tumors and some sex cord–stromal tumors tend to occur in adolescents and young women. Appropriate surgical staging and assessment, however, are necessary for determining the extent of surgery and the need for postoperative chemotherapy. With the advent of modern surgical and postsurgical techniques, response rates and survival have improved dramatically and are excellent for most types of nonepithelial ovarian tumors.

INTRODUCTION

Ovarian cancer is the most frequent cause of death from gynecologic cancer among women in the United States, accounting for an estimated 25,580 new cases and 16,090 deaths in 2004 (Jemal et al, 2004). Ninety percent of these malignancies are epithelial in origin, with the remaining 10% comprised of sex cord–stromal tumors, germ cell tumors, soft tissue tumors not specific to the ovary, unclassified tumors, and metastatic tumors. The classification of ovarian tumors has been formalized by the World Health Organization and is depicted in Table 13–1.

Table 13–1. Modified World Health Organization Comprehensive Classification of Ovarian Tumors

I. Common epithelial tumors
II. Sex cord–stromal tumors
A. Granulosa stromal cell
B. Androblastomas; Sertoli-Leydig cell tumors
C. Lipid cell tumors (steroid cell tumors)
D. Gynandroblastoma
E. Unclassified
III. Germ cell tumors
A. Dysgerminoma
B. Endodermal sinus tumor (yolk sac tumor)
C. Embryonal carcinoma
D. Polyembryoma
E. Choriocarcinoma
F. Teratomas
G. Mixed forms
H. Gonadoblastoma
IV. Soft tissue tumors not specific to the ovary
V. Unclassified tumors
VI. Metastatic (secondary) tumors
VII. Tumor-like conditions

Source: Herbst (1997).

Treatment of nonepithelial ovarian cancers is determined by many factors, including patient age, parity, and desire for future fertility; extent of disease; comorbid conditions; and karyotype. Often, the gynecologist or gynecologic oncologist is faced with a patient with an adnexal mass, the precise histologic classification of which is difficult to determine, even with the pathologic evaluation of frozen tissue sections. The surgeon must then follow general guidelines for nonepithelial ovarian tumors during the initial operative management and reevaluate the need for adjuvant or additional therapy on the basis of the final pathologic results. With close attention to all details, including histologic type, patient characteristics, and extent of disease, the need for reexploration and more extensive surgery can be minimized. This chapter will discuss the management of different nonepithelial ovarian neoplasms with regard to preoperative, intraoperative, and postoperative decision making and offer practical guidelines for appropriate management.

Sex Cord–Stromal Tumors

Sex cord–stromal tumors originate from specialized gonadal stromal cells and their precursors. Granulosa cells and Sertoli cells arise from sex cord cells, while theca cells, Leydig cells, lipid cells, and fibroblasts arise from stromal cells and their pluripotential mesenchymal precursors. Sex cord–stromal tumors can occur as a single histologic type or a combination of types, and together they account for 7% of all ovarian malignancies (Koonings et al, 1989). Since tumor cells from sex cord–stromal malignancies can be involved in steroid hormone production, physical manifestations of excess estrogen or androgen production are not infrequent at the time of diagnosis. Although the majority of these tumors are clinically indolent and are associated with a good long-term prognosis, many occur in adolescents and women of reproductive age; therefore, individualized treatment following appropriate guidelines is the key to successful outcomes, including the maintenance of fertility.

General Treatment Guidelines

Surgical Therapy

When a pelvic mass is first diagnosed, its specific histologic characteristics are unknown. Patient characteristics including age (adolescence or age in the third or fourth decade) and physical signs of excess estrogen (precocious breast enlargement, abnormal uterine bleeding) or androgen (hirsutism, virilism) can suggest the diagnosis of a sex cord–stromal tumor. A frank discussion should always be held preoperatively with any woman of childbearing age who has an adnexal mass regarding her wishes for future fertility and her desires for maintaining ovarian and/or uterine function in light of the potential operative findings. Although this is often a difficult conversation for the physician to initiate, it is better discussed preoperatively with the patient than intraoperatively with the next of kin when a malignancy is encountered.

Although occasionally patients may undergo laparoscopic evaluation for a small, solid adnexal mass or complex ovarian cyst, patients with large, solid adnexal masses or evidence of hemodynamic instability should undergo laparotomy through a vertical skin incision to allow for appropriate surgical staging, if necessary. Several characteristics can suggest a sex cord–stromal tumor upon initial inspection. A unilateral solid adnexal mass, often yellow and multilobulated or hemorrhagic with hemoperitoneum evident, can suggest a granulosa cell tumor or other sex cord–stromal tumor. Upon beginning exploration of the peritoneal cavity, the surgeon should obtain pelvic washings and evacuate any hemoperitoneum. The site of hemorrhage is most commonly the mass itself, and therefore surgical removal may stop the bleeding. A unilateral mass in a patient of any age should be removed by unilateral salpingo-oophorectomy and sent for immediate histologic evaluation. Every attempt should be made to avoid rupture of the mass, as this results in the disease being classified as a more advanced stage and may adversely affect survival (Bjorkholm and Silfversward, 1981). For this reason, the tumor should never be morcellated to effect laparoscopic removal. When laparoscopy is used initially, a Cook's bag with an extended incision should be utilized or the procedure should be converted to a laparotomy to avoid morcellating the tumor mass.

Occasionally, to remove what is thought to be a benign dermoid cyst, an ovarian cystectomy is performed in an attempt to preserve ovarian tissue. In these cases, the tumor should be sent for immediate histologic evaluation, and in the event of a sex cord–stromal tumor, the entire ovary should be removed. No support exists in the literature for ovarian cystectomy in premenopausal patients with sex cord–stromal tumors. Articles that summarize "conservative management" of these tumors invariably describe unilateral salpingo-oophorectomy with conservation of the normal contralateral ovary in patients with limited disease. Therefore, we do not perform ovarian cystectomy but instead opt for unilateral salpingo-oophorectomy as the initial step in the treatment of patients with apparent limited disease.

Once the diagnosis of a sex cord–stromal tumor is made, the entire abdominopelvic cavity should be explored, with attention paid to all peritoneal surfaces and abdominopelvic organs. A complete staging procedure should be performed, including cytologic evaluation of each hemidiaphragm, infracolic omentectomy, and peritoneal biopsies from each paracolic gutter, the vesicouterine fold, and the pouch of Douglas. Additionally, biopsies of any suspicious areas should be performed.

Pelvic and para-aortic lymph node sampling are recommended for full staging, as a small percentage of patients with apparent early-stage disease have positive lymph nodes on final pathologic review, which changes the stage, recommended treatment, and prognosis. The bowel should be inspected from the ileocecal valve to the ligament of Treitz, with specific evaluation for tumor implants and sites of obstruction. Tumor-reductive surgery should be performed in patients with advanced disease to reduce the tumor burden as much as possible, preferably leaving the patient with no macroscopic disease.

Patients who have completed childbearing should undergo total abdominal hysterectomy and bilateral salpingo-oophorectomy regardless of the stage of disease. Young patients who desire continued fertility are another issue, however. If the contralateral ovary and/or uterine serosa are grossly involved by tumor, the surgeon may have no choice but to remove the uterus and both adnexa. If the contralateral ovary and uterine serosa appear normal, conservative management with preservation of the uterus and contralateral adnexa is appropriate, as 95% of sex cord–stromal tumors are unilateral.

The treatment of patients who have had inadequate staging is a difficult issue. If the patient has documented large amounts of residual disease after a limited initial attempt at tumor reduction, repeat exploration with staging and tumor-reductive surgery is indicated. If the patient has had an inadequate exploration, such as through a small Pfannenstiel incision or through a limited laparoscopy, more information needs to be collected before a decision is made about postsurgical treatment. Options include repeat laparoscopic or open exploration with full surgical staging or, in some circumstances, physical examination, computed tomography (CT), and measurement of serum inhibin and serum CA-125 levels. If the results of all of these are negative, the decision may be made to observe the patient clinically, with or without hormonal suppression therapy using leuprolide acetate.

Postsurgical Therapy

Since sex cord–stromal tumors are rare, clinical trials designed to determine which treatment regimens are best for specific histologic subtypes are not feasible. Most published studies combine most or all subtypes of sex cord–stromal tumors, and therefore the recommendations for treatment of these tumors are based on limited data. The majority of data have been gathered from patients with adult granulosa cell tumors, but occasionally other tumor types are encountered, and we treat these in a similar manner.

Adjuvant treatment is not indicated for most patients with surgically staged stage I disease (Herbst, 1997). Patients with stage IC disease may benefit from some adjuvant therapy, and we have used either paclitaxel and carboplatin or hormonal therapy with leuprolide acetate for this group of patients. Patients with more advanced disease are typically treated with combination chemotherapy. Although many patients have been treated with 3 to 4 courses of bleomycin, etoposide, and cisplatin (BEP) (Homesley et al, 1999), we have also treated patients with 6 courses of paclitaxel and carboplatin with good results and fewer toxic effects (Brown et al, 2004a). Confirmation of equivalent outcomes between these 2 regimens awaits performance of a larger randomized trial.

Patients who have recurrent disease after a long interval are candidates for repeat tumor-reductive surgery. In our series (Brown et al, 2004a), many patients, including some with multifocal disease, enjoyed long-term survival after multiple tumor-reductive surgeries. In cases of widespread disease or disease refractory to surgery, chemotherapy and hormonal therapy are options for treatment. Although the response rate is higher earlier in the disease course and declines as the number of prior treatment regimens increases, paclitaxel in combination with carboplatin results in a 60% overall response rate with minimal toxicity (Brown et al, 2004a). Other chemotherapeutic regimens with demonstrated response include carboplatin; BEP; cisplatin, doxorubicin, and cyclophosphamide; etoposide and cisplatin; vincristine, dactinomycin, and cyclophosphamide (VAC); oral etoposide; topotecan; liposomal doxorubicin; and ifosfamide and etoposide (Brown et al, 2004b). Paclitaxel and carboplatin remain the most commonly used single agents at first and second relapse. Early in the treatment of recurrent disease, we also administer leuprolide acetate, which frequently results in the regression or stabilization of disease (Fishman et al, 1996). Commonly used dosing schedules are listed in Table 13–2. Radiation therapy is also occasionally employed in the treatment of localized or symptomatic disease.

Disease-Specific Considerations

Granulosa Cell Tumors

Granulosa cell tumors occur in 2 distinct histologic varieties, adult and juvenile. The patient profile, natural history, and recommended treatment differ between these subtypes.

Adult granulosa cell tumors can occur at any age but are most common in perimenopausal women. Patients often present with a solid adnexal mass and hemoperitoneum. Recommendations for surgical therapy are the same as those outlined above (see the section "Surgical Therapy"). If the patient has abnormal uterine bleeding, however, a preoperative endometrial biopsy or intraoperative endometrial curettage should be performed, as the excess estrogen produced by many granulosa cell tumors can lead to endometrial hyperplasia or malignancy. If malignancy is encountered, the uterus should be removed regardless of patient age.

Since only 5% of adult granulosa cell tumors are bilateral, it is appropriate to conserve a normal-appearing uterus and contralateral ovary in a reproductive-age woman with apparent early-stage disease confirmed by

Table 13–2. Common Dosing Schedules for Chemotherapy and Hormonal Therapy for the Treatment of Sex Cord–Stromal Tumors

Regimen	Agent and Dose	Route	Interval
Paclitaxel and carboplatin	Paclitaxel 175 mg/m^2	IV	Every 3 weeks
	Carboplatin AUC = 5	IV	Every 3 weeks
Paclitaxel	135-200 mg/m^2	IV	Every 3 weeks
Carboplatin	80-100 mg/m^2	IV	Weekly
BEP	Bleomycin 15 IU day 1	IV	Every 3 weeks
	Etoposide 100 mg/m^2 days 1-5	IV	Every 3 weeks
	Cisplatin 20 mg/m^2 days 1-5	IV	Every 3 weeks
PAC	Cisplatin 40-50 mg/m^2	IV	Every 4 weeks
	Doxorubicin 40-50 mg/m^2	IV	Every 4 weeks
	Cyclophosphamide 400 mg/m^2	IV	Every 4 weeks
EP	Etoposide 100 mg/m^2	IV	Every 4 weeks
	Cisplatin 75 mg/m^2	IV	Every 4 weeks
VAC	Vincristine 1.5 mg/m^2 day 1	IV	Every 2 weeks
	Dactinomycin 0.5 mg days 1-5	IV	Every 4 weeks
	Cyclophosphamide 150 mg/m^2 days 1-5	IV	Every 4 weeks
Oral etoposide	Etoposide 50 mg/m^2/day × 21 days	PO	Every 21 days
Topotecan	Topotecan 1.5 mg/m^2/day × 5 days	IV	Every 3 weeks
Doxorubicin	Doxorubicin 40 mg/m^2	IV	Every 4 weeks
Ifosfamide and etoposide	Ifosfamide 1.2 g/m^2/day × 5 days	IV	Every 3 weeks
	Etoposide 100 mg/m^2/day × 5 days	IV	Every 3 weeks
Leuprolide acetate	7.5 mg or	IM	Every 4 weeks
	22.5 mg	IM	Every 3 months

Abbreviations: AUC, area under the curve; IV, intravenous; PO, orally; IM, intramuscular.

frozen section analysis to be an adult granulosa cell tumor. Surgical staging should be performed. Additionally, serum inhibin and CA-125 levels, if not obtained preoperatively, should be obtained after surgery, as they may be helpful in postoperative follow-up to confirm the resolution of disease and identify recurrence.

Although adult granulosa cell tumors are indolent lesions, they can recur many years, even decades, following the initial diagnosis and treatment. Patients should be followed up at gradually increasing intervals with physical examinations and with serum inhibin and CA-125 measurements. Recommendations for the treatment of recurrent disease are outlined above (see the section "Postsurgical Therapy").

The majority of juvenile granulosa cell tumors present in adolescent girls. Therefore, maintaining reproductive capacity without adversely affecting survival is of paramount importance. Even though the survival rate in patients with early-stage tumors is above 95%, patients should still be surgically staged because advanced-stage juvenile granulosa cell tumors are typically more aggressive and less responsive to therapy than the adult counterpart. The same guidelines for surgical staging and preservation of childbearing capacity that apply to adult granulosa cell tumors are used for juvenile granulosa cell tumors. Any patient with greater than stage IA disease should receive platinum-based chemotherapy. Although BEP has been used historically, we typically use paclitaxel and carboplatin.

Unfortunately, when juvenile granulosa cell tumors recur, they usually do so after a shorter progression-free interval than is seen with adult granulosa cell tumors. Although many approaches to treatment have been used, including surgical cytoreduction, radiation therapy, and multiple chemotherapy regimens including high-dose chemotherapy, few sustained responses are seen in patients with recurrent juvenile granulosa cell disease. In our experience, responses have been achieved with BEP; paclitaxel and/or carboplatin; topotecan; bleomycin, vincristine, and cisplatin; etoposide and cisplatin; cisplatin, doxorubicin, and cyclophosphamide; high-dose chemotherapy; and gemcitabine. Hormonal therapy with leuprolide acetate has resulted in several cases of stable disease.

Sertoli-Leydig Cell Tumors

Sertoli-Leydig cell tumors include tumors containing only Sertoli cells and tumors containing both Sertoli and Leydig cells. Tumors composed of Sertoli cells only are uniformly stage I, and only 1 death has ever been reported. Sertoli-Leydig cell tumors, also called arrhenoblastomas, are rare, accounting for less than 0.2% of all ovarian tumors. These tumors usually occur in patients in their teens and twenties. Since over 95% of these tumors are confined to 1 ovary at the time of diagnosis, the normal-appearing uterus and contralateral ovary can be preserved. However, since stage is the most important predictor of outcome, these patients should be surgically staged. Patients with stage IC disease or greater, with poorly differentiated tumors of any stage, or with heterologous elements present have a 50% to 60% risk of recurrence. Owing to the rare nature of the disease and the lack of controlled trials, there is little scientific support for any treatment approach; however, adjuvant therapy seems reasonable given the substantial risk of recurrence. Therefore, it is our practice to administer adjuvant therapy in the form of BEP or paclitaxel and carboplatin to these patients.

Patients with Sertoli-Leydig cell tumors can be followed up with physical examination and with serum alpha-fetoprotein, inhibin, and testosterone level measurement. Of the 18% of patients who have a recurrence, two thirds do so within the first year after diagnosis. Additional platinum-based chemotherapy is the mainstay of treatment for recurrent disease.

Lipid Cell Tumors (Steroid Cell Tumors) and Gynandroblastomas

Stromal luteomas and Leydig cell tumors represent benign steroid cell tumors that do not require staging or postoperative therapy. Childbearing potential should be maintained in the occasional young patient with this diagnosis.

Steroid cell tumors not otherwise specified are a distinct category of steroid cell tumor that can be malignant and aggressive. Therefore, when a steroid cell tumor is diagnosed intraoperatively, it should be staged and aggressively cytoreduced. Lipid cell tumors that are pleomorphic, have an increased mitotic count, are large, or are at an advanced stage should be treated with additional postoperative platinum-based chemotherapy.

Gynandroblastomas are a separate, rare entity comprised of granulosa cell elements, tubules, and Leydig cells. These tumors should also be staged and aggressively cytoreduced.

Sex Cord Tumor with Annular Tubules

The group of tumors known as ovarian sex cord tumors with annular tubules (SCTAT) represents a separate category of sex cord–stromal tumors. It is controversial whether these tumors are more closely related to granulosa cell tumors or Sertoli-Leydig cell tumors, but they do seem to represent a distinct entity.

Clinically, there appear to be 2 subgroups of ovarian SCTATs. The first subgroup is associated with Peutz-Jeghers syndrome and is typically multifocal, bilateral, and almost always benign. Patients with this tumor should be carefully screened for adenoma malignum of the cervix, as 15% of patients have an occult lesion. Therefore, hysterectomy should be strongly considered in these patients.

The second subgroup of ovarian SCTATs occurs incidentally, independent from Peutz-Jeghers syndrome. These tumors have a significant potential for malignant behavior, and a percentage recur and metastasize.

GERM CELL TUMORS

Germ cell tumors arise from germ cells present in the normal ovary. These tumors comprise the second most common group of malignant ovarian neoplasms, accounting for approximately 7% of all malignant ovarian tumors. Germ cell tumors can be divided into 3 broad classes of neoplasms: benign teratomas, malignant tumors arising from teratomas, and malignant germ cell tumors. Except for malignant tumors arising from teratomas, which tend to occur in postmenopausal women, the neoplasms in this class occur most frequently in adolescents, so the issue of fertility preservation is important. Treatment of this group of neoplasms has improved in the past several years, and germ cell tumors are now largely amenable to therapy.

General Treatment Guidelines

Preoperative Evaluation

In the evaluation of a patient with an adnexal mass, several features may be suggestive of a germ cell tumor. Patient age is a consideration. Benign teratomas, also known as dermoid cysts or mature cystic teratomas, occur most commonly in young women but occasionally occur in children and in postmenopausal women. Malignant transformation of dermoid cysts occurs almost exclusively in women over 40 years of age. Most malignant germ cell tumors, however, occur in adolescent girls and young women. In the series studied at our center, the median age at diagnosis was 16 to 20 years, depending on histologic type, with a range from 6 to 31 years (Gershenson et al, 1984).

Presenting symptoms and signs include abdominal pain and a palpable mass, which are present in 85% of patients. Abdominal distention, fever, and vaginal bleeding occur in a minority of cases, and isosexual precocity due to tumor production of human chorionic gonadotropin is occasionally seen. Teratomas may also demonstrate sonographic findings suggestive of dermoids, including evidence of teeth.

Certain tumor markers can be helpful in diagnosing germ cell tumors preoperatively. In a premenarchal or adolescent girl or a woman of reproductive age with a solid mass, it is advisable to measure levels of human chorionic gonadotropin, alpha-fetoprotein, and lactate dehydrogenase prior to surgery. These tumor markers can provide insight into the diagnosis prior to surgery (Table 13–3), thereby facilitating counseling of the patient and her family, and can also be useful in following up on the patient for response or recurrence. CA-125 levels, although nonspecific, may be variably elevated in germ cell tumors and therefore may be helpful in following patient progress.

Surgical Therapy

All patients suspected of having a malignant germ cell tumor of the ovary should undergo surgical intervention for diagnosis and treatment unless

Table 13–3. Serum Tumor Markers in Malignant Germ Cell Tumors of the Ovary

Tumor	hCG	AFP	LDH
Dysgerminoma	+/–	–	+
Endodermal sinus tumor	–	+	+/–
Immature teratoma	–	+/–	+/–
Embryonal carcinoma	+	+	+/–
Choriocarcinoma	+	–	–
Polyembryoma	+/–	+/–	+/–
Mixed	+/–	+/–	+/–

Abbreviations: hCG, human chorionic gonadotropin; AFP, alpha-fetoprotein; LDH, lactate dehydrogenase.

surgery is medically contraindicated. The initial approach for patients with an adnexal mass suspected to be a germ cell tumor of the ovary is an exploratory laparotomy through a vertical midline incision. We do not routinely use laparoscopy in these cases. Once exploration of the peritoneal cavity is begun, ascites should be aspirated and sent for permanent cytologic evaluation. If no ascites is present, pelvic washings should be obtained. Visual and manual exploration of the entire abdomen and pelvis should follow, with attention directed to all peritoneal surfaces, the liver and subhepatic region, diaphragm, retroperitoneal structures, omentum, colon, small bowel, mesentery, and all pelvic contents, including both adnexa and the uterus.

Although 60% to 70% of malignant germ cell tumors are stage I at diagnosis, 25% to 30% are stage III, some of which are upstaged only because of occult metastases. Therefore, if disease appears to be confined to 1 or both ovaries, complete surgical staging is imperative, as staging affects treatment recommendations and prognosis. Cytologic evaluation of each hemidiaphragm should be performed. Biopsies should be performed of any area with suspected tumor. If no abnormalities are identified, random peritoneal samples for biopsy should be taken of each paracolic gutter, the vesicouterine fold, and the pouch of Douglas. Bilateral pelvic and para-aortic lymph node sampling should be performed, as occult metastases involving the regional lymphatics are not uncommon. An infracolic omentectomy should also be performed.

The majority of malignant germ cell tumors are unilateral and large. A review at our institution identified a median size of 15 cm, with a range from 7 to 35 cm (Gershenson et al, 1984). Following exploration, the affected ovary should be removed and sent for immediate pathologic evaluation. If the diagnosis is a malignant germ cell tumor of any histologic subtype, excluding a benign mature cystic teratoma, complete surgical staging is indicated. In the rare adult patient who has completed childbearing, total abdominal hysterectomy and salpingo-oophorectomy is performed. In the more common circumstance of a young patient who desires continued fertility, preservation of reproductive potential is attempted. The contralateral ovary is inspected and, if normal in appearance, left undisturbed. Various recommendations have been made regarding the need for biopsy of the contralateral ovary, but given the low incidence of positive results with random ovarian biopsy and the potential for disruption of reproductive potential owing to adhesions or trauma, we do not perform a biopsy on a normal-appearing contralateral ovary. If the contralateral ovary appears to contain a cyst, an ovarian cystectomy is performed and the sample is sent for immediate histologic evaluation. If this reveals malignant disease, bilateral oophorectomy is performed, but in the 5% to 10% of malignant germ cell tumors associated with a benign mature cystic teratoma in the contralateral ovary, the remainder of that ovary can be preserved.

Unless grossly involved with tumor, the uterus is left in place in young patients who desire to maintain their reproductive potential. The conventional approach of total abdominal hysterectomy with bilateral salpingo-oophorectomy is not indicated in view of current assisted reproductive techniques using donor oocytes with hormonal support. Such techniques make conception and childbearing a viable alternative for patients with a uterus but no ovaries.

Patients with advanced-stage disease should undergo cytoreductive surgery. Every attempt should be made to achieve optimal tumor reduction (no implant larger than 1 cm) and, when possible, to leave no visible tumor. Response to chemotherapy and survival are significantly improved in patients who undergo optimal or complete cytoreduction (Williams et al, 1994).

Postsurgical Therapy

Historically, the standard for adjuvant treatment of germ cell tumors has been VAC, but on the basis of trials at our institution (Gershenson et al, 1990) and those sponsored by the Gynecologic Oncology Group (Williams et al, 1994), the preferred treatment regimen has changed to BEP. Although a direct comparison between VAC and BEP was not performed, adjuvant therapy with BEP resulted in a 96% sustained response rate. This was thought to be better than surgery alone (75% to 80% recurrence rate) or VAC (38% recurrence rate). Therefore, adjuvant therapy with BEP is indicated for all patients with resected early-stage germ cell tumors of the ovary.

Prior to initiating chemotherapy, we obtain baseline hematology, chemistry, and liver function blood tests. We also perform pulmonary function testing, specifically evaluating the diffusing capacity of the lungs before beginning bleomycin. We administer 3 to 4 courses of BEP using the dosing schedule shown in Table 13-4, obtaining weekly complete blood cell counts. Prior to each course, we perform a history and physical examination and obtain serum chemistry and pulmonary function testing values; if aberrant results are found, the drug dose is adjusted appropriately. If a patient has rales on examination or demonstrates a 15% reduction in the diffusing capacity of the lungs, bleomycin is discontinued from the BEP regimen.

The only patients not treated with adjuvant chemotherapy are those with a stage IA or IB grade 1 immature teratoma or stage IA pure dysgerminoma. These patients are not given adjuvant chemotherapy and can be closely observed after surgery. There is an increasing body of literature supporting no postsurgical treatment (observation only) in patients with any stage I germ cell tumor. Future clinical trials should address and resolve this issue.

Since virtually all patients with germ cell tumors are given chemotherapy postoperatively, the role of repeat laparotomy in patients referred after an incomplete staging procedure is minimal. If it appears that the surgeon performed an adequate exploration to exclude gross residual disease,

Table 13–4. Protocol for Bleomycin, Etoposide, and Cisplatin (BEP) Chemotherapy Regimen

---

- Maintenance fluids of 5% dextrose in normal saline with 10 mEq/L potassium chloride and 8 mEq/L magnesium sulfate at 42 mL/hr are initiated on admission and continued during and 24 hours after chemotherapy.
- Thirty minutes prior to cisplatin administration each day, prehydrate with 1 L normal saline with 20 mEq potassium chloride and 16 mEq magnesium sulfate at 250 mL/hr for 4 hours, and give
    Ondansetron 8 mg in 50 mL normal saline IVPB,
    Dexamethasone 20 mg in 50 mL normal saline IVPB, and
    Diphenhydramine 50 mg in 50 mL normal saline.
- Cisplatin 20 mg/m^2/day in 1 L normal saline with 50 g mannitol IVPB over 4 hours on days 1-5.
- Etoposide 100 mg/m^2/day in 500 mL normal saline IVPB over 2 hours on days 1-5.
- Bleomycin 10 IU in 1 L normal saline IVPB over 24 hours on days 1-3.
- Follow with:
    Ondansetron 8 mg in 50 mL normal saline IVPB every 8 hours,
    Albuterol nebulizers 2.5 mg every 6 hours for 24 hours, and if needed,
    Prochlorperazine 10 mg in 50 mL normal saline IVPB every 6 hours to treat nausea.
- Regimen repeated every 28 days.

Abbreviations: IVPB, intravenous piggyback.

postoperative computed tomography of the abdomen and pelvis can be performed for confirmation, and adjuvant chemotherapy with BEP should be initiated. If evaluation of the extrapelvic contents and retroperitoneum has been insufficient, leaving open the possibility of gross residual disease, repeat laparotomy with complete surgical staging is indicated.

Patients with gross residual disease or advanced-stage disease after initial surgery should receive BEP as outlined above. These patients are followed up with CT and tumor marker analysis, and a total of 3 to 6 courses of BEP are given, providing the patient does not experience adverse effects from the chemotherapy. There is no consensus on the optimal number of treatment cycles, but for patients with elevated alpha-fetoprotein levels, it is our custom to continue giving BEP for 2 cycles after normalization of alpha-fetoprotein levels, although this is not based on scientific data. It is also prudent to supplement BEP treatment with growth factors when necessary to maintain adequate leukocyte and platelet counts. Appropriate use of growth factors obviates treatment delay.

For the rare patient with a recurrent germ cell tumor, no standard treatment regimen exists. Regimens that have been useful in our experience include etoposide, methotrexate, dactinomycin, and cisplatin; vinblastine, ifosfamide, and cisplatin; and ifosfamide, carboplatin, and etoposide. In selected patients, one should consider consolidation with high-dose chemotherapy, although its role remains unclear.

Second-look surgery is not usually recommended for patients with germ cell tumors. The only possible exception is the patient with an element of immature teratoma in whom no serum markers are positive, and second-look surgery is controversial in this setting. In patients diagnosed with immature teratomas, any residual disease after treatment usually consists of either a benign mature teratoma or a mass comprising gliosis. A CT-guided biopsy to confirm this diagnosis and follow-up using serial imaging may be preferable to a second major surgery. Likewise, patients with dysgerminoma who have a mass remaining at the conclusion of chemotherapy usually have only desmoplastic fibrosis. This can be confirmed by CT-guided biopsy and followed up with serial imaging.

Disease-Specific Considerations

Teratomas

When an adnexal mass is found to be a mature cystic teratoma, areas of squamous differentiation and small nodules in the wall of the cyst should be specifically evaluated for the presence of malignant elements. If such elements are present, the tumor should be treated as a malignant germ cell tumor, and the general surgical recommendations for germ cell tumors presented earlier in the chapter should be followed. Likewise, if immature elements—typically neural elements—are identified, the tumor is classified as an immature teratoma and is treated as a malignant germ cell tumor. If, however, no malignant elements are identified, the neoplasm is benign and can be treated with an ovarian cystectomy alone. The contralateral ovary should be evaluated, as 12% of benign cases are bilateral. A contralateral cystectomy should be performed in this case, with preservation of as much normal ovarian tissue as possible.

Dysgerminoma

Patients diagnosed with dysgerminoma on frozen section pathologic evaluation present a unique situation. A minority of these tumors have an associated gonadoblastoma and arise in a dysgenetic gonad. Patients with gonadoblastoma have abnormal karyotypes and have a significant risk of developing a future malignant germ cell tumor arising in the contralateral dysgenetic, or "streak," gonad. Therefore, any patient, regardless of age, in whom elements of a gonadoblastoma are identified should have a bilateral salpingo-oophorectomy to remove any gonadal tissue.

Upon the intraoperative diagnosis of dysgerminoma, the pathologist should be asked to carefully evaluate the specimen for any residual normal ovary and to look for any elements of gonadoblastoma. As the pathologist is evaluating the specimen further, the surgeon should inspect the contralateral adnexa to determine whether a normal ovary or dysgenetic gonad is present. Normal ovarian tissue excludes the possibility of dysgenetic gonads, thereby allowing the surgeon to conserve the contralateral ovary and preserve reproductive potential. Dysgerminoma is bilateral in 15% of cases, so in most patients, 1 ovary can be preserved if normal ovarian tissue is present.

Although patients with dysgerminoma have historically been noted to be sensitive to radiation therapy, chemotherapy with BEP is more effective, less toxic, and less likely to adversely affect reproductive potential than radiation therapy. Therefore, BEP is recommended for adjuvant and postoperative therapy at our institution.

Patients are followed up with measurement of levels of serum lactate dehydrogenase to document serologic response and to detect subclinical recurrence. Alternative chemotherapy regimens as outlined above—such as etoposide, methotrexate, dactinomycin, and cisplatin; vinblastine, ifosfamide, and cisplatin; or ifosfamide, carboplatin, and etoposide—or radiation therapy can be used to treat recurrent disease.

Choriocarcinoma

Nongestational, isolated choriocarcinoma of the ovary is exceedingly rare, for it usually co-exists with other elements. Due to the rare nature of this tumor, there is no absolute standard treatment. However, treatment options include either BEP or etoposide, dactinomycin, methotrexate, vincristine, and cyclophosphamide after surgical resection.

OVARIAN TUMORS OF LOW MALIGNANT POTENTIAL

Tumors of low malignant potential (LMP) represent a category of neoplasms distinct from benign cystadenomas and cystadenocarcinomas. First described by Taylor in 1929, they have since also been referred to as borderline tumors and atypically proliferating tumors. LMP tumors of the ovary comprise approximately 15% of all epithelial ovarian tumors. The clinical and pathologic characteristics, treatment, and prognosis of LMP tumors are significantly different from those of invasive ovarian carcinomas.

Clinical and Pathologic Characteristics

Invasive epithelial ovarian cancer is typically a disease of postmenopausal women, but LMP tumors occur in younger women, with 71% occurring in premenopausal women. The average age at presentation of women with LMP is reported to be 40 years, approximately 20 years younger than the average age of women with invasive disease. The most common presenting sign is a palpable abdominal or pelvic mass, found in approximately 90% of patients. Symptoms may also include abdominal distention, pain, and postmenopausal bleeding. Serum CA-125 levels are variably elevated.

Diagnosis of an LMP tumor by gross inspection is difficult. Pathologic criteria for diagnosis include the absence of stromal invasion in the ovary and at least 2 of the following characteristics: epithelial tufting, multilayering of the epithelium, mitotic activity, and nuclear atypia. These neoplasms arise from the surface epithelium of the ovary, and 80% to 95% are of serous or mucinous histology.

Guidelines for Therapy

When intraoperative pathologic evaluation in a patient with a pelvic mass indicates an LMP tumor, the patient should undergo complete surgical staging (Lin et al, 1999). Such staging includes pelvic washings; examination of all peritoneal surfaces; omental biopsies; and biopsies of any suspicious lesions and the paracolic gutters, pelvic sidewalls, vesicouterine fold, and pouch of Douglas. Pelvic and para-aortic lymph node sampling is also usually performed. Some controversy exists regarding the need for complete staging in patients with apparent early disease, particularly with regard to lymph node sampling, because of the low frequency of positive findings. However, we recommend complete staging with lymph node sampling because the rationale for staging clinically early disease is to exclude advanced disease (e.g., microscopic retroperitoneal lymph node metastases) and peritoneal invasive and noninvasive implants, which affect prognosis and treatment. Additionally, it is difficult to accurately determine the extent of invasion of mucinous tumors by frozen section analysis; therefore, patients with these tumors should always undergo complete staging and appendectomy.

Although it is unusual to see patients with bulky, advanced-stage extrapelvic disease, this does occur. Every attempt should be made to remove all visible disease from the abdominopelvic cavity, as LMP tumors are relatively resistant to chemotherapy.

The recommended surgical procedure for a patient who has completed childbearing is a total abdominal hysterectomy and bilateral salpingo-oophorectomy with staging and possible tumor-reductive surgery. However, in patients of reproductive age who desire continued fertility and who have clinically apparent limited disease with no involvement of the contralateral ovary or the uterus, conservative therapy with unilateral salpingo-oophorectomy and staging is appropriate and safe. Both ovaries should be carefully evaluated, but there is no role for wedge biopsy of the clinically uninvolved contralateral ovary because microscopic metastases have not been demonstrated in patients with LMP tumors and wedge biopsy increases the risk of subsequent infertility. Ovarian cystectomy performed instead of unilateral oophorectomy may not be advisable because it results in a higher incidence of recurrence (Lim-Tan et al, 1988).

If the diagnosis of an LMP tumor is made postoperatively, a decision must be made regarding whether the patient should undergo repeat surgical exploration for staging. This decision is controversial and should take into account the extent of the exploration during the initial surgery. Up to 24% of patients with apparent stage I or II disease have their disease upstaged on repeat exploration (Yazigi et al, 1988), and a percentage of patients may have invasive metastatic implants (Gershenson et al,

1998a), changing the staging and treatment recommendations. However, we attempt to avoid surgical restaging when possible, instead utilizing close surveillance with periodic history and physical examination, measurement of CA-125 levels, and CT.

Several regimens of chemotherapy have been investigated for the treatment of advanced-stage LMP tumors, but no benefit in disease-free or overall survival has been demonstrated with any regimen at any stage. Therefore, we do not administer chemotherapy to patients with LMP tumors of the ovary and noninvasive implants.

A minority of patients with LMP tumors of the ovary will have invasive implants on staging biopsies. These patients have a worse prognosis and a higher recurrence rate than patients with noninvasive implants. Scientific data to support treatment recommendations are limited, but since these invasive implants represent small foci of invasive carcinoma, we administer 6 courses of paclitaxel and carboplatin at 21-day intervals to these patients.

Prognosis

The indolent nature of LMP tumors is best demonstrated by the 95% 5-year survival rate and 80% 20-year survival rate for all stages of the disease. Although the recurrence rate is between 7% and 30%, these tumors usually recur as low-grade serous tumors (75%) or LMP tumors (25%). Thus, they are amenable to repeat surgical resection.

OTHER UNCOMMON OVARIAN TUMORS

Another type of rare nonepithelial tumor of the ovary is carcinosarcoma, or malignant mixed müllerian tumor of the ovary. This histologic variant is more commonly identified in the uterus but can occur as a primary ovarian neoplasm. Surgical therapy is the initial treatment, including a total abdominal hysterectomy, bilateral salpingo-oophorectomy, staging procedure, and tumor-reductive surgery. This is followed by postoperative chemotherapy. We often attempt to place patients with malignant mixed müllerian tumors of the ovary on sarcoma protocols, but in the absence of active protocols, we treat them with combination chemotherapy: paclitaxel and carboplatin or ifosfamide and cisplatin.

Small cell carcinoma of the ovary is an extremely rare entity for which there exists no standard protocol. Following surgical resection with total abdominal hysterectomy and bilateral salpingo-oophorectomy, staging, and tumor reduction, adjuvant therapy is administered because of the aggressive nature of this neoplasm. The literature suggests that etoposide and cisplatin or VAC are the most useful chemotherapy combinations. High-dose chemotherapy may have a role in treatment, but this has not yet been investigated. Radiation therapy may be useful for local control.

The remaining nonepithelial ovarian tumors consist of metastases to the ovary from primary tumors of other origin. The most common primary tumors include breast, colon, and stomach cancers and lymphoma. In the case of an isolated metastasis, the ovaries should be removed, but if widespread metastatic disease is present, the benefit of debulking surgery is limited. Postoperative therapy should follow guidelines for the primary tumor.

KEY PRACTICE POINTS

- Treatment of nonepithelial ovarian neoplasms is determined by many factors, including patient age and desire for future fertility, extent of disease, comorbid conditions, and karyotype.

- Exploratory surgery is indicated for solid adnexal masses, and histologic type should be determined intraoperatively when possible. Surgical therapy should include a thorough staging procedure and tumor reduction in the event of extraovarian disease.

- For most young patients with apparent limited disease, fertility-sparing surgery with unilateral salpingo-oophorectomy and complete surgical staging is appropriate. Patients who have completed childbearing should have a total abdominal hysterectomy, bilateral salpingo-oophorectomy, and complete surgical staging.

- The histologic type and stage of the neoplasm determine the need for adjuvant chemotherapy. Patients with sex cord–stromal tumors stage IC and higher may benefit from adjuvant chemotherapy with BEP or paclitaxel and carboplatin.

- Patients with granulosa cell tumors may be monitored for recurrence by measuring CA-125 and serum inhibin levels. Several treatment options exist for patients with recurrent disease.

- All patients with resected early-stage germ cell tumors are treated with BEP, except for patients with stage IA or IB grade 1 immature teratomas or stage IA dysgerminoma.

- Patients with dysgerminoma should be evaluated for the presence of gonadoblastoma. If gonadoblastoma is present, all gonadal tissue, including dysgenetic gonads, should be removed.

SUGGESTED READINGS

Bjorkholm E, Silfversward C. Prognostic factors in granulosa-cell tumors. *Gynecol Oncol* 1981;11:261–274.

Brown J, Shvartsman HS, Deavers MT, Burke TW, Munsell MF, Gershenson DM. The activity of taxanes in the treatment of sex cord–stromal ovarian tumors. *J Clin Oncol* 2004a;22:3517–3523.

Brown J, Shvartsman HS, Deavers MT, et al. Taxane-based chemotherapy compared with bleomycin, etoposide, and cisplatin for the treatment of sex cord–stromal ovarian tumors [abstract]. *Gynecol Oncol* 2004b;92:402.

Fishman A, Kudelka AP, Tresukosol D, et al. Leuprolide acetate for treating refractory or persistent ovarian granulosa cell tumor. *J Reprod Med* 1996;41:393–396.

Gershenson DM. Management of early ovarian cancer: germ cell and sex cord–stromal tumors. *Gynecol Oncol* 1994;55(suppl):S62–S72.

Gershenson DM, Del Junco G, Copeland LJ, Rutledge FN. Mixed germ cell tumors of the ovary. *Obstet Gynecol* 1984;64:200–206.

Gershenson DM, Morris M, Burke TW, Levenback C, Matthews CM, Wharton JT. Treatment of poor-prognosis sex cord–stromal tumors of the ovary with the combination of bleomycin, etoposide, and cisplatin. *Obstet Gynecol* 1996;87:527–531.

Gershenson DM, Morris M, Cangir A, et al. Treatment of malignant germ cell tumors of the ovary with bleomycin, etoposide, and cisplatin. *J Clin Oncol* 1990;8:715–720.

Gershenson DM, Silva EG, Levy L, Burke TW, Wolf JK, Tornos C. Ovarian serous borderline tumors with invasive peritoneal implants. *Cancer* 1998a;82:1096–1103.

Gershenson DM, Silva EG, Tortolero-Luna G, Levenback C, Morris M, Tornos C. Serous borderline tumors of the ovary with noninvasive peritoneal implants. *Cancer* 1998b;83:2157–2163.

Gershenson DM, Wharton JT, Kline RC, Larson DM, Kavanagh JJ, Rutledge FN. Chemotherapeutic complete remission in patients with metastatic ovarian dysgerminoma. Potential for cure and preservation of reproductive capacity. *Cancer* 1986;58:2594–2599.

Herbst AL. Neoplastic diseases of the ovary. In: Mishell DR, Stenchever MA, Droegemueller W, Herbst AL, eds. *Comprehensive Gynecology*. 3rd ed. New York, NY: Mosby-Year Book Inc.; 1997:912.

Homesley HD, Bundy BN, Hurteau JA, Roth LM. Bleomycin, etoposide, and cisplatin combination therapy of ovarian granulosa cell tumors and other stromal malignancies: a Gynecologic Oncology Group study. *Gynecol Oncol* 1999;72:131–137.

Jemal A, Tiwari RC, Murray T, et al. Cancer statistics, 2004. *CA Cancer J Clin* 2004;54:8–29.

Koonings PP, Campbell K, Mishell DR Jr, Grimes DA. Relative frequency of primary ovarian neoplasms: a 10-year review. *Obstet Gynecol* 1989;74:921–926.

Lim-Tan SK, Cajigas HE, Scully RE. Ovarian cystectomy for serous borderline tumors: a follow-up study of 35 cases. *Obstet Gynecol* 1988;72:775–781.

Lin PS, Gershenson DM, Bevers MW, Lucas KR, Burke TW, Silva EG. The current status of surgical staging of ovarian serous borderline tumors. *Cancer* 1999;85:905–911.

Serov SF, Scully RE, Robin IH. Histological typing of ovarian tumors. In: *International Histologic Classification of Tumors*, No. 9. Geneva: World Health Organization; 1973:37–42.

Taylor HC. Malignant and semimalignant tumors of the ovary. *Surg Gynecol Obstet* 1929;48:204–230.

Williams S, Blessing JA, Liao SY, Ball H, Hanjani P. Adjuvant therapy of ovarian germ cell tumors with cisplatin, etoposide, and bleomycin: a trial of the Gynecologic Oncology Group. *J Clin Oncol* 1994;12:701–706.

Yazigi R, Sandstad J, Munoz AK. Primary staging in ovarian tumors of low malignant potential. *Gynecol Oncol* 1988;31:402–408.

14 GESTATIONAL TROPHOBLASTIC DISEASE

Hui T. See, Ralph S. Freedman, Andrzej P. Kudelka,
and John J. Kavanagh

CHAPTER OUTLINE

CHAPTER OVERVIEW

Gestational trophoblastic tumors comprise a wide spectrum of neoplastic disorders that arise from placental trophoblastic tissue after abnormal fertilization. In the United States, gestational trophoblastic tumors account for fewer than 1% of all gynecologic malignancies and are potentially highly curable, even at advanced stages. With appropriate treatment, patients can not only be cured but also retain fertility, with no long-term sequelae in their offspring. Patients are classified into different prognostic groups based on factors such as the histologic subtype, the extent of disease, the level of human chorionic gonadotropin, the duration of disease, the nature of the antecedent pregnancy, and the extent of prior treatment. The probability of cure depends on the designated prognostic category. After having their disease carefully staged and being classified into a prognostic group, all patients should receive individualized care provided by a multidisciplinary team.

INTRODUCTION

Gestational trophoblastic tumors (GTTs) are a group of neoplastic diseases that arise from placental trophoblastic tissue after abnormal fertilization. GTTs are classified histologically into 4 distinct subgroups: hydatidiform mole (complete or partial), chorioadenoma destruens (invasive mole), choriocarcinoma, and placental site tumor.

The most common type of GTT is the hydatidiform mole. Hydatidiform moles can be considered a benign disease with a variable potential for malignant transformation. These molar pregnancies are characterized by the lack of a viable fetus, trophoblastic hyperplasia, edematous chorionic villi, and loss of normal villous blood vessels.

Most molar pregnancies resolve after uterine evacuation, with no lasting adverse effects. However, at any time during or after gestation, malignant transformation into invasive nonmetastatic or metastatic trophoblastic disease occurs in up to one fifth of patients. In nearly two thirds of these cases, the malignant disease is an invasive mole that is confined to the uterus (chorioadenoma destruens). In one third of cases, the malignant disease is choriocarcinoma.

Placental site tumors are uncommon neoplasms arising from intermediate trophoblast cells of the placenta. These tumors can be identified by cellular secretion of placental lactogen and small amounts of human chorionic gonadotropin (hCG) or low levels of β-hCG.

Chorioadenoma destruens, choriocarcinoma, and placental site tumors are also known as malignant GTTs, and they have the potential to lead to a fatal outcome.

In the United States, GTTs account for fewer than 1% of all gynecologic cancers. Among the GTTs, choriocarcinoma has the worst prognosis. Fifty years ago, women with choriocarcinoma had a less than 5% chance of survival. With a better understanding of the natural history and prognostic factors of the disease and the development of effective chemotherapy regimens and a reliable tumor marker (β-hCG) for diagnosis, the cure rate for patients with choriocarcinoma is now 90% to 95%, even for patients with advanced-stage disease. Also, a large proportion of women who have been treated for GTTs are able to retain fertility, with no long-term sequelae in their offspring. Studies continue to further characterize GTTs, and recently much has been revealed about the pathology, molecular biology, diagnosis, and treatment of these malignancies.

EPIDEMIOLOGY

Overall, approximately 80% of GTTs are hydatidiform moles, 15% are chorioadenomas, and 5% are choriocarcinomas.

In the United States, a hydatidiform mole develops in approximately 1 in 1,000 to 2,000 pregnancies. Molar pregnancies are reported in approximately 3,000 patients per year, and malignant transformation occurs in 6% to 19% of these cases. Complete molar pregnancies are associated with 1 in 15,000 aborted pregnancies and 1 in 150,000 nonaborted pregnancies. The estimated incidence of twin pregnancies consisting of a molar pregnancy and a normal fetus is 1 per 22,000 to 100,000 pregnancies. Choriocarcinoma is associated with an antecedent hydatidiform mole in 50% of cases, a history of abortion in 25%, previous term delivery in 20%, and previous ectopic pregnancy in 5%.

Worldwide, true estimates of the incidence of molar pregnancies are difficult to obtain owing to the vast variation in the presentation and management of normal and abnormal pregnancies. Early observations suggest a 5- to 15-fold higher incidence in the Far East and Southeast Asian countries compared to that in the United States. The incidence of molar pregnancies has been reported to be as high as 1 in 120 pregnancies in the Far East. In Singapore, the incidence of molar pregnancy has been as high as 1 in 72 pregnancies. In the past it was thought that ethnic and racial differences contributed to the variable incidence of GTTs. However, data collected in recent years have been conflicting. Studies have not been able to show that African Americans have a higher incidence of GTTs. Asian women living in the United States do not appear to have a higher rate of GTTs compared with other ethnic groups, in contrast to their counterparts in the Far East. Other studies of Far East and Middle East countries have not provided corroborative data to suggest strong ethnic and racial differences.

However, the occurrence of GTTs has been consistently associated with several factors:
- Extremes of reproductive age (younger than 20 and older than 40 years)
- Prior molar pregnancies
- Lower socioeconomic status
- Particular ABO blood groups.

Women older than 40 years have as much as a 5-fold increase in the risk of molar pregnancy. In general, women younger than 20 have a 1.5- to 2-fold higher relative risk. Younger women also seem to have longer disease-free survival than older women. Women with a history of hydatidiform mole have a 10-fold higher risk of a second molar pregnancy and a more than 1,000-fold higher risk of choriocarcinoma than do women who have had only normal pregnancies. Women in lower socioeconomic groups have a 10-fold higher rate of molar pregnancies than their more affluent counterparts. This trend is apparent not only in the Far East but also in the Middle East and United States. The relationship between GTT incidence and geographic region, culture, and socioeconomic status suggests that diet and nutrition may contribute to the etiology of the disease. The ABO blood groups of parents appear to be related to the development of choriocarcinoma. There is a particular risk for women with blood group A who are married to men with blood group O. Studies of human lymphocyte antigens have not revealed any connection to GTT incidence.

PATHOLOGY

Normal fertilization results from the union of a single sperm and egg, which is followed by rapid cellular division and creation of an embryo. Early embryonic differentiation gives rise to trophoblasts, specialized epithelial cells responsible for developing the placenta and the villi. GTTs arise from the abnormal union of sperm with the ovum. The chain of events that follows results in abnormal trophoblasts and early embryo death. A complete hydatidiform mole contains nuclear chromosomes of paternal origin and mitochondrial chromosomes of maternal origin. This occurs when a sperm fertilizes an empty ovum, which subsequently divides, or when 2 sperms unite with an ovum that is devoid of genetic material. Both methods result in a diploid complete mole. A partial mole, on the other hand, is the abnormal union of 2 sperms with 1 ovum with intact chromosomes, resulting in a triploid karyotype. It has been postulated that these genetic aberrations result in the activation of oncogenes or loss of tumor suppressor genes, leading to the development of malignant tumors. Indeed, genes such as *TP53*, *BCL2*, and *MDM2* are abnormally regulated in GTTs.

GTTs that occur after the evacuation of moles tend to be malignant but can exhibit the histologic features of either hydatidiform moles or choriocarcinoma. On the other hand, persistent GTTs after a nonmolar pregnancy almost always have the histologic pattern of choriocarcinoma. Hydatidiform moles have distinctive morphologic, pathologic, and karyotypic features, which are outlined in Table 14–1. Choriocarcinoma is characterized by sheets of anaplastic syncytiotrophoblasts and cytotro-

Table 14–1. Features of Complete and Partial Hydatidiform Moles

Feature	Complete Moles	Partial Moles
Fetal or embryonic tissue	Absent	Present
Hydatidiform swelling of chorionic villi	Diffuse	Focal
Trophoblastic hyperplasia	Diffuse	Focal
Trophoblastic stromal inclusions	Absent	Present
Genetic parentage	Paternal	Biparental
Karyotype	46XX; 46XY	69XXY; 69XYY
Persistent hCG	20% of cases	0.5% of cases

phoblasts with no preserved chorionic villous structures. Placental site tumors are extremely rare GTTs that predominantly consist of intermediate trophoblasts and a few syncytial elements.

CLINICAL PRESENTATION

Complete Mole

The most common presenting symptom in a complete molar pregnancy is vaginal bleeding. The classic signs of a molar pregnancy, in addition to vaginal bleeding, are the absence of fetal heart sounds and physical evidence of a uterus that is larger than expected for the gestational age. Patients also may present with abdominal pain due to an enlarged uterus. Intrauterine blood clots may also liquefy, resulting in pathognomonic prune juice–like vaginal discharge. Owing to recurrent bleeding, patients may also present with an iron deficiency more severe than that expected due to pregnancy. Twenty percent to 30% of patients also present with early toxemia, with a rare possibility of toxemic convulsions. Ten percent of patients present with hyperemesis gravidarum, and 7% of patients present with hyperthyroidism, presumably due to the structural similarities between β-hCG and the β subunit of thyroid-stimulating hormone. In rare cases, thyroid storms have been reported. Other rare presentations include respiratory distress, disseminated intravascular coagulation, and microangiopathic hemolytic anemia.

Partial Mole

Unlike complete moles, partial moles do not usually result in an enlarged uterus. However, it is important to note that intact fetuses can coexist with partial moles, albeit in fewer than 1 in 100,000 pregnancies. Patients with partial moles usually do not have the hormonal symptoms that patients with complete moles suffer, and only rarely does toxemia occur. In general, patients with partial moles present with the signs and symptoms of a missed or incomplete abortion, and a partial mole is diagnosed only after histologic review of curettage specimens.

Malignant GTTs

Fifty percent of all malignant GTTs occur after molar pregnancies, while 25% occur after normal pregnancies and 25% occur after ectopic pregnancy or abortion. Patients treated for molar pregnancies are followed up closely for any signs or symptoms of malignant transformation. Details of follow-up for patients who have had a molar pregnancy are outlined in the section "Follow-up" below.

Persistent invasive nonmetastatic GTT usually presents with a recurrence of symptoms such as irregular vaginal bleeding, theca lutein cysts, asymmetric uterine enlargement, and persistently elevated serum β-hCG levels. The tumor may even perforate the myometrium, causing intraperitoneal bleeding, or the uterine vessels, causing vaginal hemorrhage. Patients can also present with sepsis and abdominal pain, as the uterine tumor presents a nidus for infection.

Placental site tumors are extremely rare GTTs that present like an invasive mole and produce small amounts of β-hCG for their size. Both chorioadenoma destruens and placental site tumors tend to be confined to the uterus and to metastasize late.

Metastatic GTT occurs in 4% of patients after the evacuation of a complete mole. Metastatic disease is more commonly associated with choriocarcinoma than with chorioadenoma destruens and placental site tumors. Choriocarcinomas are highly vascular tumors that tend to metastasize extensively, and the symptoms of metastasis may include spontaneous hemorrhage at the metastatic foci. Metastases occur most often in the lungs, followed by the vagina, pelvic tissue, brain, liver, and other sites (bowel, kidney, spleen). Serologic recurrence (raised hCG level only) occurs in fewer than 5% of cases.

DIAGNOSIS

Ultrasonography is a reliable and sensitive technique for the diagnosis of complete molar pregnancy. It is therefore the first imaging modality used. Often, the classic "snowstorm" appearance on the sonographic picture is due to the numerous chorionic villi exhibiting diffuse hydatidiform swelling (Figure 14–1). Serum β-hCG, a product of the syncytiotrophoblast, is elevated in GTTs, and its level is measured in all patients with suspected disease. Serum β-hCG measurement is used not only to aid in diagnosis but also as a treatment and follow-up marker of disease. The ratio of serum β-hCG to β-hCG in the cerebral spinal fluid has also been used to detect occult brain metastases, although it is no longer routinely used. At M. D. Anderson Cancer Center, all β-hCG levels are measured using a sensitive bioassay. A urine pregnancy test alone is not considered adequate for measuring β-hCG levels, although it is sometimes used to validate a positive blood test. CA-125 has occasionally been used as a

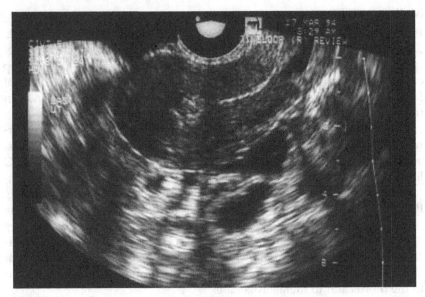

Figure 14–1. Diagnostic ultrasonography of a uterus shows gestational trophoblastic disease.

marker, and elevated CA-125 levels have been associated with persistent GTT. Because 70% to 80% of patients with metastatic GTT have lung involvement, a chest x-ray is obtained in all patients. Magnetic resonance imaging (MRI) or computed tomography (CT) is also frequently performed to confirm or rule out the presence of disease in areas such as the lungs, pleura, brain, abdomen, or pelvis. At M. D. Anderson, MRI is the preferred modality for identifying localized disease in the pelvis or the brain. MRI is considered the best imaging modality for determining the invasiveness of local disease as well as vascularity within the tumor (Figure 14–2).

Staging and Prognosticating Systems

Hydatidiform moles are confined to the uterine cavity. Chorioadenoma destruens is a locally invasive, rarely metastatic lesion. Choriocarcinomas are highly malignant and tend to metastasize extensively. There are many staging and prognosticating systems used for GTTs. All were created in an attempt to define prognostic groups that can direct a rational therapeutic strategy aimed at the highest possible cure rate. The International Federation of Gynecology and Obstetrics (FIGO) staging system (Table 14–2) is used to define low- and high-risk categories of GTT. This system is capable of predicting how patients will respond to single-agent chemotherapy.

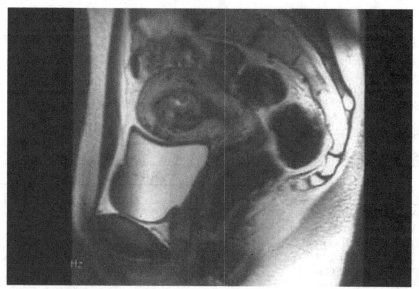

Figure 14–2. Magnetic resonance imaging scan of a uterus in a patient with gestational trophoblastic disease.

TREATMENT

The treatment of GTTs is mainly surgical. For malignant GTTs, the treatment depends on the cell type, stage, serum β-hCG level, duration of the disease, specific sites of metastasis, if any, and extent of prior treatment. Each patient's care is considered individually and managed by a multidisciplinary team. Figure 14–3 outlines succinctly the general diagnostic and therapeutic approaches used at M. D. Anderson.

Molar Pregnancy

Hydatidiform moles are 100% curable. The management of these moles is determined on the basis of the patient's desire to preserve reproductive capability. All patients are evaluated for medical conditions secondary to the mole, and these conditions are managed appropriately before surgery. If a patient does not wish to retain the ability to conceive, a hysterectomy is performed with the mole in situ. In younger patients, the ovaries are preserved. Patients who wish to remain fertile are counseled about the possibility of another molar pregnancy and malignant transformation. If the decision is made to retain the uterus, a suction curettage is performed to remove the mole.

Depending on the trophoblastic elements present, the amount of bleeding during surgery can vary widely. Oxytocin infusion immediately prior

Table 14–2. International Federation of Gynecology and Obstetrics 2000
Staging and Prognostic Scoring for Gestational Trophoblastic Disease

Staging

Stage I	Disease confined to the uterus
Stage II	Tumor extends outside of the uterus, but is limited to the genital structures (adnexa, vagina, broad ligament)
Stage III	Tumor extends to the lungs, with or without genital tract involvement
Stage IV	All other metastatic sites

Scoring

	Score*			
Prognostic Factor	0	1	2	4
Age (years)	<40	≥40	–	–
Antecedent pregnancy	Mole	Abortion	Term	–
Interval (months) from index pregnancy	<4	4–≤7	7–<13	≥13
Pretreatment hCG level (IU/L)	<10³	10³–≤10⁴	10⁴–<10⁵	≥10⁵
Largest tumor size, including uterus (cm)	<3	3–<5	≥5	–
Site of metastases	Lung	Spleen, kidney	Gastrointes- tinal	Liver, brain
Number of metastases	–	1–4	5–8	>8
Previous failed chemotherapy regimens	–	–	Single drug	≥2 drugs

*Low-risk disease is defined as a total score of 0–6, and high-risk disease as a total score of >6.
Reprinted with permission from Ngan (2004).

to surgery can be used to limit the volume of blood loss, although caution is exercised in patients with medical comorbidities such as heart failure. This is because of concerns regarding hyponatremia and fluid overload associated with the infusion. Specimens from the surgery are sent for pathologic evaluation.

Eighty percent of patients need no further treatment. The other 20% will go on to develop a malignant sequela, which is no longer considered a molar pregnancy but a malignant GTT. These patients are identified on the basis of the following criteria:

- Rising β-hCG levels for 2 weeks (taken at 3 separate intervals)
- Tissue diagnosis of choriocarcinoma
- Failure to reach normal titers of β-hCG
- Evidence of metastatic disease
- Elevation of the β-hCG level after a normal value
- Postevacuation bleeding not due to retained tissues.

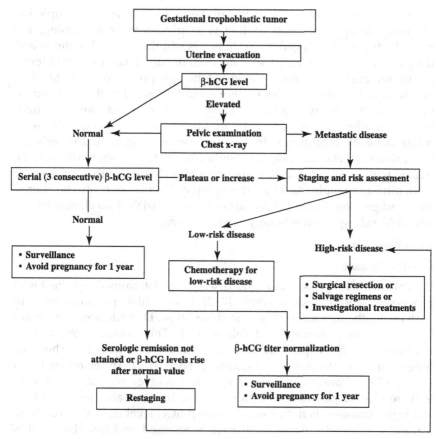

Figure 14–3. Diagnostic and therapeutic approach to gestational trophoblastic disease, as practiced at M. D. Anderson. Modified from Kudelka AP, Freedman RS, Kavanagh JJ. Gestational trophoblastic tumors. In: Pazdur R, Coia LR, Hoskins WJ, Wagman LD. *Cancer Management: A Multidisciplinary Approach.* 7th ed. New York: The Oncology Group; 2003:502.

Nonmetastatic Malignant GTTs

For patients who do not wish to preserve fertility, hysterectomy is the treatment of choice for nonmetastatic malignant GTTs. Single-agent chemotherapy given after surgery is sometimes considered but is not standard treatment. The rationale behind chemotherapy is that it may reduce the likelihood of dissemination of viable tumor cells at surgery and during the immediate postoperative period as well as eliminate any occult metastases. However, clinical trial data are controversial regarding the benefit of prophylactic chemotherapy.

For patients who wish to retain fertility, chemotherapy is offered as primary treatment for low-risk disease. The first-choice regimen at M. D. Anderson is the combination of methotrexate and folinic acid. Other chemotherapy regimens are listed in Table 14–3. If at the completion of chemotherapy the level of β-hCG is persistent or increasing, the patient's tumor is restaged. If the tumor is still limited to the uterus and the patient is over the age of 40 years and/or has no wish to retain fertility, hysterectomy is offered. Patients who still prefer to retain fertility, and who fit into the low-risk category, can be treated with other combination chemotherapy regimens. Even in cases of resistance to first-line chemotherapy, a cure rate of almost 100% is achieved with combination chemotherapy. In the rare case of a tumor that is resistant to combination chemotherapy, patients who wish to retain fertility can be treated with localized resection after careful evaluation with perioperative MRI, ultrasonography, and/or arteriography. Patients may also be offered an investigational treatment as part of a clinical trial. If no clinical trial is available, salvage chemotherapy is administered.

Metastatic GTTs

Low-Risk Disease

Patients with low-risk metastatic disease, as determined by the FIGO prognostic scoring system (Table 14–2), have a high potential for cure with chemotherapy alone. The first choice at M. D. Anderson is the combination of methotrexate and folinic acid. This combination induces remission in 90% of patients with low-risk disease, with few short- or long-term toxic effects. Other regimens used at M. D. Anderson are listed in Table 14–3. Patients are treated for 2 to 3 courses after attaining serologic remission (i.e., normal β-hCG levels). In very rare cases in which serologic remission is not attained or the β-hCG level rises after reaching a normal value, the patient's disease is restaged and her risk level is reevaluated. At this point, it is prudent to check with the laboratory to make sure that the rising β-hCG level is not a false-positive result from phantom hCG (see the section "Phantom hCG Syndrome" later in this

Table 14–3. Chemotherapy Regimens for Low-Risk* Gestational Trophoblastic Disease

Drug	Administration	Cycle†
Methotrexate and folinic acid	1 mg/kg (up to 70 mg) IM or IV days 1, 3, 5, 7 0.1 mg/kg IM or IV days 2, 4, 6, 8	14 days
Methotrexate	0.4 mg/kg IM or IV daily for 5 days	14 days
Methotrexate	30 to 50 mg/m² IM	7 days
Dactinomycin	10 µg/kg (up to 0.5 mg) IV daily for 5 days	14 days
Dactinomycin	1.25 mg/m²	14 days

Abbreviations: IM, intramuscular; IV, intravenous.
*Based on International Federation of Gynecology and Obstetrics (FIGO) risk criteria.
†Withhold treatment for marrow recovery, if necessary.
Reprinted with permission from Kudelka AP, Freedman RS, Kavanagh JJ. Gestational trophoblastic tumors. In: Pazdur R, Coia LR, Hoskins WJ, Wagman LD. *Cancer Management: A Multidisciplinary Approach.* 7th ed. New York: The Oncology Group; 2003:503.

chapter). In the event of confirmed persistent GTT, either experimental therapy or salvage chemotherapy is given. Salvage chemotherapy is discussed in the section "Salvage Therapy" below.

High-Risk Disease

The discovery that etoposide is an effective agent against trophoblastic disease led to the development of the etoposide, methotrexate, dactinomycin, cyclophosphamide, and vincristine (EMA-CO) regimen by Bagshawe (1976), who reported an 83% survival rate in patients with high-risk metastatic GTT. Data from centers around the United States have confirmed a cure rate of as high as 100%. The regimen is described in Table 14–4. Although originally developed for high-risk disease, EMA-CO is the preferred regimen at M. D. Anderson for both high-risk and medium-risk GTTs. EMA-CO is well tolerated, with a very low incidence of life-threatening toxic effects. Anemia, neutropenia, and stomatitis are mild; however, alopecia is universal. Reproductive function is preserved

Table 14–4. EMA-CO Regimen for Middle- and High-Risk* Gestational Trophoblastic Disease

EMA-CO regiment	Administration
Course I	
Day 1	
Etoposide	100 mg/m² IV over 30 minutes
Methotrexate	100 mg/m² IV bolus
Methotrexate‡	200 mg/m² IV as 12-hour continuous infusion
Dactinomycin	0.5 mg IV bolus
Day 2	
Etoposide	100 mg/m² IV over 30 minutes
Folinic acid	15 mg IV/IM/PO every 6 hours for 4 doses, beginning 24 hours after start of methotrexate
Dactinomycin	0.5 mg IV bolus
Course II	
Day 8	
Cyclophosphamide	600 mg/m² IV over 30 minutes
Vincristine	1 mg/m² (up to 2 mg) IV bolus

Abbreviations: EMA-CO, etoposide, methotrexate, dactinomycin, cyclophosphamide, and vincristine; IV, intravenous; IM, intramuscular; PO, orally.
*Based on the International Federation of Gynecology and Obstetrics (FIGO) risk criteria.
†Repeat the regimen every 14 days as toxicity permits.
‡In case of central nervous system metastases, the dose of infused methotrexate is increased to 1,000 mg/m² IV over 12 hours after alkalinization of the urine, and the number of folinic acid doses is increased to 8 given every 6 hours. This regimen is called high-dose methotrexate EMA-CO.
Modified from Kudelka AP, Freedman RS, Kavanagh JJ. Gestational trophoblastic tumors. In: Pazdur R, Coia LR, Hoskins WJ, Wagman LD. *Cancer Management: A Multidisciplinary Approach.* 7th ed. New York: The Oncology Group; 2003:505.

in 75% of patients. In patients with significant tumor volume, extreme care should be taken to watch for signs of rapid necrosis of tumor, which may lead to hemorrhage. In particular, patients with extensive pulmonary metastases and central nervous system metastases are closely monitored, sometimes in the intensive care setting, for signs of rapid tumor necrosis. When intrapulmonary or intracerebral metastases are very extensive, chemotherapy may be given at 50% of the calculated dose for body surface area. In 25% of patients with high-risk disease, a complete remission is not attained. These patients are offered experimental therapy, if available, or given salvage chemotherapy (see the section "Salvage Therapy" below).

Management of First Remission

Patients in first remission who are thought to have a high risk of recurrence are followed up closely with serum β-hCG measurements and post-therapy radiologic imaging. Patients who had lung metastases before treatment should undergo repeat high-resolution CT at the end of chemotherapy to serve as a baseline for follow-up. This is because many patients have residual nodules in the lung field on CT or chest x-ray, signifying fibrous scar tissue. Patients who had brain metastases should undergo MRI of the head, and patients who had liver metastases should have CT of the liver. If the uterus is in place and there was previously disease at that site, consideration is also given to obtaining a baseline MRI of the uterus. The rationale is that modest increases in the β-hCG level signifying relapse may be accompanied by subtle changes in the sterile lesions noted on baseline imaging of the uterus. In these situations, surgery may be considered for the residual disease.

If imaging reveals suspicious nodules or masses and the β-hCG level is normal, a positron emission tomography scan is sometimes obtained to serve as a baseline. If the β-hCG level subsequently rises during follow-up, this scan is helpful in delineating the presence of active disease.

Salvage Therapy

There is no standard regimen for patients with refractory high-risk metastatic GTTs, and all such patients are treated individually. The essential strategy is salvage chemotherapy and the identification of chemotherapy-resistant sites for consideration of surgical resection. At M. D. Anderson, numerous salvage chemotherapy regimens have been administered. Cisplatin-containing regimens are not used as primary therapy because of their significant nephrotoxicity. However, in salvage therapy, cisplatin serves as a very effective part of combination regimens. At M. D. Anderson, Gordon et al (1986) reported that 2 of 10 patients treated with cisplatin, vinblastine, and bleomycin had a sustained remission. Other salvage regimens used at M. D. Anderson include chemotherapy drugs that were not employed in the patient's first-line treatment. High-dose chemotherapy has also been reported to be a useful salvage therapy, although it is not standard treatment for patients at M. D. Anderson.

Placental Site Tumors

For patients with rare placental site tumors, hysterectomy is the preferred treatment. This is because these tumors are highly curable in the early stages, but advanced-stage disease is resistant to chemotherapy and can be fatal. This tumor rarely produces increased levels of β-hCG.

GTTs Coexisting with Normal Pregnancies

Very rarely, GTTs have been known to coexist with normal intrauterine pregnancies, including both spontaneous and in-vitro-fertilization gestations. The GTTs described have been either molar pregnancies or malignant neoplasms, including metastatic malignant GTTs. The incidence of twin pregnancies consisting of a molar pregnancy and a normal fetus may increase as the number of patients who undergo assisted fertility increases. Patients with this rare condition pose a therapeutic dilemma. At M. D. Anderson, all such patients are carefully evaluated to judge the threat of the disease to the mother and child. This is especially true in patients with paraneoplastic endocrine and hematologic symptoms. In many cases, a definitive diagnosis can only be made after a therapeutic abortion. The decision regarding which follow-up strategy to use is made only after consultation with the patient, a perinatologist, and a gynecologic oncologist.

Follow-up

After primary surgical treatment for molar pregnancies and primary chemotherapy for patients with malignant GTTs, all patients are monitored with weekly serum β-hCG measurements until the level returns to normal on 3 consecutive assays (i.e., until complete remission is attained). At this time it is prudent to be mindful of phantom hCG syndrome (see the section "Phantom hCG Syndrome" below). Once serologic remission has occurred, β-hCG levels should be checked monthly for 12 months, every 4 months for the following year, and then yearly after that. At M. D. Anderson, β-hCG levels are measured with a sensitive bioassay, as urine pregnancy tests alone are considered inadequate. β-hCG levels typically normalize within 8 weeks, but in 20% of patients, normalization may take up to 14 to 16 weeks.

Patients are followed up long term with regular complete blood cell counts and β-hCG measurements. Patients treated with combination chemotherapy with etoposide are counseled regarding the increased risk of leukemia associated with this type of regimen. GTT survivors are also followed up with the management of any psychosocial problems that may be associated with GTTs and their treatment.

Future Childbearing

After successful treatment of a molar pregnancy, the risk of a future molar pregnancy is 1% to 2% of all pregnancies. Standard chemotherapy seems to have a minimal impact on patients' subsequent ability to reproduce. However, during the period of treatment and for 1 year after achieving serologic remission, patients are advised not to get pregnant and to use effective hormonal or barrier contraception. Intrauterine contraceptive devices are not used because of the risk of uterine perforation.

Most patients are able to have a normal gestation with a live birth after a molar pregnancy. There does not seem to be an increase in adverse events such as first- or second-trimester abortions, still births, premature births, or caesarean deliveries, nor is there an increase in anomalies in the offspring. Nevertheless, patients treated for molar pregnancies at M. D. Anderson are still monitored closely throughout any subsequent pregnancy, especially in the first trimester. Patients who have difficulty conceiving are considered for fertility treatment.

Phantom hCG Syndrome

Phantom hCG syndrome is also called phantom choriocarcinoma or pseudohypergonadotropinemia. It refers to the persistent mild elevation of hCG in the absence of true hCG and trophoblastic tissue. hCG is a glycoprotein composed of 2 subunits, an α subunit and a β subunit, held together by charge and hydrophobic interactions. Over 40 different professional laboratory serum hCG assays are available, most of which use the multiantibody "sandwich assay" method using labeled-enzyme or radioimmunoassay techniques developed in the 1950s. The mechanism by which heterophilic antibodies cause false-positive results relates to the nature of this immunometric assay. One antibody, commonly a mouse monoclonal immunoglobulin G (IgG), immobilizes hCG by binding 1 site on the molecule; a second antibody, commonly a polyclonal antibody, labeled with an enzyme or chemiluminescent agent, proceeds to mark the first antibody. Heterophilic antibodies usually bind the assay of IgG at sites common to humans and other species. They are bivalent and therefore link the capture and tracer antibodies, mimicking hCG immunoactivity. The binding of human antibodies to mouse IgG is the most common form of interference, although antibodies that bind rabbit, sheep, goat, and bovine IgG have been identified. This interference is not a problem with testing hCG in pregnancy, as hCG is consistently the principal molecule present. However, in patients with trophoblastic disease and molar pregnancies, different hCG variants may be present. In healthy individuals from 1 series, the incidence of these heterophilic antibodies was found to be 3.4%.

A urine hCG test can be used to support or refute a phantom hCG test. If the urine test is positive as well, it is prudent to begin searching for occult disease. If the urine test is negative, it is possible to use different assay systems to confirm the first serum test result, assuming there are no clear radiologic sites of disease.

This issue of phantom hCG emphasizes the clinical dilemma that arises when the care of patients is based primarily on laboratory data. False-positive hCG test results can lead to patients being unnecessarily treated during the follow-up period after primary surgery for molar pregnancies or chemotherapy for malignant disease. It is the clinician's responsibility, therefore, to interpret all test results with caution.

KEY PRACTICE POINTS

- Gestational trophoblastic disease is a highly curable disease, even at advanced stages.

- Most malignant trophoblastic disease occurs after molar pregnancies, but it can also occur after normal pregnancies, ectopic pregnancies, and abortions.

- Surgical treatment of molar pregnancies, localized chorioadenoma (invasive mole), and localized choriocarcinoma is based on whether the patient desires preservation of fertility.

- Placental site tumors are rare tumors that are relatively chemoresistant, and treatment is usually a hysterectomy. Metastases occur late in the course.

- Metastatic gestational trophoblastic disease is stratified according to the FIGO 2000 scoring system.

- The chemotherapy regimen of choice for low-risk disease is methotrexate and folinic acid, which has a cure rate of more than 90%.

- The chemotherapy regimen of choice for both medium- and high-risk disease is EMA-CO, which has a cure rate of 75% in patients with high-risk disease.

- In 80% of patients, β-hCG levels normalize within 8 weeks after treatment, but it may take up to 14 to 16 weeks for levels to normalize.

- Individualized salvage chemotherapy that utilizes a platinum-based regimen can cure most patients with refractory disease.

- Patients with high-risk metastatic disease who have a high volume of disease are monitored closely during treatment for life-threatening complications of rapid tumor necrosis.

Suggested Readings

Amir SM, Osathanondh R, Berkowitz RS, Goldstein DP. Human chorionic gonadotropin and thyroid function in patients with hydatidiform mole. *Am J Obstet Gynecol* 1984;150:723–728.

Bagshawe KD. Risk and prognostic factors in trophoblastic neoplasia. *Cancer* 1976;38:1373–1385.

Bakri YN, Berkowitz RS, Khan J, Goldstein DP, von Sinner W, Jabbar FA. Pulmonary metastases of gestational trophoblastic tumor. Risk factors for early respiratory failure. *J Reprod Med* 1994;39:175–178.

Benson CB, Genest DR, Bernstein MR, Soto-Wright V, Goldstein DP, Berkowitz RS. Sonographic appearance of first trimester complete hydatidiform moles. *Ultrasound Obstet Gynecol* 2000;16:188–191.

Berkowitz RS, Bernstein MR, Laborde O, Goldstein DP. Subsequent pregnancy experience in patients with gestational trophoblastic disease. New England Trophoblastic Disease Center, 1965–1992. *J Reprod Med* 1994;39:228–232.

Berkowitz RS, Goldstein DP, Bernstein MR. Ten year's experience with methotrexate and folinic acid as primary therapy for gestational trophoblastic disease. *Gynecol Oncol* 1986;23:111–118.

Berkowitz RS, Im SS, Bernstein MR, Goldstein DP. Gestational trophoblastic disease. Subsequent pregnancy outcome, including repeat molar pregnancy. *J Reprod Med* 1998;43:81–86.

Buckley JD. The epidemiology of molar pregnancy and choriocarcinoma. *Clin Obstet Gynecol* 1984;27:153–159.

DiSaia PJ, Creasman WT. Gestational trophoblastic neoplasia. In: DiSaia PJ, Creasman WT, eds. *Clinical Gynecologic Oncology*, 6th ed. St Louis, Missouri: Mosby; 2002:185–210.

Dobkin GR, Berkowitz RS, Goldstein DP, Bernstein MR, Doubilet PM. Duplex ultrasonography for persistent gestational trophoblastic tumor. *J Reprod Med* 1991;36:14–16.

DuBeshter B, Berkowitz RS, Goldstein DP, Bernstein MR. Analysis of treatment failure in high-risk metastatic gestational trophoblastic disease. *Gynecol Oncol* 1988;29:199–207.

Garner EI, Lipson E, Bernstein MR, Goldstein DP, Berkowitz RS. Subsequent pregnancy experience in patients with molar pregnancy and gestational trophoblastic tumor. *J Reprod Med* 2002;47:380–386.

Garrett AP, Garner EO, Goldstein DP, Berkowitz RS. Methotrexate infusion and folinic acid as primary therapy for nonmetastatic and low-risk metastatic gestational trophoblastic tumors. 15 years of experience. *J Reprod Med* 2002;47:355–362.

Gordon AN, Kavanagh JJ, Gershenson DM, Saul PB, Copeland LJ, Stringer CA. Cisplatin, vinblastine, and bleomycin combination therapy in resistant gestational trophoblastic disease. *Cancer* 1986;58:1407–1410.

Ha HK, Jung JK, Jee MK, et al. Gestational trophoblastic tumors of the uterus: MR imaging—pathologic correlation. *Gynecol Oncol* 1995;57:340–350.

Kohorn EI, Goldstein DP, Hancock BW, et al. Combining the staging system of the International Federation of Gynecology and Obstetrics with the scoring system of the World Health Organization for trophoblastic neoplasia. Report of the

Working Committee of the International Society for the Study of Trophoblastic Disease and the International Gynecologic Cancer Society. *Int J Gynecol Cancer* 2000;10:84–88.

Li HW, Tsao SW, Cheung AN. Current understandings of the molecular genetics of gestational trophoblastic diseases. *Placenta* 2002;23:20–31.

Ngan HY. The practicability of FIGO 2000 staging for gestational trophoblastic neoplasia. *Int J Gynecol Cancer* 2004;14:202–205.

Page RD, Kudelka AP, Freedman RS, Kavanagh JJ. Gestational trophoblastic tumors. In: Pazdur R, ed. *Medical Oncology, A Comprehensive Review*. Huntington, NY: PRR; 1995:377–391.

Palmer JR, Driscoll SG, Rosenberg L, et al. Oral contraceptive use and risk of gestational trophoblastic tumors. *J Natl Cancer Inst* 1999;91:635–640.

Rotmensch S, Cole LA. False diagnosis and needless therapy of presumed malignant disease in women with false-positive human chorionic gonadotropin concentrations. *Lancet* 2000;355:712–715.

Schorge JO, Goldstein DP, Bernstein MR, Berkowitz RS. Recent advances in gestational trophoblastic disease. *J Reprod Med* 2000;45:692–700.

Steigrad SJ, Cheung AP, Osborn RA. Choriocarcinoma co-existent with an intact pregnancy: case report and review of the literature. *J Obstet Gynaecol Res* 1999;25:197–203.

Wenzel L, Berkowitz RS, Newlands E, et al. Quality of life after gestational trophoblastic disease. *J Reprod Med* 2002;47:387–394.

Wenzel LB, Berkowitz RS, Robinson S, Goldstein DP, Bernstein MR. Psychological, social and sexual effects of gestational trophoblastic disease on patients and their partners. *J Reprod Med* 1994;39:163–167.

15 FERTILITY-SPARING OPTIONS FOR TREATMENT OF WOMEN WITH GYNECOLOGIC CANCERS

Pedro T. Ramirez

CHAPTER OUTLINE

CHAPTER OVERVIEW

Preservation of fertility is an extremely important issue for many women diagnosed with a gynecologic malignancy. As we continue to expand our knowledge of the biological behavior and patterns of spread of gynecologic tumors and to improve our surgical practice, women will be offered more treatment options that will not compromise their fertility. Gynecologic cancers represent 12% to 15% of all cancers suffered by women. Approximately 21% of gynecologic malignancies will present in women of reproductive age who wish to complete or start a family.

Patients with early-stage cervical cancer have several treatment options that may not require hysterectomy or radiotherapy. Similarly, patients interested in reproduction who develop low-grade endometrial cancer can opt for medical management and close surveillance rather than a hysterectomy. Women of reproductive age who are diagnosed with an early-stage ovarian tumor will also be able to consider treatment options that will allow them to maintain fertility.

The chapter will also briefly discuss very novel techniques being studied for young patients with malignancies who are required to undergo treatment with chemotherapy or radiotherapy. These novel approaches explore the potential for ovarian transplantation to maintain not only ovarian hormonal function but also the capacity for ovulation and subsequent pregnancy.

CERVIX

Preinvasive Lesions

Approximately 50 million Papanicolaou tests are done in the United States each year. Nearly 3.5 million (7%) are interpreted as abnormal. Of these, almost 250,000 are considered indicative of high-grade squamous intraepithelial lesions. Typically, the natural history of high-grade squamous intraepithelial lesions is such that 30% to 45% of patients will have regression of their lesion, 35% to 55% will have persistent disease, and 12% to 22% will have lesions that ultimately progress to invasive cancer.

All patients diagnosed with cervical dysplasia should undergo colposcopic evaluation, along with directed biopsies, if indicated. If diagnostic evaluation confirms the presence of cervical dysplasia, a procedure such as a loop electrosurgical excision procedure (LEEP) is recommended in nonpregnant patients. If the patient is pregnant, close surveillance with a Pap test and colposcopy every 3 months is recommended. Cold knife conization (CKC) of the cervix is another option; however, it has the risks of infection, hemorrhage, cervical stenosis, and cervical incompetence. Previous studies have evaluated whether LEEP is as effective as CKC in the removal of cervical dysplasia. One study showed that there was no significant difference between LEEP and CKC in the proportion of cases with negative residual disease (Huang and Hwang, 1999). The operating time in the LEEP group was shorter than in the CKC group. One factor that may present a drawback to LEEP is the fact that thermal artifacts may sometimes limit the histologic interpretation of the specimen. The impact of LEEP on future fertility has been previously studied, and there appear to be no significant detrimental effects on pregnancy.

Unlike patients with cervical adenocarcinoma in situ, who will be discussed below, patients with squamous carcinoma in situ have a low risk of persistent or recurrent disease after CKC. Nearly 80% of patients will remain free of disease during follow-up, even when the surgical margins are positive for squamous carcinoma in situ. However, it should be noted that persistent or recurrent disease is more common in patients in whom both the endocervical and ectocervical margins are involved than in those in whom only the ectocervical or the endocervical margin is involved.

In summary, any patient with a squamous intraepithelial lesion can be safely treated and followed up without compromising her future fertility. Patients with positive surgical margins and those with persistent disease should be counseled and followed up closely, without the need for hysterectomy. Our recommendation is for these patients to undergo pelvic examination with Pap testing and colposcopy every 3 months for at least 2 years. If the lesions resolve, the patient may be followed up every 6 months or yearly, depending on the patient's risk factors and physician discretion.

Adenocarcinoma In Situ

Adenocarcinoma in situ of the cervix is a rare entity that has been reported with increasing frequency in recent years. The median age of patients with this lesion is in the fourth decade of life. It is characterized pathologically by the presence of pseudostratified epithelial cells with enlarged and hyperchromatic nuclei and frequent mitotic figures but with no stromal invasion. Adenocarcinoma in situ is believed to be a precursor of invasive adenocarcinoma.

The average age of patients with clinically detected adenocarcinoma in situ is approximately 5 years younger than that of patients with early invasive adenocarcinoma. Adenocarcinoma in situ is typically diagnosed by colposcopically directed biopsies; however, the disease typically lacks distinguishing clinical or colposcopic features. It is usually located high within the endocervix or deep in the endocervical glands. Recent studies have shown that the sensitivity of the Pap test alone for detecting a glandular abnormality before a cone biopsy diagnosis of adenocarcinoma in situ is 69% (85% with the addition of cervical biopsy and endocervical curettage) (Shin et al, 2002).

In the past, many clinicians favored an extrafascial hysterectomy as the standard treatment for adenocarcinoma in situ. The rationale was that the anatomic distribution of such lesions in the endocervical glands was highly variable. Similarly, it was believed that standard conization did not achieve a complete excision of all preinvasive foci.

Our recommendation for women diagnosed with adenocarcinoma in situ who are no longer interested in childbearing is to undergo a simple hysterectomy. This procedure may be performed as an abdominal hysterectomy, vaginal hysterectomy, or laparoscopic-assisted vaginal hysterectomy. Patients who are strongly interested in childbearing are counseled extensively regarding the potential risks associated with conservative management. There are increasing data in the literature to support the treatment of adenocarcinoma in situ with cervical conization alone rather than simple hysterectomy. However, it should be stressed that with this approach there is a 10% to 15% risk of recurrence. One of the major concerns regarding treatment limited to conization alone is the fact that studies have shown up to a 53% risk of residual disease in the hysterectomy specimen in women with positive margins on the cone biopsy and a 33% risk of residual disease in those with negative cone margins (Wolf et al, 1996). The same study also showed that 57% of patients who underwent cervical conization by LEEP had residual disease in the uterus.

We recommend that women with known or suspected adenocarcinoma in situ from an abnormal Pap test be evaluated with colposcopically directed biopsies and endocervical curettage. If biopsies confirm adenocarcinoma in situ, a cone biopsy should be performed to exclude invasive adenocarcinoma. Patients who refuse hysterectomy should be counseled carefully regarding the potential risks of recurrent disease. The follow-up for patients who refuse hysterectomy and are interested in maintaining fertility should include a Pap test with a cytobrush every 3 to 4 months for at least 2 years.

Microinvasive Disease (Stage IA1)

The latest International Federation of Gynecology and Obstetrics classification defines microinvasive cervical cancer (stage IA1 tumor) as any lesion invading the cervical stroma no deeper than 3 mm and no wider than 7 mm (Pecorelli and Odicino, 2003). The current literature supports a strong correlation between depth of invasion and the risk of nodal metastasis. Spread of disease to the lymph nodes has been universally accepted as the single most important prognostic factor for early invasive squamous cell carcinoma of the cervix. Patients with 3 mm or less of stromal invasion and no evidence of lymph-vascular space invasion have a very low incidence of nodal metastasis and risk of recurrence. Therefore, patients with these findings are candidates for fertility-sparing therapy.

Most women with microinvasive cervical cancer do not have any signs or symptoms, and thus, most cases are detected by routine cervical screening. Whenever a patient has a Pap test result showing the possibility of invasive cancer, but no lesion is visible, colposcopy and directed biopsy are indicated. Ultimately, the diagnosis is confirmed by cone biopsy. A simple punch biopsy is not sufficient. The cone specimen should be systematically sectioned and thoroughly evaluated. Most pathologists recommend a minimum of 12 cone sections, with step sectioning of those specimens involved with microinvasion.

The consideration of conization alone in patients with microinvasive cervical cancer requires careful patient selection and pathologic evaluation. The ideal patient is one who strongly desires fertility, whose cone margins are negative for invasion and high-grade dysplasia, and whose pathologic evaluation conforms to accepted standards. Conization can be considered a safe approach both for squamous and adenocarcinoma microinvasion in cases of free resection margins, no vascular or lymphatic invasion, and negative endocervical curetings. In such cases, the risk of nodal metastasis is less than 1%.

It is important to note that even in patients with tumors invading less than 3 mm, the risk of nodal metastasis may increase if there is evidence of lymph-vascular space invasion. Previous studies have shown that as the tumors invade more deeply into the stroma, the incidence of lymph-vascular space invasion increases—from 4% with lesions less than or equal to 1 mm deep to almost 20% for lesions 3 to 5 mm deep. In this patient population, patient selection for fertility-sparing recommendations becomes even more critical, given the potential for an increased rate of recurrence if the patient is treated conservatively. The treatment options for these patients include cervical conization along with pelvic lymphadenectomy. The latter procedure should preferably be performed laparoscopically. If the nodes are negative and the cone margins are clear, fertility may be maintained and no further therapy is indicated at that time.

Another option for patients with early-stage cervical cancers who wish to preserve their fertility is a procedure that was first proposed by Dargent et al in 1994. The procedure comprises a laparoscopic pelvic lymph node dissection, followed by a vaginal approach for resection of the cervix, the parametrial tissue, and 2 cm of the upper vagina. The novelty of this approach is that at the same time as receiving adequate cancer management, these women are given a chance to maintain fertility. However, it is important to highlight the fact that the procedure is limited by the lack of long-term outcomes. The actuarial recurrence rate in this group of patients is 4.2%, and the mortality rate is 3% (Plante et al, 2004). In a review of 6 radical trachelectomy series, the authors found that 73% of pregnancies resulted in full-term deliveries. The percentage of live births was 67% (Steed and Covens, 2003).

An area of increased debate is the treatment of patients with microinvasive cervical adenocarcinoma. For years the standard of care was that any patient with microinvasive cervical adenocarcinoma should undergo a radical hysterectomy and nodal dissection. However, studies of more than 100 women have shown that no disease recurrences were detected in patients with lesions identifiable only microscopically and having a depth of invasion of up to 3 mm and a tumor width of up to 7 mm (Ostor et al, 1997; Schorge et al, 1999). Given the lack of data on the subject, patients with stage IA1 cervical adenocarcinoma who strongly desire to maintain fertility should be advised that conization alone may be a feasible option; however, they should be fully informed that the risk for disease recurrence is unknown and be followed up carefully.

The follow-up recommendations at our institution for patients who undergo conization alone for microinvasive disease are a pelvic examination with a Pap test, endocervical curettage, and colposcopy every 3 months for at least 2 years. After 2 years, surveillance may be less frequent. The same criteria for follow-up should apply to patients who opt to be treated with radical trachelectomy.

Stage IA2 and IB1 Disease

The International Federation of Gynecology and Obstetrics classification defines a stage IA2 tumor as any tumor for which the depth of stromal invasion is more than 3 mm but not greater than 5 mm and the horizontal spread is not greater than 7 mm. The definition of a stage IB1 tumor is a clinical lesion no greater than 4 cm in greatest dimension confined to the cervix. The risk of nodal metastasis with a stage IA2 lesion can be up to 5%, and the risk with a stage IB1 lesion is approximately 10% to 15%. Therefore, the typical recommendation is a radical hysterectomy with bilateral lymphadenectomy.

As previously described, in 1994 Dargent et al proposed for the first time a radical trachelectomy plus laparoscopic pelvic lymphadenectomy for the treatment of women with early-stage cervical cancers who desire to maintain fertility. To date, several groups have reported on the procedure and have concluded that the overall morbidity and complication rates are low and the lymph node count is satisfactory. They also have shown that successful pregnancies are possible after this procedure. To date, with more than 300 cases reported in the literature, recurrence rates are comparable to those noted with radical hysterectomy. Ideal candidates for this procedure are patients who have no clinical evidence of impaired fertility, stage IA2 to IB1 disease, lesions smaller than 2 cm, limited endocervical involvement at colposcopy, and no evidence of pelvic lymph node metastasis after laparoscopic lymphadenectomy. At our own institution, we still recommend the standard of care for patients with stage IA2 to IB1 disease, which is a radical hysterectomy and bilateral pelvic and para-aortic lymphadenectomy; however, we also give patients who are interested in fertility preservation the option to undergo the radical trachelectomy procedure.

UTERUS

It is estimated that 3% to 5% of all endometrial cancers occur in women under the age of 45 years. A well-known risk factor for endometrial cancer is the presence of atypical hyperplasia. Approximately 25% of cases of atypical endometrial hyperplasia will progress to endometrial cancer. The diagnosis of endometrial hyperplasia is typically made by performing an endometrial biopsy in the office setting. Further investigation with endometrial curettage is indicated in patients with complex hyperplasia with atypia, given the fact that coexisting endometrial carcinoma may be found at the time of the diagnosis in 25% of patients who undergo hysterectomy. The prognosis of a patient with a well-differentiated endometrial adenocarcinoma without myometrial invasion is excellent, and the 5-year survival rate after primary therapy exceeds 95%. The patient usually undergoes a total abdominal or vaginal hysterectomy with bilateral lymphadenectomy, if indicated.

Women who are diagnosed with a well-differentiated endometrial adenocarcinoma, who are suspected of having little or no myometrial invasion, and who are interested in maintaining fertility are candidates for conservative management. There is increasing evidence in the literature that these women may be safely treated with progestins. Medroxyprogesterone acetate is the progestin most commonly used. It is associated with a response rate of approximately 75%, and the median length of treatment required in 1 study was 9 months (Randall and Kurman, 1997). In addition to medroxyprogesterone acetate, other progestins have been used and reported in the literature. These include hydroxyprogesterone caproate, clomiphene, and megestrol acetate. In the United States, oral megestrol acetate (Megace) at a dose of 40 to 160 mg per day is the most commonly used regimen. Oral progestins appear to be well tolerated, with thrombophlebitis being the most frequent adverse effect, occurring in approximately 5% of patients (Thigpen et al, 1999).

A recent review of the literature evaluated 81 patients with grade 1 endometrial adenocarcinoma treated with progestins (Ramirez et al, 2004). The authors showed that 76% of the patients responded to treatment. The median time to response was 12 weeks. Twenty-four percent of the patients who initially responded to treatment had recurrent disease. The median time to recurrence was 19 months. Twenty patients were able to become pregnant at least once after completing treatment. The median follow-up in that study was 36 weeks. No patients died of their disease.

It is very important to assess the degree of myometrial invasion in patients who are to undergo conservative management with progestins. It has been shown that the 5-year survival rate for patients with deeply invasive lesions is approximately 60% to 70%. Methods that have been found to be effective in assessing myometrial invasion include magnetic resonance imaging and ultrasonography. These imaging techniques also aid in detecting any possible ovarian involvement. The sensitivity of these studies in detecting myometrial invasion is about 90%, while the specificity is approximately 85%. The overall accuracy is nearly 90%.

The usual recommendation for follow-up once a patient has been started on a progestin regimen is for a pelvic examination and repeat endometrial biopsy or, preferably, dilatation and curettage 3 months after starting therapy. If at that time there is persistent disease, we strongly encourage the patient to proceed with a hysterectomy. On the contrary, if there is no further evidence of disease, the patient is encouraged to begin pursuing pregnancy. There are a number of isolated reports of successful pregnancies after conservative treatment of endometrial cancer.

One should note that the treatment of endometrial adenocarcinoma with progestins is not without risks, and patients must be counseled extensively about the potential for progression of disease while on treatment. There have been reports of patients who did not respond to treatment and upon undergoing hysterectomy were found to have more advanced disease than initially estimated, which necessitated adjuvant treatment in the form of radiotherapy. On the basis of the current literature, treatment with progestational agents is not recommended for patients with less differentiated tumors, such as grade 2 or 3 adenocarcinoma. Lastly, one should never underestimate the potential risk for synchronous ovarian and endometrial involvement, which would be detrimental for a young patient who opts for conservative management.

OVARY

It has been previously reported that between 3% and 17% of patients with ovarian cancer are younger than 40 years of age at the time of their diagnosis and that 7% to 8% of all stage I epithelial ovarian cancers occur in women younger than 35 years (McHale and DiSaia, 1999). The usual recommendation for most patients who are suspected of having an ovarian malignancy is to undergo an exploratory laparotomy and frozen section analysis of the ovarian mass. If this is identified as an invasive carcinoma, the surgeon will proceed with a total abdominal hysterectomy, bilateral salpingo-oophorectomy, tumor debulking, omentectomy, pelvic and para-aortic lymph node biopsies, and multiple peritoneal biopsies and washings of the pelvis and abdomen. This is generally followed by adjuvant combination chemotherapy with carboplatin and paclitaxel.

There are a number of prognostic factors that should be considered when proposing a conservative approach to patients with ovarian cancer. These include tumor grade and ploidy, histologic subtype, International Federation of Gynecology and Obstetrics stage, serum CA-125 level, and the patient's age and overall performance status. Unfortunately, the majority of these factors will only be available after the final pathology has been confirmed, typically several days postoperatively. Thus, a clear and concise plan that takes into account patient preference as well as the physician's surgical plan must be determined prior to surgical exploration. Generally, patients who are deemed suitable candidates for conservative management include those with tumors of low malignant potential, grade 1 mucinous or endometrioid tumors, negative peritoneal washings, and tumors that are encapsulated and free of adhesions and patients who are nulligravid or have low parity.

Ovarian Low-Malignant-Potential Tumors

It is very important to define and differentiate between tumors of low malignant potential, or borderline tumors, and frankly invasive carcinomas. A tumor of low malignant potential is diagnosed when the following histopathologic characteristics are identified: stratification of the epithelial lining of the papillae, epithelial pleomorphism, atypicality, mitotic activity, and no stromal invasion. These tumors constitute approximately 10% to 15% of all epithelial ovarian malignancies. The prognosis for patients with low-malignant-potential (LMP) tumors is generally excellent, and patients who have not completed childbearing can be treated with conservative surgery to preserve fertility (Gotlieb et al, 1998).

A recent study by Camatte et al (2002) evaluating patients with advanced-stage LMP tumors showed very interesting findings. The authors reported a series of patients who were treated with conservative surgery for stage II and III LMP ovarian tumors to determine if pregnancies could be successfully achieved and to determine the effect that conservative management might have on ultimate outcomes. The patients were followed up for a median of 60 months. Eight pregnancies occurred in 7 patients at a median of 8 months after surgery. Six of the 8 pregnancies occurred spontaneously, 1 followed ovarian stimulation using clomiphene, and 1 followed an in vitro fertilization procedure. Nine women had recurrences, 7 of which were LMP tumors in the remaining ovary and 2 of which were recurrences of peritoneal implants. No deaths were recorded during the follow-up period. Although this series was too small to ascertain the long-term outcomes of treatment, it does offer information that could be helpful for patients and physicians trying to decide whether the potential for fertility should be maintained in patients with advanced-stage LMP tumors.

Patients with LMP ovarian tumors who undergo conservative surgery occasionally require ovulation induction to become pregnant. However, the data regarding the safety of assisted reproductive technologies in these scenarios remain anecdotal. Many women will accept the potential increased risk of assisted reproduction to improve their chances of conception. A recent study analyzed the experiences of a series of women who were diagnosed with LMP ovarian tumors and underwent conservative treatment (Beiner et al, 2001). The study found that 19 (44%) of 43 patients delivered a total of 25 healthy children after a diagnosis of an LMP ovarian tumor; 7 of these patients underwent in vitro fertilization after diagnosis. Of these 43 women, 9 had recurrences. Five of the 9 patients with recurrences were treated with cystectomy alone at the time of recurrence, and all 5 were without evidence of disease at a mean follow-up of 75 months. This study supports the fact that ovulation induction may be feasible after conservative management of ovarian LMP tumors.

Invasive Ovarian Carcinoma

In the current literature, it has been argued that younger age is an independent favorable prognostic factor in patients diagnosed with ovarian cancer. More careful analysis of the data has revealed that the findings are most likely secondary to the fact that younger patients have a higher pre-disposition to being diagnosed with ovarian LMP tumors, and if these tumors are not selectively excluded when the data are evaluated, a better prognosis is detected in the younger population. Most clinicians would agree that young women with invasive ovarian carcinoma should be treated as aggressively as older women. However, many young women will be interested in preserving their fertility, despite the diagnosis of ovarian cancer.

When a young patient presents with a pelvic mass, there are several factors that help the physician determine his or her level of suspicion for the mass being malignant. The first approach should be a detailed history. Symptoms suggestive of a malignancy include abdominal pain or bloat-ing, increasing abdominal girth, and weight loss. Equally important in the patient's initial evaluation is a thorough family history, particularly inquiring about any family history of ovarian, breast, endometrial, or colon cancer. On physical examination, one should be attentive to any evi-dence of lymphadenopathy, abdominal distention, or firm palpable masses, and on pelvic examination, any evidence of a firm, fixed, irregu-lar, and nodular mass should be considered suggestive of a malignancy. The initial evaluation should include pelvic ultrasonography to deter-mine the characteristics of the mass. Findings such as solid components, septations, excrescences, and low resistant index are all suggestive of a malignant process. A serum CA-125 measurement is also helpful, although CA-125 is only elevated in approximately 50% of patients with early ovarian cancer. If indicated, a computed tomography scan will pro-vide additional information about the patient's upper abdomen and pelvis. It is generally suggested that the patient undergo chest radiogra-phy prior to surgery to rule out any distant disease.

Having made the decision to proceed with surgical intervention, the patient must be counseled regarding the surgical plan. It is important for the patient and physician to engage in a detailed discussion addressing the potential risks of conservative management in the event a carcinoma is detected on frozen-section evaluation. The patient must be informed about the possibility of a diagnosis of an LMP ovarian tumor and, in the case of such a diagnosis, be counseled on how to proceed with regard to the contralateral ovary. Another scenario is that of a diagnosis of an ovar-ian carcinoma confined grossly to 1 ovary, with no other gross evidence of disease. In this setting, the patient should undergo a unilateral salpingo-oophorectomy and staging. The preoperative visit is of extreme impor-tance in that all potential findings may be discussed and an effective plan formulated.

Another important decision is that which deals with the surgical approach. The advantages of laparoscopy over laparotomy for the man-agement of an adnexal mass have been extensively reported; however, many physicians argue strongly against the use of laparoscopy in the management of ovarian malignancies. The drawbacks of laparoscopy in this setting include the potential for rupture of an adnexal mass, causing the spillage of cyst contents, with malignant cells, into the abdominal and pelvic cavities. The accidental rupture of cystic masses occurs in approximately 10% of ovarian surgical cases, and this figure may be higher in laparoscopic cases. Previous studies have shown that of cases of ovarian cancer that were laparoscopically excised, only 30% were removed intact (Maiman et al, 1991). It remains controversial whether spilling the contents of an ovarian mass during excision of the mass has an adverse impact on overall survival. However, most patients who have had spillage of the mass have undergone treatment with adjuvant chemotherapy. Another argument against laparoscopy is that it does not allow one to perform a thorough staging, given that the capacity to palpate structures or reach certain locations in the upper abdomen may be limited with the laparoscopic approach. In our institution, if the preoperative evaluation is suggestive that the mass may be benign or an LMP tumor, laparoscopy is offered as an option, provided that the tumor is no larger than 5 to 7 cm in diameter. However, when there is suspicion that a mass is malignant, we recommend an exploratory laparotomy.

The exploratory laparotomy should begin with a midline vertical incision to ensure adequate exposure of the upper abdomen. Upon entering the abdominal and pelvic cavity, the surgeon should obtain washings for cytologic evaluation. Every attempt should be made to remove the ovary intact. Once the pathologist confirms the diagnosis of ovarian cancer, the contralateral ovary should be evaluated. This is very important, particularly in serous tumors where the incidence of bilateral disease is 33%, compared with 15% for mucinous tumors. In the past, a sample of the contralateral ovary was obtained by making a bivalvular incision in the ovary. This practice is no longer performed because it has not been found to provide additional useful information and may lead to future infertility secondary to adhesion formation. As mentioned earlier, even when the patient has opted for conservative management, it is crucial that a complete staging procedure be performed. This includes sampling of the omentum, abdominal and pelvic peritoneum, and pelvic and para-aortic lymph nodes. This is recommended because approximately 15% of patients with apparent stage I epithelial ovarian cancers have occult lymph node involvement.

The results of unilateral salpingo-oophorectomy have been compared with those of total abdominal hysterectomy and bilateral salpingo-oophorectomy in multiple studies. The 5-year survival rate is approximately 75% in both groups. Another study found that the recurrence rates in patients treated conservatively and those treated with a more radical approach were 9% and 11.6%, respectively (Zanetta et al, 1997). A recent multi-institutional study assessed the recurrence rate, survival rate, and pregnancy outcomes in 52 patients with stage IA or IC invasive epithelial ovarian cancer treated with unilateral adnexectomy (Schilder et al, 2002). The median duration of follow-up was 68 months. The authors found that 5 patients had recurrent disease, and the estimated survival rate was 98% at 5 years and 93% at 10 years. Twenty-four patients attempted pregnancy, and 17 (71%) conceived. These 17 patients had 26 full-term deliveries, with no congenital anomalies noted. The authors concluded that the long-term survival of patients with stage IA and IC epithelial ovarian cancer treated with unilateral adnexectomy is excellent. Although this study was limited by its retrospective nature and the fact that the majority of the patients had stage IA, grade 1 tumors, it provides additional evidence that patients with early-stage ovarian cancer can be treated conservatively, preserving their potential for fertility. There are very limited data concerning what recommendations should be made regarding the uterus and remaining ovary after childbearing is completed. This is a decision that is individualized to each patient, given the lack of definitive data.

In patients diagnosed with ovarian germ cell tumors and sex cord–stromal tumors , fertility conservation is the standard practice, given the fact that these tumors typically arise in young adolescent women and that the likelihood of bilateral ovarian involvement is rare. In addition, the majority of these tumors respond very well to adjuvant chemotherapy, therefore offering no compromise to the patient's potential for childbearing. For most patients, unilateral salpingo-oophorectomy with preservation of the contralateral ovary and uterus is appropriate. One of the most common adjuvant regimens recommended for patients with ovarian germ cell tumors is bleomycin, etoposide, and cisplatin. This combination results in a cure rate of at least 95% for early-stage disease and at least 75% for advanced-stage disease.

It should be emphasized that patients with clear evidence of advanced epithelial ovarian cancer should not be candidates for conservative surgery. These patients should undergo complete tumor-reductive surgery, including a total abdominal hysterectomy and bilateral salpingo-oophorectomy. Another group of patients who should not be considered candidates for conservative management are those who have already had difficulty with fertility and have failed to conceive after multiple attempts.

In our practice, we are frequently asked to counsel patients who have undergone exploratory laparotomy or laparoscopy with excision of an adnexal mass that is subsequently found postoperatively to be a carcinoma. The majority of these patients have not had appropriate disease staging. Typically, the exploratory surgery was performed through a low transverse Pfannenstiel incision, which significantly limits access to the upper abdomen. The operative reports often describe that the contralateral ovary and the remainder of the abdomen and pelvis "looked normal." It is important to discuss with the patient her options at that point. In our practice, these include re-exploration, with adequate biopsies and staging, and possible resection of the contralateral ovary and uterus or conservative management, based on normal postoperative computed tomography of the abdomen and pelvis, chest radiography, and serum CA-125 levels. The re-exploration may be performed by laparotomy or laparoscopy.

A recent study evaluated the benefits of comprehensive surgical staging in the management of apparent clinically early-stage ovarian cancer (Le et al, 2002). The authors found that 36% of patients had extraovarian metastases, and these were subsequently treated with adjuvant chemotherapy. Six (10%) of the 60 patients in the study with surgically proven stage I disease that was treated expectantly had recurrent disease, whereas 7 (28%) of the 25 patients with clinical stage I disease treated expectantly because of a lack of risk factors had disease recurrence. The investigators concluded that the absence of surgical-pathologic high-risk factors is inferior to comprehensive staging laparotomy findings in guiding recommendations for subsequent adjuvant therapy. All patients with presumed early-stage ovarian cancer should be considered for comprehensive staging surgery prior to further treatment recommendations.

OVARIAN CRYOPRESERVATION AND TRANSPLANTATION

Approximately 2% of all malignancies, totaling 8,600 new cases per year in the United States, occur during infancy and childhood. The most common childhood cancers that place female patients at risk for ovarian failure due to chemotherapy, radiotherapy, or both are leukemia, neuroblastoma, Hodgkin's lymphoma, osteosarcoma, Ewing's sarcoma, rhabdomyosarcoma, Wilms' tumor, and non-Hodgkin's lymphoma. In women of reproductive age, nearly 5% of all invasive breast cancers occur in those under the age of 40 years. It has been reported that 42% of patients with cancer treated with combined modalities reach menopause by age 31, compared with 5% of controls.

Several options exist for cancer patients who wish to preserve fertility, including chemoprotection, transposition of the ovaries, and cryopreservation of the gametes, ovaries, or embryos. However, a novel technique is emerging and active research is under way in the field of cryopreservation of ovarian tissue. This option offers an advantage over both oocyte and embryo freezing. In this procedure, hundreds of immature oocytes are cryopreserved without the necessity of ovarian stimulation or a delay in initiating cancer treatment. The success of this technique will allow young cancer survivors to not only maintain fertility but also benefit from a continued endogenous source of estrogen to protect against osteoporosis and vasomotor symptoms.

Research in the cryopreservation and transplantation of ovarian tissue is still in its early phases of development, and many questions remain unanswered. Optimization of the freeze-thaw process method is crucial, the issues related to ischemia and reperfusion injury remain unresolved, the most practical and effective graft sites have not been found, and there are issues of safety and ethics, in particular assuring that tissue with potential cancer cells is not reimplanted into a young patient who has achieved complete clinical remission. Nevertheless, ovarian tissue cryopreservation and transplantation may prove to be a useful method of restoring fertility and endocrine function (Kim et al, 2001; Oktay and Buyuk, 2004).

CONCLUSION

Over the past several years, there has been increasing interest in most areas of oncology to strive towards reducing the radicalism of therapeutic approaches. In gynecologic oncology, we are committed to providing young women with an opportunity to maintain their fertility without compromising the effectiveness of the therapy. As we learn more about the pathophysiology of gynecologic malignancies, we are able to offer women less invasive procedures and at the same time implement therapeutic modalities that do not require surgical intervention in order to maintain uterine and ovarian function intact. Novel techniques such as ovarian cryopreservation and transplantation may allow for ovarian viability to be restored after treatment in young women who need to undergo treatments such as chemotherapy or radiotherapy.

KEY PRACTICE POINTS

- Approximately 21% of gynecologic malignancies will present in women of reproductive age who still wish to complete or start a family.

- Any patient with a squamous intraepithelial lesion can be safely treated and followed up without compromising fertility.

- The ideal patient for conservative management of a cervical stage IA1 tumor is one who strongly desires fertility, whose cone margins are negative for invasion and high-grade dysplasia, and whose pathologic evaluation has conformed to accepted standards.

- Patients with stage IA1 cervical adenocarcinoma who strongly desire to maintain fertility should be advised that conization alone may be a feasible option, but they should be fully informed of the risks for disease recurrence.

- Ideal candidates for radical trachelectomy are patients who have no clinical evidence of impaired fertility, stage IA2 to IB1 disease, lesions smaller than 2 cm, limited endocervical involvement at colposcopy, and no evidence of pelvic node metastases after laparoscopic lymphadenectomy.

- Women who are interested in future fertility who are diagnosed with a well-differentiated endometrial adenocarcinoma that is suspected of having little or no myometrial invasion are candidates for conservative management.

- There are a number of prognostic factors that should be considered when proposing a conservative approach to patients with ovarian cancer. These include tumor grade and ploidy, histologic subtype, International Federation of Gynecology and Obstetrics stage, serum CA-125 level, and the patient's age and overall performance status.

- The prognosis for patients with LMP tumors is generally excellent, and patients with such tumors who have not completed childbearing can be treated with conservative surgery to preserve fertility.

- Long-term survival of patients with stage IA and IC epithelial ovarian cancer treated with unilateral adnexectomy is excellent.

- The success of ovarian tissue cryopreservation and transplantation will allow young cancer survivors to not only maintain fertility but also benefit from a continued endogenous source of estrogen to protect against osteoporosis and vasomotor symptoms.

Suggested Readings

Beiner ME, Gotlieb WH, Davidson B, et al. Infertility treatment after conservativemanagement of borderline ovarian tumors. *Cancer* 2001;92:320–325.

Burnett AF, Roman LD, O'Meara AT, Morrow CP. Radical vaginal trachelectomy and pelvic lymphadenectomy for preservation of fertility in early cervical carcinoma. *Gynecol Oncol* 2003;88:419–423.

Camatte S, Morice P, Pautier P, et al. Fertility results after conservative treatment of advanced stage serous borderline tumor of the ovary. *Br J Obstet Gynecol* 2002;109:376–380.

Dargent D, Brun JL, Roy M, et al. La tracheolectomie elargie (T.E.), une alternative a l'hysterectomie radicale dans le traitement des cancers infiltrants developpes sur la face externe du col uterin. *J Obstet Gynecol* 1994;2:285–292.

Gotlieb WH, Flikker S, Davidson B, et al. Borderline tumors of the ovary: fertility treatment, conservative management, and pregnancy outcome. *Cancer* 1998;82:141–146.

Huang LW, Hwang JL. A comparison between loop electrosurgical excision procedure and cold knife conization for treatment of cervical dysplasia: residual disease in a subsequent hysterectomy specimen. *Gynecol Oncol* 1999;73:12–15.

Kim SS, Battaglia DE, Soules MR. The future of human ovarian cryopreservation and transplantation: fertility and beyond. *Fertil Steril* 2001;75:1049–1056.

Le T, Adolph A, Krepart GV, et al. The benefits of comprehensive surgical staging in the management of early-stage epithelial ovarian carcinoma. *Gynecol Oncol* 2002;85:351–355.

Maiman M, Seltzer V, Boyce J. Laparoscopic excision of ovarian neoplasms subsequently found to be malignant. *Obstet Gynecol* 1991;77:563–565.

McHale MT, DiSaia PJ. Fertility-sparing treatment of patients with ovarian cancer. *Compr Ther* 1999;25:144–150.

Oktay K. Ovarian tissue cryopreservation and transplantation: preliminary findings and implications for cancer patients. *Hum Reprod Update* 2001;7:526–534.

Oktay K, Buyuk E. Fertility preservation in women undergoing cancer treatment. *Lancet* 2004;363:1830.

Ostor A, Rome R, Quinn M. Microinvasive adenocarcinoma of the cervix: a clinicopathologic study of 77 women. *Obstet Gynecol* 1997;89:88–93.

Pecorelli S, Odicino F. Cervical cancer staging. *Cancer J* 2003;9:390–394.

Plante M, Renaud MC, Francois H, Roy M. Vaginal radical trachelectomy: an oncologically safe fertility-preserving surgery. An updated series of 72 cases and review of the literature. *Gynecol Oncol* 2004;94:614–623.

Ramirez PT, Frumovitz M, Bodurka DC, Sun CC, Levenback C. Hormonal therapy for the management of grade 1 endometrial adenocarcinoma: a literature review. *Gynecol Oncol* 2004;95:133–138.

Randall TC, Kurman RJ. Progestin treatment of atypical hyperplasia and well-differentiated carcinoma of the endometrium in women under age 40. *Obstet Gynecol* 1997;90:434–440.

Schilder JM, Thompson AM, DePriest PD, et al. Outcome of reproductive age women with stage IA or IC invasive epithelial ovarian cancer treated with fertility-sparing therapy. *Gynecol Oncol* 2002;87:1–7.

Schorge JO, Lee KR, Flynn CE, et al. Stage IA1 cervical adenocarcinoma: definition and treatment. *Obstet Gynecol* 1999;93:219–222.

Shin CH, Schorge JO, Lee KR, et al. Cytologic and biopsy findings leading to conization in adenocarcinoma in situ of the cervix. *Obstet Gynecol* 2002;100:271–276.

Steed H, Covens A. Radical vaginal trachelectomy and laparoscopic pelvic lymphadenectomy for preservation of fertility. *Postgrad Obstet Gynecol* 2003;23:1–6.

Thigpen JT, Brady MF, Alvarez RD, et al. Oral medroxyprogesterone acetate in the treatment of advanced or recurrent endometrial carcinoma: a dose-response study by the Gynecologic Oncology Group. *J Clin Oncol* 1999;17:1736–1744.

Wolf JK, Levenback C, Malpica A, et al. Adenocarcinoma in situ of the cervix: significance of cone biopsy margins. *Obstet Gynecol* 1996;88:82–86.

Zanetta G, Chiari S, Rota S, et al. Conservative surgery for stage I ovarian carcinoma in women of childbearing age. *Br J Obstet Gynecol* 1997;104:1030–1035.

16 QUALITY OF LIFE AND SEXUAL FUNCTIONING

Diane C. Bodurka and Charlotte C. Sun

CHAPTER OUTLINE

CHAPTER OVERVIEW

Quality-of-life issues, which range from psychosocial issues to fertility concerns to end-of-life care, are an extremely important part of the treatment of women with gynecologic malignancies. Therefore, it is critical to assess patients' quality of life, especially when treatment offers no chance of cure and little survival benefit. Asking patients about specific treat-ment-related side effects can ensure that they receive adequate support-ive care. Psychosocial concerns such as depression and anxiety can often be alleviated with therapeutic interventions ranging from one-on-one counseling to support groups to exercise therapy. For many women with gynecologic cancers, life with and after cancer includes learning to cope with serious, long-term sexual problems. Communication between patients and health care providers is essential to managing sexual side effects through counseling, vaginal dilation, and the use of hormone therapy. Complementary therapies, such as exercise, yoga, biofeedback, and hypnosis, are now being integrated with conventional treatments for gynecologic cancers. Decisions regarding the use of palliative chemother-apy and surgery should take into account quality-of-life issues. The appropriate care of patients at the end of life is a critical area for training, research, and practice in gynecologic oncology. Good end-of-life care encompasses physical concerns such as symptom control as well as emo-tional and psychosocial issues such as family concerns, financial issues, and spiritual needs.

INTRODUCTION

Quality of life (QOL) is a difficult concept to define. It can mean different things to different individuals at the same point in time. It can also mean different things to the same person at different points in time. As health care providers to women with gynecologic malignancies, we must con-sider the trade-offs patients make regarding quality versus quantity of life. These difficult choices are often made with the needs of the patient's loved ones in mind. It is critical that we recognize that issues that are important to us as health care providers may not be significant to our patients, and vice versa.

MEASURING QUALITY OF LIFE

QOL is usually defined as a subjective, multidimensional concept that emphasizes the subjective experience of various aspects of one's life, including such factors as access to health care and health services, the safety of the environment, and social status. The term "health-related QOL" is used to describe QOL as it relates to diseases or their treatment. This concept usually includes the psychological, physical, and social func-tioning of patients but excludes perceptions of the environment, housing, or other external dimensions.

A central question in oncology is whether a specific treatment provides sufficient benefit to compensate for the negative impact it may have on

QOL. In some situations, treatment may improve QOL; this occurs when treatment successfully eliminates the cancer in a patient with a significant symptom or tumor burden. It is important to recognize, however, that cancer treatment may also worsen QOL, as when chemotherapy-induced peripheral neuropathy does not abate after therapy has been discontinued. Assessment of the patient's QOL is most critical when treatment is being considered that may worsen QOL, especially when the treatment offers little survival benefit.

At M. D. Anderson Cancer Center, we evaluate patients' QOL using a variety of different tools in a variety of clinical settings. Studies have been performed to quantify the levels of anxiety and depression as well as sexual functioning in patients with epithelial ovarian cancer. Studies also are under way to evaluate the role of exercise in relation to the QOL of endometrial cancer survivors. QOL endpoints are the focus of these studies.

We have also made a conscientious effort to include QOL and symptom assessment in other clinical trials and prevention studies. While these data may be secondary endpoints, the information we continue to gather gives us valuable insight into the impact of our treatments on patients' QOL. Every attempt is made to use reliable, validated questionnaires, as this is crucial to data interpretation. Examples of instruments we frequently use include the Functional Assessment of Cancer Therapy—Ovarian, Memorial Symptom Assessment Scale, and the Center for Epidemiologic Studies—Depression scale. We have performed QOL assessments in the clinic, while patients received standard and high-dose chemotherapy, and at the bedside.

TREATMENT-RELATED SIDE EFFECTS

The treatment of gynecologic malignancies can involve several different modalities, including surgery, chemotherapy, and radiation therapy. Patients may therefore experience a variety of side effects related to the cancer and its treatment. One particularly helpful method of proactively managing side effects is to establish good communication between the patient and her health care team.

At each M. D. Anderson clinic visit, patients are asked about specific side effects by a nurse and the attending physician. Patients are encouraged to report all side effects of therapy, as some may be alleviated by supportive care measures and others might require more evaluation and further treatment. Patients on protocol often keep a diary containing information about side effects, as required by the specific study. Questions we ask the patient include:

1. What type of side effect are you experiencing?
2. When does it occur?

3. How frequently does it occur?
4. How severe is it?
5. How bothersome is it in your day-to-day life?
6. Does anything make it better or worse?
7. How have you tried to manage the problem?

Neutropenia and Anemia

Although chemotherapy can certainly cause pancytopenia, tremendous advances have occurred in the supportive care field to help manage such side effects. Our patients undergo extensive counseling prior to the initiation of a new chemotherapy regimen to inform them of its possible side effects. They are given written information about pertinent side effects and after-hours contact information. Patients are also introduced to the possibility of needing filgrastim or pegfilgrastim for neutropenia as well as epoetin alfa or darbepoetin alfa for anemia. Written information about these supportive care measures is provided as needed. Our Gynecologic Oncology Center provides patients receiving chemotherapy with guidelines for the treatment of fever and neutropenia. The M. D. Anderson Pharmacy also provides specific guidelines regarding the use of growth factors in patients receiving chemotherapy. Clinic nurses give instructions to the individuals who will be giving patients subcutaneous injections. Lastly, patients are reminded to call the clinic or the physician on call if they have a temperature higher than 100.5°F or any other symptoms that might indicate a serious problem. Through the use of our electronic medical records, we are able to quickly retrieve pertinent medical information and tell the patient the appropriate steps to take.

Neurotoxicity

Patients receiving chemotherapy, especially those treated with taxanes, platinum-based agents, and vinca alkaloids, are at increased risk of neurotoxicity. Peripheral neuropathy occurs when sensory nerves are damaged; motor nerves may also be affected. Ototoxicity can occur with the administration of cisplatin. Although symptoms can sometimes resolve, this is not the case in all patients. Therefore, the discussion of symptoms is an important part of every chemotherapy visit. Gabapentin and vitamin B6 may be helpful in decreasing peripheral neuropathy.

Urinary Issues

Urinary incontinence, defined by the International Continence Society as any involuntary leakage of urine, has been estimated to affect more than 20 million American women. Radical hysterectomy may predispose patients to incontinence secondary to radical dissection and nerve injury. Radiation therapy is associated with bladder overactivity, decreased bladder capacity secondary to fibrosis, and fistula formation. Recent data indicate that urinary incontinence affects 41% of gynecologic oncology patients and that patients with cervix cancer are at the highest risk. Patients with gynecologic malignancies who are bothered by urinary incontinence often do not raise the issue with physicians (Botros et al, January 2005, unpublished data). Since patients with gynecologic malignancies are at high risk for urinary incontinence, they should be screened and evaluated routinely for urinary incontinence symptoms.

Chemotherapy-Induced Nausea and Vomiting

The majority of chemotherapy agents are associated with some degree of anorexia, nausea, and vomiting. Whereas some chemotherapy regimens cause nausea and vomiting within the first 12 to 24 hours after chemotherapy administration, other regimens cause delayed nausea, as is typical of carboplatin. In our interviews of large numbers of patients receiving chemotherapy, we found that most patients have an aversion to and dread of nausea and vomiting. Patients consistently rank nausea and vomiting among the worst side effects associated with chemotherapy and among those they would most like to avoid.

We tailor our antiemetic regimens to the emetogenic potential of the chemotherapy regimen. Preprinted orders reflect this practice and are available for each chemotherapy regimen. As noted at the beginning of this section, good doctor-patient communication is an integral part of each patient's care. Patients are asked about their nausea and vomiting at every chemotherapy visit, and antiemetics are adjusted as indicated. Patients are also given antiemetics for break-through nausea and vomiting prior to discharge from the chemotherapy unit, as well as specific instructions regarding the use of antiemetics after chemotherapy.

It is important to remember that chemotherapy and antiemetics such as ondansetron may also interrupt normal bowel function, resulting in either constipation or diarrhea. For women experiencing constipation, we recommend a high-fiber diet with a generous fluid intake (i.e., water, fruit juices). Laxatives such as Senokot may be prescribed for persistent constipation, although the possibility of bowel obstruction should be considered when clinically appropriate. Patients with persistent diarrhea should be evaluated for possible infection, electrolyte imbalances, and dehydration. Diphenoxylate and atropine or loperamide are prescribed when indicated to control diarrhea.

Alopecia

Alopecia is a significant concern of many women receiving chemotherapy, who often feel that their hair loss sets them apart from others and draws more attention to their malignancy. Although we have not been able to prevent alopecia, we do our best to help patients cope with this side effect. At M. D. Anderson, we have a wig shop and a shop that offers patients items such as hats and scarves. Most insurance companies will pay for a wig as long as the prescription identifies it as a "hair prosthesis."

Psychosocial Concerns

In addition to battling cancer, many women with gynecologic malignancies deal with depression and anxiety. We recently surveyed 172 patients with epithelial ovarian cancer and found that 21% of the women had symptoms warranting a full clinical evaluation for depression, compared with approximately 15% of the general population (Bodurka-Bevers et al, 2000). The prevalence of depression in women with a poor performance status (Zubrod >2) was double that of the general population and 4 times that of women with epithelial cancer who were asymptomatic. In this same group of women, 29% had high levels of anxiety, compared with 25% of the general population. As in the case of depression, patients with a poor performance status were twice as likely to be anxious as were women in the general population.

The impact of psychosocial risk factors on patients with ovarian cancer is also emerging as an important issue. Data show that behavioral factors such as social support and distress are associated with changes in cellular immune responses. Behavioral factors are also known to be associated with angiogenic mechanisms in blood and in the tumor microenvironment. Based on these data, there are myriad possibilities for innovative therapeutic interventions ranging from one-on-one counseling to support groups to exercise therapy.

At M. D. Anderson, the Department of Psychiatry is a wonderful resource for helping our patients deal with psychosocial concerns. We are able to schedule consultations and counseling sessions with psychiatrists for our patients, and immediate assistance is available in crisis situations.

Each care center also has at least 1 inpatient and 1 outpatient social worker. This person helps patients with financial concerns, job-related issues, and establishing advance directives. Lodging questions, transportation issues, and even meal tickets are usually taken care of by the social worker. The social worker also collaborates closely with the departments of Psychiatry and Chaplaincy on an as-needed basis.

Spirituality

Spirituality has been defined as a person's sense of peace, purpose, and connection to other people. It also influences how a person interprets the meaning of life. Although religious practice may be a way of expressing spirituality, a person may be spiritual but not religious. A woman's spiritual perspective may help her cope with a life-changing event such as the diagnosis of cancer. Cancer affects every part of a woman's life—at home, at work, with family, and with friends.

Some experts believe that spiritual and religious well being may improve a woman's mental outlook. This, in turn, may help her better cope with the disease and treatment process. At M. D. Anderson, we respect patients' religious and spiritual views. The Department of Chaplaincy at M. D. Anderson offers regular chapel services, sacramental ministry, intercessory prayers, and pastoral support. Catholic, Protestant, and Jewish worship services and an interfaith service are all offered. Worship services are also televised in patient rooms. In addition to a chapel, there are several prayer and meditation rooms available throughout the hospital. Chaplains are on call to meet the needs of patients and their families. Through collaboration with the Department of Chaplaincy and others, we are able to provide support to those with spiritual concerns during their illness.

SEXUAL FUNCTIONING

For many women with gynecologic cancers, life with and after cancer includes learning to cope with serious, long-term sexual problems. Sexual dysfunction is the most enduringly compromised QOL issue experienced by women treated for gynecologic malignancies and affects up to 50% of our patients. Unfortunately, given the sensitive nature of this topic, many patients are hesitant to discuss sexual concerns with their health care providers.

We recently interviewed 232 women with epithelial ovarian cancer; 47% were receiving treatment and 53% were under surveillance (Carmack Taylor et al, 2004). Half of the women had engaged in sexual activity in the past month. Reasons for lack of sexual activity included no partner (46%), lack of interest (38%), physical problems (16%), and fatigue (10%). Women were more likely to be sexually active if they were married, younger than 56 years of age, and undergoing surveillance rather than active treatment for cancer and if they liked the appearance of their bodies. Depression was the only factor that significantly predicted sexual frequency. Women who had lower levels of depression and liked the appearance of their bodies experienced less discomfort during sexual activity.

Although it has been demonstrated at least since the early 1980s that sexual dysfunction is perhaps the most significant side effect of treatment for cervical cancer, little progress has been made in determining the impact on sexual function of surgery versus radiation therapy or in studying the broader impact of sexual dysfunction on the QOL of cervical cancer survivors. One problem with this type of research is that virtually all studies have excluded non-English-speaking patients. Another issue is that women belonging to minority groups and those with low incomes and educational levels are more likely to be diagnosed with the disease. These women, however, are less likely to participate in trials because they have more pressing concerns such as lack of transportation or funding for medical care.

A prospective evaluation of sexual function, frequency, and behavior, as well as marital happiness and psychological distress, was conducted in

61 patients treated for early-stage cervical cancer in 1984 (Schover et al, 1989). Although the groups appeared similar immediately after treatment and at 6-month follow-up, by 1 year, women treated with radiation had more dyspareunia and problems with sexual desire and arousal than did women who underwent radical hysterectomy. Pelvic examinations were performed, and a rating scale used to assess vaginal atrophy correlated with women's reports of dyspareunia, but no specific vaginal measurements were obtained. This study remains one of the few to compare the impact of surgery versus radiation therapy on sexual function.

Women who undergo bilateral salpingo-oophorectomy for ovarian cancer or pelvic radiation therapy for cervical cancer become menopausal. They frequently experience vaginal dryness and recurrent hot flashes that sometimes awaken them throughout the night. While some women elect to take hormone replacement therapy, others decline this option. Conversations held with the patient about hormone replacement therapy should take into account the patient's personal and family history of breast cancer and whether the patient has an aversion to hormone replacement therapy. It is important to document such conversations in patients' medical records and to inform patients of the risks and benefits of hormone replacement therapy. Some patients wish to continue hormone replacement therapy, regardless of the risks. Others elect treatment with venlafaxine (37.5 mg/day) or the vaginal estring. Still others are interested in vaginal lubricants such as K-Y Jelly or Astroglide. If the patient has received pelvic radiation therapy and desires hormone replacement therapy, we recommend a combination of Premarin and Provera, as this avoids the small risk of endometrial cancer due to unopposed estrogen, even if the uterus has been irradiated. We also caution our patients about "natural" hormones and hormone supplements, as the systemic absorption of estrogen in these products is not usually well quantified or documented. Patients with a personal history of breast cancer should further discuss this issue with their breast oncologist.

Patients treated for gynecologic malignancies also frequently complain of a loss of libido. Women who are not averse to hormones should consider the use of Estratest or other androgen-estrogen combinations. Loss of libido may also signify other problems, and referral to a sex therapist is reasonable in this setting.

Women who have been treated with pelvic radiation therapy often have vaginal stenosis. Therefore, we counsel our patients regarding the importance of using a vaginal dilator. After the completion of treatment, patients are given a dilator and specific instructions regarding its use. We recommend dilator use (10 minutes/session) or sexual intercourse 3 times per week for at least 3 years after treatment. We also advise that plenty of lubricant be placed on the dilator or sexual partner.

At M. D. Anderson, we are studying the relationship between vaginal length and distensability and sexual functioning. Using a series of validated questionnaires and vaginal measurements, we are attempting to test a conceptual model of the predictors of QOL in patients with cervix cancer. Our ultimate goal is to develop culturally sensitive interventions to improve the sexual functioning and QOL of cervix cancer survivors.

Yet another important consideration for women with gynecologic malignancies is the loss of fertility, which can be one of the most difficult issues these women face. Women who have not completed childbearing or have not yet started their families may experience the loss of fertility in different ways. Support groups such as Resolve: The National Infertility Association (www.resolve.org) offer resources to women and their partners. Fertile Hope (www.fertilehope.com) is a nonprofit advocacy group that tries to improve health care and insurance coverage for cancer-related infertility. Please also refer to chapter 15 in this book for information about fertility-sparing surgery.

We often perform vaginal reconstruction in patients undergoing pelvic exenteration. Of 95 women who underwent gracilis-myocutaneous-flap vaginal reconstruction in conjunction with pelvic exenteration, a subgroup of 44 patients who returned for routine follow-up care to the Gynecologic Oncology Center were prospectively studied (Ratliff et al, 1996). All participants completed the Sexual Adjustment Questionnaire, and a vaginal assessment was performed by the attending physician. Half of the patients who completed the questionnaire did not resume sexual activity after surgery. The most common problems noted by patients in terms of adjusting to sexual activity after surgery were self-consciousness about the colostomy or urostomy and about being seen in the nude by their partner, vaginal dryness, and vaginal discharge. Sexual adjustment for these women was significantly poorer after surgery than before, even though 70% of the women were thought to have a potentially functional neovagina. This important study illustrates the sexual problems associated with pelvic exenteration and gracilis-myocutaneous-flap vaginal reconstruction. The authors suggested that modifications in surgical technique, aggressive postoperative support, and more realistic patient counseling might help minimize such problems.

Recently, we have begun to use a modification of the vertical rectus abdominis myocutaneous flap for neovagina creation (Sood et al, 2005). This technique allows for pelvic reconstruction with all the advantages of a myocutaneous flap but without the difficulty of closing a large abdominal wall defect.

COMPLEMENTARY AND ALTERNATIVE MEDICINE

Complementary and alternative medicines have recently received more attention from both patients and physicians. In a recent study performed in the Breast and Gynecologic Oncology centers at M. D. Anderson, 500 women were asked about their use of complementary and alternative medicines (Navo et al, 2004). Forty-nine percent of the women reported using complementary or alternative therapies, and only 53% had spoken to a health care provider regarding the use of those therapies.

The 2 terms, "complementary" and "alternative," should not be used interchangeably. Complementary therapies, such as exercise, yoga, biofeedback, and hypnosis, are used in addition to standard treatment. Alternative medicine refers to a treatment modality that is used in place of standard treatment. By definition, alternative treatments are not part of conventional medicine. Complementary and alternative therapies are not cures for cancer. Many alternative therapies claim to be cancer cures even though they have not undergone rigorous scientific testing. Although a small number of supplements and alternative drugs have shown some promise in federally regulated clinical trials, to date none has received Food and Drug Administration approval. Many physicians are now replacing the term "complementary and alternative medicine" with "integrative medicine." Rather than focusing on specific nonconventional treatment modalities, this term describes an approach to treating patients that tries to integrate the best complementary and conventional modalities using a multidisciplinary care approach.

At M. D. Anderson, we recognize that physical healing solves only part of the cancer puzzle. The Place...of Wellness, which opened in 1998, is the first complementary therapy facility built on the campus of a comprehensive cancer center. The Place...of Wellness offers more than 75 complementary therapy programs to current and former patients, family members, and caregivers. These programs, in conjunction with standard therapies, help participants manage symptoms, relieve stress, and enhance QOL. Programs include sessions in yoga, tai chi, and nutrition; a lecture series on complementary and integrative techniques; opportunities for individual meditation; and daily counseling, support groups, networking, and family discussion groups.

PALLIATIVE CHEMOTHERAPY

The term "palliative chemotherapy" is frequently used to describe chemotherapy prescribed for incurable disease. Many women with recurrent gynecologic malignancies have limited treatment options and are faced with the choice between palliative chemotherapy and no further treatment. Although the purpose of this therapy is both the palliation of symptoms and the maintenance of QOL, the toxicity associated with some palliative regimens may be significant. Justification for such treatments therefore requires some benefit, such as symptom management or improved QOL. While some studies have begun to incorporate QOL measures as study endpoints, few investigators have studied the effect of chemotherapy on QOL in gynecologic cancer patients. We also have no data comparing palliative chemotherapy with the best supportive care regimen in this group of patients.

Very little is known about patient expectations regarding palliative chemotherapy. Doyle and associates (2001) recently reported on patient expectations and resource utilization in 27 women with refractory or recurrent ovarian cancer. They developed a questionnaire to assess patient expectations regarding outcomes associated with palliative chemotherapy. Despite the fact that all patients met with their own oncologists before the first cycle of chemotherapy and were counseled about the noncurative intent of this treatment, 65% of the patients expected that the chemotherapy would extend their lifespan and 42% expected that this palliative chemotherapy would cure them. This discrepancy exists because patients may not wish to acknowledge the possibility of dying from their disease and may have high expectations as a mechanism for coping with stress. Also, this disconnect between reality and expectations may be the result of poor doctor-patient communication. QOL was assessed after 2 cycles of chemotherapy; an improvement in overall function was seen in 11 of 21 women. Although the numbers are small, these data are interesting because they demonstrate an improvement in QOL in half the study population receiving palliative chemotherapy.

This study raises an unanswered question: Which outcome of palliative chemotherapy do patients most value: relief of symptoms, tumor response, or improvement in QOL? Depending on the answer, how often are patient expectations regarding palliative chemotherapy met? Once again, discussions about hope and realistic expectations for treatment outcome are key aspects of successful doctor-patient communication. This is especially important when offering enrollment in chemotherapy trials to patients with recurrent, and often incurable, disease.

PALLIATIVE SURGERY

The term "palliative surgery" is often used to describe surgery to relieve bowel obstructions due to tumor progression in patients with ovarian cancer. As many as 51% of women with ovarian cancer will develop a bowel obstruction during the course of the illness. Once ovarian cancer progresses, the goal of treatment changes from curing the patient to prolonging her life, with an emphasis on providing the best possible QOL during the remaining time. The management of a bowel obstruction may include surgery (e.g., colostomy, ileostomy) or medical treatment.

Palliative surgical procedures are performed to restore the functioning of the gastrointestinal tract. "Surgical benefit" has traditionally been defined as 8 weeks of survival after surgery. The overall surgical mortality rate for procedures to alleviate acute bowel obstruction from all malignant causes is approximately 20%. This rate increases slightly to 23% when surgery is palliative and dramatically increases to 72% in patients who are emaciated or malnourished. In addition to the risk of death, surgically treated patients have a high likelihood of living with a colostomy or ileostomy for the rest of their lives. Some patients undergo surgical exploration and are found to have unresectable disease, and a significant number develop serious complications after surgery.

There is a paucity of data evaluating the medical management of bowel obstruction in patients with ovarian cancer. To our knowledge, the study conducted by Baines and colleagues (1985) is the only prospective clinical study to date of the medical management of malignant bowel obstruction. In that study, 30% of the study population (14 patients) had ovarian cancer. The authors reported an improvement in symptoms associated with bowel obstruction (e.g., intestinal colic, vomiting, diarrhea) with intensive medical management and the use of various medications; however, the mean survival time was only 3.7 months.

Attempts have been made to develop a predictive model for the appropriate management of bowel obstruction, but these instruments have not been prospectively validated. They also have not included QOL as an endpoint.

Medical and surgical treatment strategies for bowel obstruction both yield disappointing clinical outcomes and can have a negative impact on QOL. In the setting of advanced cancer and bowel obstruction, members of the health care team must work with patients to set appropriate goals for care. Clinicians must understand their patients' perspectives on QOL issues associated with treatment for bowel obstruction, as well as symptoms of recurrent ovarian cancer and bowel obstruction. Patients must be allowed to consider the trade-offs they are willing to make to arrive at the clinical outcomes they value most.

Support Services

The health care team at M. D. Anderson comprises a diverse group of people dedicated to providing the best care possible for patients. In addition to physicians and nurses, many other individuals work to provide excellent and compassionate patient care. These include social workers, whose role was discussed at the end of the section "Psychosocial Concerns," as well as other individuals whose roles are described below.

Case Managers

Case managers are assigned to hospitalized patients and help to schedule needed outpatient services, coordinate insurance applications, and facilitate discharge from the hospital. They also help patients deal with such practical issues as getting a home health nurse, renting a wheelchair, or scheduling physical therapy appointments.

Patient Advocates

All new patients who enter M. D. Anderson are assigned a patient advocate. These individuals know the "ins and outs" of the institution, and their primary function is to help patients navigate the system. Patient advocates can help patients obtain pathology reports or reschedule chemotherapy appointments or just listen to patients' concerns about their care. Having 1 person to turn to who knows the system can significantly decrease patient anxiety and help them focus on becoming well.

Anderson Network Volunteers

The Anderson Network is a volunteer organization of current and former M. D. Anderson patients. The mission of this group is to "offer hope, resources, support, and understanding to all others affected by the cancer diagnosis, treatments, and issues of survivorship." Anderson Network programs include staffing a hospitality room and providing a speakers bureau and community outreach groups. The Anderson Network also sponsors an annual conference, "Living Fully with Cancer," which is attended by more than 700 cancer survivors and their supporters. The organization also sponsors telephone "Warm Lines" connecting patients with similar diagnoses and circumstances; "Warmnet," an email support/news group; a quarterly newsletter; and Partners in Knowledge, News in Cancer (PIKNIC) weekly lunchtime forums for patients and family members. This tremendous organization has helped to improve the QOL of thousands of cancer patients and their loved ones.

Ostomy Nurses

M. D. Anderson has several enterostomal therapy nurses dedicated to the care of women with ostomies. These nurses also help take care of wounds and are proficient in the use of Wound-Vacs. Ostomy nurses are an essential part of our team, as they provide much-needed information to patients with ostomies, helping them adapt to this tremendous change in their lives. They also have organized a network of patients who volunteer to speak with other patients who are about to undergo ostomy surgery.

Nutritionists

Nutritionists provide valuable information about each patient's diet and nutritional needs and have special expertise in dealing with patients who have had surgery, especially those with ostomies. Nutrition consultations are available at the bedside and also in the Gynecologic Oncology Center. The Learning Center, which is available to patients and their family members, has additional pertinent nutritional information.

Physical and Occupational Therapists

Physical and occupational therapists are invaluable to patients recovering from surgery, experiencing cancer-related symptoms, or having treatment-related side effects. They also help patients who have undergone extensive surgery relearn skills that are integral to their recovery, such as walking and performing household tasks. Therapy services are offered on an inpatient as well as an outpatient basis.

END-OF-LIFE ISSUES

Despite advances in early diagnosis and treatment, many women with gynecologic cancers die of their disease. For this reason, the appropriate care of patients at the end of life is a critical area for training, research, and practice in gynecologic oncology.

Recent trends in the philosophy of end-of-life care have emphasized reducing the aggressiveness of measures taken to extend life and have focused on enhancing the patient's QOL as much as possible through symptom control measures and home care, if possible. Good end-of-life care encompasses physical concerns such as symptom control as well as emotional and psychosocial issues such as family concerns, economic issues, and spiritual needs. Providing good end-of-life care is complicated, however, by the fact that cancer patients typically face a more sudden decline in function before death than do people with other life-ending chronic diseases. This sometimes makes it difficult to know when the appropriate time has come to reduce the emphasis on curative or life-extending therapy. Curative therapy and supportive care should not be viewed as mutually exclusive, however, and there should be a strong emphasis on supportive care throughout the illness. Excellent symptom control should be as high a priority for patients receiving potentially curative therapy as it is for patients at the end of their lives.

End-of-life care for gynecologic cancer patients appears to be improving. At our institution, several indicators have shown improvement in end-of-life care over time (Dalrymple et al, 2002). For example, the average length of time between the placement of a do-not-resuscitate (DNR) order and the patient's death increased from 19.2 days between 1992 and 1994 to 49.4 days between 1995 and 1997. The presence of a DNR order indicates that the physician and patient have discussed the terminal nature of the disease and the patient does not wish to be resuscitated in the event of cardiopulmonary arrest. A DNR order also attempts to eliminate unnecessary procedures and changes the focus of care from cure to comfort. However, there is still room for improvement. Despite the increase in advance discussions about DNR orders, the percentage of patients who had no DNR order when they were admitted to the hospital did not change between the 2 time periods. Over the entire study period, 72% of the DNR orders were placed in the chart within 2 weeks of death, and 35% were placed within 72 hours of death.

There can be reluctance on the part of health care providers and patients to discuss end-of-life issues. In the study above, the average time between diagnosis of an incurable condition and death was 11 months, but patients were informed of the incurable nature of their condition an average of only 44 days before death. This result stands in stark contrast to those of other studies indicating that patients with gynecologic cancer prefer honest communication about the severity of their disease from their physician and that communication with the health care team at the end of life is associated with better "quality of dying and death," as rated by family members (Curtis et al, 2002).

Not all patients, however, wish to engage in frank discussions about their disease. A substantial proportion of patients who are dying do not want to address the specifics of end-of-life care, such as whether they want a DNR order. Many patients with gynecologic cancer remain determined to fight their disease even after it has been deemed incurable. Communication about end-of-life issues with gynecologic cancer patients needs to integrate both realism and hope. However, hope does not have to focus solely on curing the disease or extending life; it can also encompass overcoming suffering.

The needs of family members must be considered in the provision of end-of-life care. One of the most important aspects of high-quality end-of-life care from the perspective of family members is knowing that their relative is consistently receiving appropriate care. The ability to trust the health care team to take appropriate actions in the care of their loved one greatly relieves the family's own suffering and frees them from the role of advocate for their relative's needs. Teno and colleagues (2001) describe a "patient-focused, family-centered" model of quality medical care for patients at the end of life. The model includes 6 components: (1) physical and emotional support for the patient at the level desired; (2) encouragement of shared decision-making; (3) focus on the individual patient in her social context, with respect for the dignity of the patient and the importance of closure in social relationships; (4) attention to the needs of the family for emotional support before and after the death; (5) coordination of care; and (6) provision of information and skills to family members to enable them to care for the patient. This model illustrates the broad nature of care needed by gynecologic oncology patients at the end of life; the emphasis of care must change from specific disease processes to general symptom relief and QOL and from treating a patient to caring for the patient within the context of the family.

KEY PRACTICE POINTS

- Assessment of patients' QOL is critical when the cancer treatment considered may affect QOL negatively and offers little survival benefit.
- Reliable and validated tools are available to evaluate QOL in a variety of settings.
- Patients consistently rank nausea and vomiting among the worst side effects associated with chemotherapy and among those they would most like to avoid.
- It is important to tailor antiemetic regimens to the emetogenic potential of the chemotherapy regimen.
- Depression and anxiety are significant concerns in women with ovarian cancer.
- Up to 50% of women treated for gynecologic malignancies have sexual dysfunction.
- Antidepressants, vaginal lubrication, and the estring may help ease menopausal symptoms.
- Complementary therapies are used in addition to standard treatment. Alternative medicine refers to a treatment modality used in place of standard treatment.
- Patients often expect that palliative chemotherapy will cure them even when they are counseled regarding the palliative nature of the treatment.
- One of the most important aspects of high-quality end-of-life care from the perspective of family members is knowing that their relative is consistently receiving appropriate care, relieving them of the role of advocate for the relative's needs.

ACKNOWLEDGMENT

The authors are grateful to Lori F. Smith for her assistance in the preparation of the manuscript.

SUGGESTED READINGS

Abrams P, Cardozo L, Fall M, et al. The standardization of terminology of lower urinary tract function: report from the Standardization Sub-committee of the International Continence Society. Neurourol Urodyn 2002;21:167–178.

Baines M, Oliver DJ, Carter RL. Medical management of intestinal obstruction in patients with advanced malignant disease. A clinical and pathological study. Lancet 1985;8:990–993.

Basen-Engquist K, Bodurka-Bevers D, Fitzgerald MA, et al. Reliability and validity of the functional assessment of cancer therapy-ovarian. *J Clin Oncol* 2001;19:1809–1817.

Bodurka DC, Sun CC, Basen-Engquist KM. Quality of life in the gynecologic cancer patient. In: Gershenson DM, McGuire WP, Gore M, Quinn MA, Thomas G, eds. *Gynecologic Cancer: Controversies in Management.* Philadelphia, Pa: Elsevier Ltd.; 2004:785–794.

Bodurka-Bevers D, Basen-Engquist K, Carmack CL, et al. Depression, anxiety, and quality of life in patients with epithelial ovarian cancer. *Gynecol Oncol* 2000;78:302–308.

Carmack Taylor CL, Basen-Engquist K, Shinn EH, Bodurka DC. Predictors of sexual functioning in ovarian cancer patients. *J Clin Oncol* 2004;22:881–889.

Cella DF, Tulsky DS, Gray G, et al. The Functional Assessment of Cancer Therapy scale: development and validation of the general measure. *J Clin Oncol* 1993;11:570–579.

Curtis JR, Patrick DL, Engelberg RA, Norris K, Asp C, Byock I. A measure of the quality of dying and death. Initial validation using after-death interviews with family members. *J Pain Symptom Manage* 2002;24:17–31.

Dalrymple JL, Levenback C, Wolf JK, Bodurka DC, Garcia M, Gershenson DM. Trends among gynecologic oncology inpatient deaths: is end-of-life care improving? *Gynecol Oncol* 2002;85:356–361.

Doyle C, Crump M, Pintilie M, Oza AM. Does palliative chemotherapy palliate? Evaluation of expectations, outcomes, and costs in women receiving chemotherapy for advanced ovarian cancer. *J Clin Oncol* 2001;19:1266–1274.

Krebs HB, Goplerud DR. Surgical management of bowel obstruction in advanced ovarian carcinoma. *Obstet Gynecol* 1983;61:327–330.

Lutgendorf SK, Anderson B, Rothrock N, Buller RE, Sood AK, Sorosky JI. Quality of life and mood in women receiving extensive chemotherapy for gynecologic cancer. *Cancer* 2000;89:1402–1411.

Navo MA, Phan J, Vaughan C, et al. An assessment of the utilization of complementary and alternative medication in women with gynecologic or breast malignancies. *J Clin Oncol* 2004;22:671–677.

Portenoy RK, Thaler HT, Kornblith AB, et al. The Memorial Symptom Assessment Scale: an instrument for the evaluation of symptom prevalence, characteristics and distress. *Eur J Cancer* 1994;30A:1326–1336.

Radloff LS. The CES-D scale: a self report depression scale for research in the general population. *Applied Psychological Measurement* 1977;1:385–401.

Ratliff CR, Gershenson DM, Morris M, et al. Sexual adjustment of patients undergoing gracilis myocutaneous flap vaginal reconstruction in conjunction with pelvic exenteration. *Cancer* 1996;78:2229–2235.

Schover LR, Fife M, Gershenson DM. Sexual dysfunction and treatment for early stage cervical cancer. *Cancer* 1989;63:204–212.

Sood AK, Cooper BC, Sorosky JI, Ramirez PT, Levenback C. Novel modification of the vertical rectus abdominis myocutaneous flap for neovagina creation. *Obstet Gynecol* 2005;105:514–518.

Sun CC, Bodurka DC, Donato ML, et al. Patient preferences regarding side effects of chemotherapy for ovarian cancer: do they change over time? *Gynecol Oncol* 2002;87:118–128.

Teno JM, Casey VA, Welch LC, Edgman-Levitan S. Patient-focused, family-centered end-of-life medical care: views of the guidelines and bereaved family members. *J Pain Symptom Manage* 2001;22:738–751.

Tunca JC, Buchler DA, Mack EA, Ruzicka FF, Crowley JJ, Carr WF. The management of ovarian-cancer-caused bowel obstruction. *Gynecol Oncol* 1981;12:186–192.

17 PALLIATIVE CARE FOR GYNECOLOGIC MALIGNANCIES

Florian Strasser, Michael W. Bevers,
and Eduardo Bruera

CHAPTER OUTLINE

CHAPTER OVERVIEW

In the cancer setting, palliative care encompasses programs that address the well-being of the whole patient and her family members, the so-called unit of care, from the time of diagnosis of advanced, incurable disease until the patient's death and beyond. Such care involves early recognition, assessment, and treatment of distressing symptoms and syndromes (e.g., delirium, cachexia, and pain), dissemination of essential information, and communication that addresses physical, psychosocial, and end-of-life issues. Symptom assessment is an ongoing process of evaluating the patient's physical, psychosocial, and existential discomforts; cognition; and risk factors for altered symptom expression. Symptom management involves accurate diagnosis and appropriate treatment strategies, both of which depend on a thorough assessment. Effective communication skills enable the clinician to provide the patient and family members with information about the patient's disease and prognosis and about technical issues and procedures; this information will be useful when they are required to make treatment decisions. In addition to the patient's need for physical care, patients with an advanced, incurable disease and their family members usually require psychosocial and existential support, advice about personal and spiritual concerns, and guidance with regard to end-of-life issues, such as advance directives. To address these concerns and to assist in the transition to palliative or end-of-life care, the multidisciplinary palliative care team should include health care professionals with expertise in specialized areas, such as a social worker, psychiatric nurse, and case manager.

INTRODUCTION

At M. D. Anderson Cancer Center, palliative care is provided through an outpatient clinic, an acute-care clinic, and a mobile care unit. The outpatient clinic is a multidisciplinary clinic with 10 health care professionals who assess and treat complex multidimensional symptoms. The acute-care clinic is a specialized inpatient tertiary-care unit for patients who have severe symptoms, who are transitioning to hospice care, or who require end-of-life care. The mobile care unit is a team of palliative care specialists that travels to inpatient sites and consults with the primary care oncology team. The mobile care unit also coordinates care plans with local hospices. These palliative care services provide patients with immediate access to illness-oriented care, challenging the concept that palliative care is strictly a terminal-care service. Figure 17–1 illustrates the role of palliative care at different stages in the development of advanced cancer.

This chapter discusses the general principles of palliative care for patients with advanced cancer and aspects of palliative care related specifically to gynecologic cancer.

Palliative Care Assessment

Administration of effective palliative care interventions depends on the continual, disciplined, and multidimensional assessment of patients and family members. These assessments are used by clinicians when making treatment decisions. At M. D. Anderson, we use simple assessment instruments that do not require those administering them to have specialized skills and that can be used routinely without disrupting clinical practice.

Assessments done to determine a patient's palliative care needs generally involve (1) documentation of 10 common cancer-related symptoms; (2) screening tools to assess cognitive impairment, risk factors for altered symptom expression, psychosocial and existential distress, gastrointestinal dysfunction (i.e., constipation), and social, family, and lifestyle

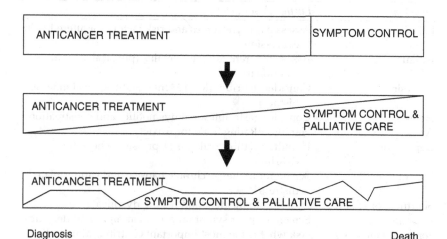

Figure 17–1. Model of the role of palliative care throughout the course of cancer.

disruptions; and (3) discussions to determine the patient's understanding of her disease and prognosis. These 3 elements reflect the basic screening battery used at M. D. Anderson to improve palliative cancer care. The instruments used to accomplish these assessments are described below.

If necessary, more comprehensive assessments focus on specific cancer syndromes (e.g., pain, cachexia, delirium), organ function, treatment side effects, and the dynamics of the cancer within the context of the individual patient.

Patient's Self-Report of Symptoms

At M. D. Anderson, patients are asked to report their symptoms daily using a questionnaire that enables them to document the occurrence and severity of 10 common cancer-related symptoms on a scale of 0 to 10, with 10 being the worst manifestation of the symptom. This instrument was adapted from the Edmonton Symptom Assessment Scale developed by Dr. Eduardo Bruera (Bruera et al, 1995). Sometimes, the instrument is completed by the patient before the examination; other times, the patient responds to the questionnaire verbally during the examination. In some cases, further assessment is needed before a treatment plan can be formulated (Table 17–1).

Assessment of Important Syndromes and Conditions Using Clinically Administered Screening Instruments

Several instruments are used by clinicians to evaluate patients' palliative care needs. Some are standard, widely accepted tools and others are adaptations of these, such as those developed specifically for use at

Table 17–1. Further Assessment of Symptoms Commonly Expressed by Patients with Advanced Cancer

Symptom	Further Assessment
Pain	Assess pain syndromes and risk factors for altered pain expression
Fatigue	Assess different fatigue domains (physical, cognitive, emotional)
Drowsiness	Consider delirium (Mini Mental Status Questionnaire, history)
Nausea	Consider gastrointestinal dysmotility and constipation
Anxiety	Hamilton Rating Scale for Anxiety
Depression	Hamilton Rating Scale for Depression, check for delirium
Loss of appetite	Screen for cachexia, chronic nausea, and eating-related distress
Shortness of breath	Assess both incident and resting dyspnea
Insomnia	Screen for poor symptom control at night and delirium
Sense of well-being	Ask what is the most important contributor, including physical, emotional, social, and existential factors

M. D. Anderson to assess for problems common among cancer patients (Table 17–2).

Cognitive Impairment

Cognitive impairment can easily be underestimated when the patient is merely asked, How have you been doing? or Can you tell me who you are and where you are? For many patients, cognitive impairment goes undiagnosed, either because it is misdiagnosed as depression or because the patient knowingly or unknowingly compensates for the deficits it imposes. Screening tools used to assess for cognitive impairment include objective evaluations of temporal and local orientation, short-term memory, and the ability to carry out a simple command. At M. D. Anderson, we routinely use the Mini Mental Status Questionnaire to assess patients' cognitive abilities.

Psychosocial and Existential Distress

To screen for emotional distress (psychosocial or existential), an interviewer will make a verbal statement to prompt the patient to express his feelings (e.g., I wish this situation were less difficult for you or I am sorry to see how much you and your family are going through). Some clinicians might consider this discussion form of assessment to be a disruption of

Table 17–2. Instruments Used to Screen for Conditions and Syndromes in Patients with Advanced Cancer

Condition or Syndrome	Instrument
Cognitive impairment	MMSQ or other objective, simple test
Altered symptom expression	MMSQ for cognitive impairment
	CAGE for alcoholism
Psychological and existential distress	Verbal prompts to elicit responses
	Attentive listening
Gastrointestinal dysfunction	Questions to determine frequency, volume, and consistency of stool
	Flat radiography to locate and quantify stool content (includes a formula for determining the amount of stool in each quadrant of the colon)
	Questions to determine nutritional status (record of food intake and history of weight changes)
Social, family, and lifestyle adjustments	Sample questions: Where do you live? Who lives with you? Who are your caregivers? How are household chores distributed among residents? Where do you work and what is your working enviroment like?

Abbreviations: MMSQ, Mini Mental Status Questionnaire; CAGE, Cut-down, Annoyed, Guilty, Eye opener.

clinical practice. They might be tempted to avoid such questions because they fear entering into a difficult-to-handle situation with an emotional patient. However, skillful screening for emotional distress can stimulate patient care–team interactions.

Risks for Altered Symptom Expression

Symptoms can be produced by a variety of conditions, can change over time, and are ultimately expressed by the patient in her own words. The expression of a symptom can be affected by the patient's coping style, cognitive impairment, history of alcohol abuse (e.g., habitual use, response to a stressful life event, or response to fears about the cancer diagnosis), and emotional distress. In addition to assessing cognitive impairment and emotional distress, we use the CAGE (Cut-down, Annoyed, Guilty, Eye-opener) questionnaire to screen for alcoholism.

Gastrointestinal Dysfunction

Constipation is a syndrome rather than a symptom. It can occur without symptoms or eventually worsen and cause symptoms such as nausea, bloating, abdominal pain, vomiting, delirium, and urinary retention. It is customary at M. D. Anderson to ask patients daily about the frequency, overall volume, and quality of bowel movements and the size and consistency of stool. Physicians will often ask the nursing staff to confirm information provided by the patient. It is also standard practice to perform flat radiography of the abdomen to quantify the stool content of the bowels (Figure 17–2). This information guides the administration of oral and rectal laxative treatment and is useful in the diagnosis of partial bowel obstruction.

Assessment of nutritional status is often underemphasized. A few simple questions can be asked to generate responses that will alert the clinician to a possible problem, including questions about weight loss over time or the presence and severity of anorexia. In addition, it should be routine practice to assess the loss of muscle and fat tissue by estimating the degree of loss (none, minimal, moderate, or severe) and to assess the volume of oral intake by asking the patient to recount the meals consumed within the previous 1 to 3 days.

Social, Family, and Lifestyle Disruptions

A brief history of the patient's social background, including information about her profession, work environment, family relations, primary caregiver, and living arrangements, is required to determine areas of stress for the patient and for others involved. The questions should be simple, and responses from the patient and family members might indicate the need for referral to social services. Questions about spiritual beliefs and perceived meaning of life are useful in assessing the need for referral to a chaplain for spiritual counseling.

Patient Knowledge of the Disease and Prognosis

An assessment of the patient's understanding of her disease can be made by asking a few simple questions that prompt the patient to discuss the cancer in her own words. This type of questioning is not popular, however, because of concerns that it will initiate a prolonged conversation or

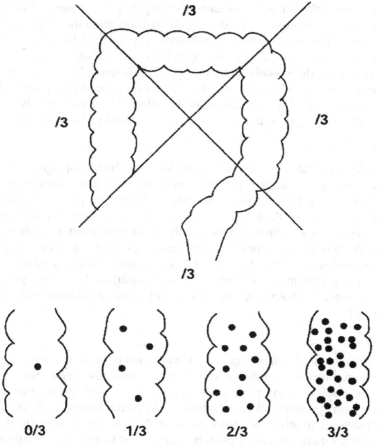

Figure 17–2. Calculation of a "constipation score" using flat abdominal radiography. On the radiograph, draw 2 diagonal lines intersecting at the umbilicus, as shown. This transects the abdomen into 4 quadrants corresponding to the ascending, transverse, descending, and rectosigmoid colons. Then, assess the amount of stool in each of the 4 quadrants using the following scoring system: 0 = no stool; 1 = stool occupying less than 50% of the lumen of the colon; 2 = stool occupying more than 50% but less than 100% of the lumen; 3 = stool completely occupying the lumen. The total score will therefore range from 0 to 12. A score of 7 or higher indicates severe constipation and requires immediate intervention. Source: Driver LC, Bruera E. *The M. D. Anderson Palliative Care Handbook.* Houston: The University of Texas M. D. Anderson Cancer Center.

that the patient will ask questions about end-of-life care that the clinician is uncomfortable discussing.

MANAGEMENT OF SELECTED SYMPTOMS AND SYNDROMES IN PATIENTS WITH ADVANCED CANCER

A symptom is the subjective evidence of the patient's disease or condition, whereas a syndrome is a complicated clinical condition that may produce symptoms. The most common syndromes experienced by patients with advanced cancer are pain, anorexia/cachexia, constipation, chronic nausea, delirium, depression and anxiety, and dyspnea. In the following sections, these syndromes and the treatment approaches practiced at M. D. Anderson to manage them are described. The syndromes typically associated with gynecologic cancers are described in a later section.

Pain

In the United States, pain is now considered the fifth vital sign, and pain assessment is a mandatory requirement of the Joint Commission on Accreditation of Healthcare Organizations. Successful pain management requires an accurate diagnosis of the exact pain syndrome. It is important to describe for the patient and the family members the difference between constant pain and incident pain syndromes. Constant pain is always present, regardless of what the patient does, whereas incident pain occurs only during certain movements. It is also important to explain possible pain management approaches and the outcome associated with each approach.

Assessment

The assessment of pain integrates an evaluation of nociceptive input, factors mediating pain conduction to the brain, and risk factors for altered pain expression. Many patients with advanced cancer experience more than 1 pain syndrome; these syndromes might not be easily distinguishable from one another, and thus, some of them might go unnoticed. For the optimal management of pain, it is important to assess each pain syndrome separately, including identifying their anatomical locations.

An assessment of nociceptive input might include the following questions: Where is the pain located? How would you describe the pain? Does the pain radiate? What actions on your part improve or worsen the pain? In addition, it is important to determine whether the physical examination and imaging studies identify a correlate to the pain complaint and whether the physical examination reveals neurologic deficits or muscle atrophy. Factors that might alter the pain experience include the use of psychotropic medications and organ failure (i.e., liver, kidney, or heart failure). Risk factors for altered pain expression include cognitive impairment, psychosocial or existential distress, and maladaptive coping mechanisms (e.g., alcoholism).

The Palliative Pain Service at M. D. Anderson routinely uses a staging system to identify patients with cancer who are at risk for poor pain control. Factors predictive of poor pain control are neuropathic pain, incident pain, cognitive impairment, psychosocial distress, maladaptive coping, and opiate tolerance (Fainsinger et al, 2005). The management of cancer pain should be discussed in a multidisciplinary setting involving clinicians in the areas of palliative care, anesthesiology, radiation oncology, medical oncology, neurosurgery, orthopedic surgery, and rehabilitation.

Pharmacologic Treatment

The pharmacologic treatment of cancer pain is guided by the 3-step World Health Organization analgesic ladder: (1) nonopioid analgesics (i.e., paracetamol, nonsteroidal anti-inflammatory agents), (2) weak opioids, and (3) strong opioids. In clinical practice, the majority of patients with cancer pain require opiate treatment. At M. D. Anderson, we often go directly to step 3 (strong opioids) and have observed good response and minimal toxic effects. Factors that compromise opiate-induced pain control include the following misconceptions: (1) patients who use strong opioids become addicted, (2) opiate treatment is of limited efficacy and should be reserved for patients whose condition is terminal, and (3) opiate treatment is always dangerous and causes respiratory depression and arterial hypotension.

The usual starting dosage of morphine sulfate for the average adult patient is 5 mg every 4 hours around the clock for constant pain and 5 mg every 1 to 2 hours for breakthrough pain. For patients with constant pain who need more than 10% to 20% of the around-the-clock dosage prescribed for breakthrough pain, the dosage should be titrated. The day after the day on which the breakthrough dose is initiated, the breakthrough dosage is added to the around-the-clock dose. This principle does not apply to patients with an incident pain syndrome because in these patients breakthrough pain presents as incident pain caused by body motion. Titration of the around-the-clock dose for treatment of incident pain would result in overdose and toxic effects. There is no upper dose limit for most strong opioids if the patient's dosage has been carefully titrated and if the diagnosis of a pain syndrome is appropriate considering risk factors for altered pain expression. In addition to morphine, other routinely used strong opiates include hydromorphone, oxycodone, fentanyl citrate or buprenorphine (transdermal or oral transmucosal), and methadone.

All strong opiates are agonists of the μ-opioid-receptor family, and they differ with respect to potency, pharmacokinetics, and pharmacodynamics. Methadone and fentanyl are synthetic opioids with fewer metabolites than natural opioids. In addition, methadone has NMDA-receptor activity, which might provide better control of neuropathic pain. Economic factors might also be a consideration when choosing an opioid.

Opiate treatment must be monitored, and adjustments are indicated if pain management is inadequate or if opioid toxicity (e.g., sedation, hallucinations, myoclonus, or nausea) is present despite adequate adjuvant medications (such as methylphenidate for sedation, haloperidol for hallucinations, and metoclopramide for nausea). Before an analgesic treatment is adjusted, the pain syndrome and the risk factors for altered pain expression should be reviewed. In most patients, opioid rotation is an adequate adjustment; however, some patients benefit from neuraxial treatments or neurolytic blockades.

Equianalgesic tables should be consulted when performing an opioid rotation. These tables are used to convert the dose of the initial opioid to that of the replacement opioid. If opioid rotation is performed because of insufficient pain control, the dose of the new opioid will be 70% to 80% of the dose of the discontinued opioid. If opioid rotation is performed because of side effects, the dose of the new opioid will be 50% of the dose of the discontinued opioid. The morphine equivalent daily dose (MEDD) is the oral dose of morphine to which all strong opioids are converted when a new dose is calculated. For example, 1 mg oral hydromorphone equals 5 mg oral morphine, and 100 μg per hour transdermal fentanyl equals 300 mg oral morphine.

The potency of methadone depends on the previous opioid dose. A conversion rate of 1:5 is used if the previous opiate dose was 1 to 60 mg MEDD per day, a rate of 1:15 is used for a prior MEDD of 61 to 300 mg per day, and a rate of 1:30 is used for a prior MEDD higher than 300 mg per day. Methadone is rarely given at a dose higher than 60 mg per day; when it is given at such a dose, however, supervision by a palliative care pain specialist is required. In addition, the variability of methadone pharmacokinetics is high, which accentuates the need for a careful conversion. Methadone levels in the blood can be altered by concomitant medications, such as antiepileptics, fluconazole, selective serotonin reuptake inhibitors, or histamine-2 blockers.

Side Effects of Opioids

It is mandatory that patients be questioned routinely to screen for opioid-related side effects. Constipation, sedation, and nausea are common side effects of opioid use. Constipation is inevitable with opioid use, and the effect is not dose dependent. Factors that aggravate constipation need to be considered, such as immobility, dehydration, hypercalcemia, hypokalemia, spinal cord compression and other neurologic dysfunctions, anal pain, and other medications (such as tricyclic antidepressants). Patients should be educated about the importance of daily bowel movements and the use of laxatives on a daily basis.

Opioid-induced sedation occurs in 2 forms: mild sedation and opioid toxicity. Mild sedation normally goes away 2 to 4 days after dose escalation or opioid rotation. Patients should be informed of this side effect to avoid opioid phobia and misdiagnosis of opioid allergy. This transient sedation must be distinguished from opioid toxicity, of which typical symptoms are hallucinations (tactile or visual), delusional thoughts, myoclonus, and seizures. Patients should be questioned about the experience of hallucinations, for example, Do you ever have a sense that someone is with you or touching you, but when you look there is no one there?

Nausea is another frequent opioid side effect. Prophylactic metoclopramide is commonly prescribed to prevent the occurrence of nausea. Nausea can be associated with constipation, in which case treatment with a laxative would be required. 5-HT$_3$ antagonists (e.g., ondansetron) are not effective against opioid-induced nausea.

Adjuvant Medications for Pain Control

Adjuvant medications used to control pain include drugs administered for purposes other than analgesia and drugs designed specifically for pain control. Acetaminophen and nonsteroidal anti-inflammatory drugs usually provide sufficient control of mild muscular and skeletal pain syndromes. The new cyclooxygenase-2 inhibitors have minimized concerns about gastrointestinal toxicity typically associated with nonsteroidal anti-inflammatory use; however, they should be used cautiously in patients with renal insufficiency, platelet abnormalities, or heart disease. Among antidepressants, amitriptyline is the most widely studied. Selective serotonin reuptake inhibitors are not used as analgesics, but they may be effective for patients with altered pain expression caused by emotional distress. However, evidence is lacking to support their use for antinociception.

Treatment of Bone and Neuropathic Pain

Bone pain is a distinct pain syndrome that, if recognized, might be treatable with certain interventions. If cancer-related bone pain occurs because the tumor involves the bone, radiation therapy should be considered. When the tumor involves the vertebrae, including cases of vertebral fracture, vertebroplasty with injection of cement might be considered, if available. Bisphosphonates have been shown to decrease bone morbidity and are recommended for bone pain even in the absence of evidence considering oncologic endpoints that supports their use. The use of radioactive isotopes, which have a systemic effect rather than a localized effect, might be beneficial because this approach limits irreversible bone marrow toxicities that impede anticancer treatment and improves pain control.

Neuropathic pain is an important pain syndrome. It is diagnosed using the combination of patient-provided pain descriptors and objective neurologic findings. Simple clinical questions (e.g., Do you feel a burning sensation? Do you feel the sensation of a pin prick or an electrical shock? Do you have a weird sensation resembling pain?) can guide clinical suspicion and help to objectively confirm a neurologic abnormality. Simple touching and skin-prick tests may reveal a deficit in sensation or muscle atrophy. In addition, an anatomic correlate of the neurologic pain syndrome is possible, such as deep tumor invasion in the pelvis or spinal cord. Many patients experience postchemotherapy or postradiation therapy pain syndromes that manifest as neuropathic pain. Neuropathic pain can be successfully managed with single-agent opioid treatment in about 50% to 70% of patients. Many patients benefit from the addition of antiepileptic or antidepressant medicines, the most common of which are gabapentin and amitriptyline, respectively. The typical starting dose of gabapentin is 100 mg every night followed the next day by 100 mg 3 times a day and then 100% up-titration every 3 to 5 days until a clinical plateau or a dose of approximately 2700 mg/day is reached. There are several new antiepileptic drugs on the market that may also be of benefit in treating neuropathic pain.

Short-term neuropathic pain relief is often achieved with moderate-dose corticosteroids (e.g., dexamethasone at 4 mg orally or intravenously every 8 hours for 3 days and tapered over 2 weeks). Some patients with superficial neuropathic pain may benefit from transdermal lidocain. It is advisable to initiate or modify only 1 treatment per consultation (either the opioid or the adjuvant analgesic). Selected patients with localized refractory neuropathic pain syndromes might benefit from neurolytic blocks or neuraxial analgesia.

Difficult-to-Manage Pain

Incident pain syndromes are often underdiagnosed. To elicit evidence for the presence of incident pain, we ask the patient the following questions: How severe is the pain right now? How severe was your worst pain experience during the previous 24 hours? What caused the severe pain? Was the pain exacerbated with movement (of the body, lungs, or bowels)? Amplification of pain expression may occur secondary to cognitive impairment. Patients with delirium or dementia sometimes lose inhibitory functions of the central nervous system, and more pain is expressed from the same nociceptive input. Clinically, there is a fine balance between recognizing and treating pain and overtreating it owing to altered pain expression resulting from cognitive impairment.

Pain expression can increase when the patient experiences psychosocial, existential, or spiritual distress. Patients with cancer undergo various periods of adjustment; must cope with multiple emotions, such as fear, anger, and depression; and experience a diminished self-image due to, for example, loss of autonomy or loss of dignity. Many patients express suffering in the manner they consider socially acceptable. For some patients, it may be easier to say, "I feel pain" than to say, "I fear dying." Sophisticated opiate treatment and interventional anesthesiology might be futile if a key component of the patient's pain expression is nonphysical suffering. In such cases, psychological counseling, emotional support, and attentive listening are recommended.

Cancer patients frequently self-medicate with alcohol or other psychotropic substances as a form of maladaptive coping. Even after many years of controlling their alcohol consumption, some patients with cancer who have a history of overusing alcohol retreat to the practice to cope with their diagnosis. It is important to recognize this risk factor for pain expression because such patients typically experience a series of opioid-induced neurotoxic effects that lead to frequent visits to the emergency room. At M. D. Anderson, these patients are often treated successfully with opioids but must first be educated about the use of these medications and agree to well-defined boundaries.

At M. D. Anderson, we are privileged to have access to 3 different pain services: the palliative pain management team, the chronic cancer pain team, and the acute postoperative pain team. All of these services emphasize that pain control is a multidisciplinary endeavor.

Anorexia/Cachexia

Most patients with advanced cancer experience involuntary weight loss. In the 1980s, it was believed that nutritional support could replenish the body with nutrients that were depleted by the cancer. It was later found that the paraneoplastic anorexia/cachexia syndrome impedes the anabolic response to eating. This section discusses the characteristics of and treatment options for this anorexia/cachexia syndrome.

Characteristics

Paraneoplastic anorexia/cachexia is a catabolic syndrome characterized by metabolic, neuroendocrine, and anabolic alterations triggered by an activated immune system and tumor-derived catabolic factors. In most patients with advanced cancer, however, other aggravating factors can lead to decreased oral intake or weight loss, referred to as secondary anorexia/cachexia. These factors include starvation, which results from decreased oral intake of food due to alterations in taste, mucositis, dysphagia, odynophagia, constipation, bowel obstruction, or severe symptoms, such as pain or shortness of breath. Starvation can also be caused by loss of nutrients due to diarrhea, malabsorption, or frequent paracentesis of body fluids. Other mechanisms of secondary anorexia/cachexia are prolonged bed rest leading to loss of muscle mass and catabolic states independent of cancer, such as chronic infections or chronic heart failure.

In reality, the paraneoplastic anorexia/cachexia and secondary anorexia/cachexia syndromes are present synchronously in most patients. Management of involuntary weight loss and associated symptoms should be based on a careful assessment of the different mechanisms of these syndromes. Some mechanisms of secondary anorexia/cachexia, including severe symptom distress, odynophagia, taste alterations, and constipation, are often reversible.

Treatment

The currently available treatments for paraneoplastic anorexia/cachexia syndrome are of limited efficacy. In more than a dozen randomized trials, progestins (megestrol acetate and medroxyprogesterone) have been found to increase appetite in about 30% to 50% of patients. Fat and water, rather than lean body mass, account for the bulk of the weight gain, however. Whether progestins reduce fatigue and improve quality of life for patients with paraneoplastic anorexia/cachexia is somewhat controversial. Caution should be taken when considering the use of progestins for patients with known thromboembolic complications.

Corticosteroids have been found to increase appetite, improve quality of life, and decrease fatigue in most patients with advanced cancer; however, these benefits are short-term, often enduring less than 1 week. Treatment with these drugs should be tapered after the first 3 days and stopped after 3 to 4 weeks.

Prokinetics have been shown to improve chronic nausea. In the United States, the most commonly used prokinetic is metoclopramide. This drug is often given at a dose of 10 mg every 4 hours around the clock and then 10 mg every 2 hours as required. The side effects of metoclopramide are akathisia, which sometimes masquerades as an anxiety attack, and other extrapyramidal symptoms.

Nutritional support may be beneficial for patients with involuntary weight loss caused by secondary anorexia/cachexia, particularly for patients with disruptions in the upper or lower gastrointestinal tract. The decision to provide artificial nutrition is difficult because patients rarely experience pure secondary anorexia/cachexia (starvation), and additional nutrition is not beneficial for the catabolic paraneoplastic anorexia/cachexia syndrome. Factors to consider when making this decision are whether the treatment will disrupt the patient's autonomy and integrity, the cost, and the likelihood of an anabolic response in a patient who is in a catabolic paraneoplastic state. Patients with slow-growing tumors and bowel obstruction may benefit most from artificial nutrition. It takes several weeks for nutritional support to improve symptoms, and whether short-term benefits are achieved is controversial.

Constipation

As discussed earlier in the subsection Gastrointestinal Dysfunction, it is necessary to monitor patients for constipation daily. The assessment should take into consideration the number of bowel movements, the amount of stool, and the consistency of the stool. The diagnosis is made by careful evaluation of the patient's medical history and examination of a flat radiograph of the abdomen enabling the clinician to quantify the stool content (Figure 17–2). In addition, the diagnosis of distal constipation or fecal impaction is made by careful digital examination.

It is mandatory that every patient taking opioids be given prophylactic laxatives around the clock. In addition, patients and family members should be encouraged to titrate the laxative treatment, which most often involves administration of a stimulant, such as Senna, and a stool softener. Because it takes more than 12 hours for a stimulant and stool softener to work, patients must be instructed to use these drugs regularly rather than reactively. There is no standard upper dose; in fact, patients are often underdosed. Lactulose is a stool softener that works within a few hours but might cause flatulence, which can cause pain. Suppositories primarily stimulate the distal rectum. Enemas can be beneficial, especially in patients with distal constipation.

Fecal impaction is an often-unrecognized complication of constipation, and symptoms (i.e., urinary incontinence, nausea and vomiting, and delirium) can occur without the patient's awareness of constipation.

Chronic Nausea

Chronic nausea probably comprises a subgroup of symptoms of the paraneoplastic anorexia/cachexia syndrome, with concurrent dysmotility of the upper gastrointestinal tract. Treatment for chronic nausea is different from treatment for nausea caused by antineoplastic treatments. $5-HT_3$ antagonists (such as ondansetron) can be used effectively to treat chemotherapy-induced vomiting but have little effect on chronic nausea or opioid-induced constipation; in fact, $5-HT_3$ antagonists might cause even more constipation and lead to chronic nausea.

Delirium

Delirium is an important but often unrecognized syndrome. It typically develops over a short period of time, usually hours to days, and cognition fluctuates during the course of the day. Delirium should be suspected in patients with fluctuating symptoms of depression, patients who have anxiety or who become unexpectedly "difficult," and patients in the terminal stage of illness. The routine use of an instrument such as the Mini Mental Status Questionnaire to assess cognition is essential.

Delirium is diagnosed on the basis of an assessment of alterations in the patient's cognition (whether the condition has an acute onset or a fluctuating course); impairments in the patient's consciousness and attention; or neuropsychiatric symptoms. Delirium can present with either hyperactive symptoms (e.g., agitation or restlessness) or hypoactive symptoms (e.g., catatonia or stupor). Altered cognition can present as disorientation, language disturbance, or perceptional disturbance (e.g., tactile or visual hallucinations). The patient may exhibit disturbance of consciousness, with reduced awareness of the environment and a reduced ability to sustain or shift attention. Neuropsychiatric symptoms may include anxiety, sleep disturbance, irritability or restlessness, or affective symptoms, such as sadness, anger, euphoria, or emotional lability.

Delirium can occur as a side effect of treatment with opioids and other psychotropic medications, such as neuroleptics, benzodiazepines, antiepileptics, and cytokines, and can result from dehydration, hypercalcemia, hyponatremia, renal or liver failure, or infection. It can also occur following withdrawal of nicotine, alcohol, or other addictive drugs and owing to unrecognized leptomeningeal disease or brain metastases. It is not yet possible to quickly identify the exact cause of delirium on the basis of hyperactive or hypoactive presentations.

Clinically, it is important to distinguish delirium from dementia and depression. Dementia typically does not fluctuate and develops over weeks to months. The patient's medical history, as provided by family members and caregivers, is vital in diagnosing dementia. Patients who show signs of a depressive state should always be assessed for cognitive impairment. The reversibility rate of delirium is only 30% to 50% in cancer patients referred for specialized palliative care services; however, with accurate and timely diagnosis and treatment, full cognition and quality of life can be restored in many of these patients. The management of delirium involves treatment of the underlying cause of the condition and of its symptoms. At M. D. Anderson, we perform an opioid rotation in most patients, correct electrolyte imbalances, and administer a rehydration regimen (50 to 100 cm^3 normal saline/hour for a patient weighing 70 kg who does not have chronic heart failure). Patients might benefit from empiric antibiotic treatments if infections are the suspected cause of delirium. Corticosteroids (4 mg dexamethasone every 6 hours around the clock and tapered after a few days) are often beneficial in patients who have a tumor that is suspected to involve the leptomeningeal area or the brain.

Haloperidol (0.5 to 1 mg orally or intravenously every 6 to 8 hours around the clock) can be used to treat symptoms of delirium. These doses are typically not sufficient to induce sedation and can improve alertness. Haloperidol and other neuroleptics (e.g., olanzapine) probably provide the most efficient treatment for delirium that presents with symptoms of hyperactivity. Benzodiazepines should be avoided as first-line therapy in patients with delirium because their use might be necessary to sedate patients with refractory hyperactive delirium.

In delirium management, it is important to educate the family about the presence of a delirium syndrome and to screen the patient for cognitive impairment in their presence. It is helpful for the family to understand the cause of the patient's disturbing perceptions, emotions such as anger or depression, irritability, or often-expressed strong, and unrealistic, wishes to go home.

Depression and Anxiety

In the United States, major depression occurs in about 10% to 15% of patients treated for cancer, but depressive symptoms are much more frequent. The clinical features of depression are depressed mood, dysphoria (the loss of joy and interest in life), loss of energy, feelings of hopelessness or inappropriate/excessive guilt, difficulty concentrating or inability to make decisions, perceived worthlessness, passive or active thoughts of death, and suicidal ideation. The physical signs typically associated with depression are not reliable for diagnosing this condition in patients with advanced cancer because they are common in this patient group. Sadness, an adjustment disorder with depressed mood, or major depression can affect family members and the care team as well as the patient, and all parties should be assessed. Depression in men may manifest with atypical signs, such as increased pain expression, acting out, and dissocial behavior.

With sadness and adjustment disorders, counseling and normalization of reactions to these conditions are generally sufficient treatments for patients and family members. Being given the opportunity to express emotions can provide great emotional relief. The benefit of antidepressants and selective serotonin reuptake inhibitors as treatment for these conditions, however, is somewhat controversial. Patients with major depression should be attended to by a psychiatrist.

Dyspnea

Patients often perceive shortness of breath as lacking adequate air to breathe or as labored breathing that imposes extra work on the respiratory muscles. The patient's perception (which is a symptom) often differs from the health care professional's observation of increased respiration rate or decreased oxygen saturation (which are syndromes). It is important to question the patient about the experience of dyspnea during rest and during exertion.

Assessment

The assessment of dyspnea includes a thorough history, clinical examination (e.g., to detect signs of pleural effusions, wheezing, etc.), and chest radiography. The causes of dyspnea that are directly related to cancer include restrictive changes in the lungs due to pulmonary involvement of tumor, loss of pulmonary tissue due to surgery, pleural effusions, lymphangiosis carcinomatosa, and phrenic nerve paresis. The causes indirectly related to cancer are anemia, infections, obstructive lung disease, loss of respiratory muscle tissue due to cachexia, and most importantly, pulmonary embolism.

Treatment

Management of dyspnea involves treating the underlying cause of the condition and its symptoms. In the clinical decision-making process, it is important to clearly define the goal of any intervention: How likely is it that the patient will gain symptomatic benefit from the intervention, even if correction of the pathology is accomplished?

Obstructive symptoms are often treated with inhalation or systemic application of corticosteroids and β-mimetics. Treatment of a pulmonary embolism might improve the symptom of dyspnea (the perception of difficult breathing). Anemia should be treated, but only patients who improve after the first blood transfusion should receive other transfusions. A short course of corticosteroids can decrease inflammation and open the airway spaces. Opioids have been proven to decrease the sensation of dyspnea in most patients. Alternatively, benzodiazepines might be used to treat dyspnea in selected patients with anxiety.

It is important to address the issue of respiration when educating relatives of dying patients. It is crucial to describe the respiratory sounds that the dying patient is likely to make and to explain that dying is a physiologic process rather than intractable suffering. For example, the sound resulting from a partially closed larynx might be perceived as moaning or groaning and the "death rattle" might resemble choking.

MANAGEMENT OF SYNDROMES SPECIFIC TO GYNECOLOGIC CANCER

In addition to the syndromes typically associated with advanced cancer, there are several syndromes related specifically to gynecologic cancer. These include lymphedema, bleeding complications, infections, fistulas, distorted body image (which may occur because of colostomy), and bowel obstruction. This section describes the approaches used in the management of these syndromes.

Lymphedema

In the gynecologic cancer setting, lymphedema most often presents as secondary edema caused by a focal lymphatic obstruction resulting from direct tumor involvement, scars from a prior surgery, or irradiation of lymph nodes. Lymphedema often presents with an infection caused by *staphylococcus* or *streptococcus* bacteria, which can be treated with empirical antibiotics.

It is important for patients to recognize circumstances and activities that might exacerbate lymphedema, such as heavy lifting; sustained activity or inactivity of the affected limb; constriction of the limb, such as during blood pressure measurements or when wearing tight clothing; inflammation caused by infection; skin breakdown; or exposure to excessive heat and humidity.

Therapeutic interventions include wrapping the limb in bandages, elevating the limb, performing static limb compression (from proximal to distal, which is counterintuitive yet correct for lymphedema) using a combination of physical therapies, and managing infections. These interventions emphasize the importance of a multidisciplinary team approach to treatment.

It is important to distinguish lymphedema from deep venous thrombosis. The distinction can typically be made by a careful review of the patient's medical history. It is also important to monitor for distortions in the patient's body image; some patients may not readily report swelling.

Bleeding Complications

Bleeding complications, though rare (occurring in only 3% to 10% of patients), can be a very frightening experience. The risk of spontaneous bleeding increases when a patient's platelet count falls below 20,000/mL. It is important to educate the patient, family members, and caregivers about the possibility of bleeding. Such a discussion might be difficult, however, because it involves discussing the dangers associated with bleeding, including its association with limited life span. The patient and her family members should be advised to use dark towels and bed sheets during episodes of bleeding and told that the patient should sit or lie down to avoid fainting during bleeding episodes.

Patients who experience bleeding are often given emergency palliative sedation with 2.5 to 5 mg midazolam or 5 to 20 mg lorazepam as a rapid intravenous infusion or injection. Midazolam can be stored at room temperature in a dark area for up to 30 days, whereas lorazepam requires constant refrigeration.

If the bleeding is mild, antithrombolytic agents such as thromboplastine or tranexamic acid can halt the bleeding.

Infections

Infections may manifest with the classic signs of fever and elevated white blood cell count, triggering empirical or specific antibiotic treatments. However, more important are clinically unrecognized infections, such as smoldering infections of the pelvis or chronic infections due to fistula or wounds. Patients with such infections may present with severe pain rather than with signs of infection. The pain is caused by nociceptive input from locally inflamed tissue. Patients with unrecognized infections sometimes complain of an offensive smell or increased secretions from the fistula, which can cause hygiene problems. Antibiotic treatment can be used for symptom control (i.e., pain, smell, and secretions) but often will not eradicate the microbe, which might not be detectable owing to the depth of the infection.

Fistula

Fistula can cause serious distress for patients and family members owing to associated hygiene problems, decreasing autonomy, altered body image, and disruptions in social life. Vaginal-intestinal fistulas are common and can produce a foul-smelling discharge. Metronidazole, administered topically or systemically, may control the odor, which is caused primarily by an anaerobic organism. Silver sulfadiazine cream (1%) can be used for wound care. Patients may express anger about the social consequences of fistula and about altered body function and thus might benefit from psychological and practical (wound care) counseling.

Bowel Obstruction

Bowel obstruction can be caused by a mechanical obstruction (extrinsic or intrinsic), occlusion, or paralytic dysfunction of the bowels. Occlusion can occur secondary to (1) infections, (2) tumors infiltrating the nervous system or causing a direct block, (3) neuropathy, such as in patients with lung cancer (paraneoplastic autonomic dysfunction), or (4) chronic obstruction (e.g., due to diabetes, prior surgery, or radiation therapy).

Important risk factors for partial bowel obstruction are fecal impaction and constipation, dehydration, and transient inflammatory edema. Patients may complain of vomiting (intermittent or continual) and nausea. Patients typically have colicky pain with tenesmus due to tension on the proximal side of the obstruction, but the intensity might be variable. In addition, patients might have continuous pain and experience symptoms such as dry mouth, constipation, and partial-overflow diarrhea.

Treatment for bowel obstruction involves maintaining a fine balance between aggressive interventions and primary symptom control. It is important to rule out significant constipation as a major factor in bowel obstruction, with implications for a diagnosis of dehydration. Also, routine flat radiography of the abdomen to quantify bowel content is crucial (Figure 17–2).

Surgical intervention should not be performed routinely, although it should be considered in most patients. With emergency colostomy, the surgery-related mortality rate is about 33% and the complication rate is up to 90%. Patients with bowel obstruction who are most likely to receive a benefit from surgery are (1) those in whom the cause of the obstruction is not the malignancy, (2) those who do not have peritoneal carcinomatosis, (3) those who do not have nutritional deficits or cachexia, and (4) those who have only 1 level of obstruction.

A venting gastrostomy tube with suction is often successful in reducing secretions, colicky pain, and abdominal distension. A percutaneous endoscopic gastrostomy tube (in contrast to the nasogastric tube) is suitable for long-term decompression of the obstructed gastrointestinal tract; however, patients and family members must be trained in its use.

Interventions for bowel obstruction often focus on the management of symptoms such as pain, vomiting, and psychosocial issues. These symptoms cannot be treated with oral medications. For colicky pain, anticholinergics such as hyoscine butylbromide, hyoscine hydrobromide, or glycopyrrolate are often administered in addition to opioids. Vomiting should be treated with antiemetics that act on the central nervous system (such as metoclopramide) and drugs that reduce secretions. Anticholinergics also are used to reduce gastrointestinal secretions. Hyoscine butylbromide has low lipid solubility, in contrast to atropine and hyoscine hydrobromide, which penetrate the blood-brain barrier. Typical daily doses of these anticholinergics are (1) hyoscine butylbromide, 40 to 120 mg subcutaneously or intravenously either in 4 or 6 doses or continuously; (2) glycopyrrolate, 0.1 to 0.2 mg 3 times a day subcutaneously or intravenously; and (3) hyoscine hydrobromide, 1.8 to 2.0 mg intravenously in 3 doses.

The somatostatin analogue octreotide is an antisecretory agent that has been shown in 2 clinical trials to be superior to hyoscine butylbromide with regard to effectiveness and speed in reducing gastrointestinal secretions, reducing nausea, and preventing vomiting. In addition, octreotide appears to be effective in patients with upper abdominal obstruction in whom hyoscine hydrobromide has failed to produce relief. In patients with partial bowel obstruction, octreotide may prevent irreversible bowel obstruction. The regular dose is 0.2 to 0.9 mg/day. Its use might be limited, however, by its high cost.

Antiemetic treatment with the prokinetic metoclopramide can be given, but only for patients with partial obstruction and no colicky pain, which can worsen with kinetic activity. Other drugs that can be used as antiemetics are (1) neuroleptic agents, such as haloperidol at 5 to 15 mg/day subcutaneously or intravenously or chlorpromazine at 50 mg every 8 hours rectally or intramuscularly, and (2) antihistaminic agents such as diphenhydramine at 50 to 100 mg/day subcutaneously.

When deciding on treatment for patients with bowel obstruction, it is helpful to involve the medical oncologist, palliative care specialist, surgeon, and other clinicians, as appropriate.

TALKING ABOUT CANCER

The success of palliative care interventions depends on effective communication between the patient and family members and the health care providers. In discussions between these parties, information about prognosis, end-of-life issues, diagnostic and treatment procedures, and supportive care for psychosocial, existential, and spiritual concerns is disseminated. In the cancer setting, communication oftentimes involves "breaking bad news." There are several strategies clinicians can use to ensure that the patient is adequately informed and the information is presented in a respectful manner.

It is important for the clinician to use appropriate interpersonal and social skills to put the patient and family members at ease and to assure them that their needs and concerns are a priority. Consultations should take place in a comfortable setting, and the clinician should be relaxed and unhurried. It is also important for the clinician to get the patient and family members involved in the discussion by asking questions, such as How much do you know about this disease?

The patient should also be allowed to ask questions. In some instances, however, patients have difficulty composing a question that will generate the desired information. This situation can be addressed with the use of a prompt sheet, which is a list of statements the patient can use as a guide when asking questions. A common mistake of clinicians is providing a lot of information rather than directly answering the patient's questions. This practice can produce information overload and can result in the patient's questions not being answered appropriately. In the multidisciplinary palliative care outpatient clinic at M. D. Anderson, we provide patients and family members with audiotapes of consultations with physicians that can be reviewed at a later time in a more relaxed setting. This practice facilitates information recall.

In addition to being a method of obtaining essential information, communication is also the avenue through which patients express their emotions about their cancer diagnosis and through which their emotions are acknowledged by clinicians. It is important to assure the patient that her emotions are common reactions to a threatening experience and that the health care team will provide the necessary support to help her cope. At M. D. Anderson, we encourage patients and family members to express their emotions freely in person, on paper, by e-mail, or through any other method they are comfortable with. Such an open communication strategy is often perceived by busy oncologists as a disruption of their clinical practice, partly because their time is limited and partly because they fear that such discussions place them at risk for loss of control. However, the goal of this strategy is to present information in a manner that is useful. This can be accomplished as effectively in a brief discussion as in a prolonged discussion.

At M. D. Anderson, the guidelines for "breaking bad news" are outlined in a system called SPIKES (Setting, Permission, Information, Knowledge, Emotions, and Support). This system is defined in Table 17–3.

Occasionally, physicians may underestimate the severity of a disease or erroneously establish a patient's prognosis. When this happens, do-not-resuscitate orders are typically not discussed in a timely manner. For example, in the absence of an outpatient do-not-resuscitate order, a patient treated in an emergency situation could die in the emergency room or in an ambulance on the way to the hospital. If a do-not-resuscitate order had been on file, however, the patient could have died with more dignity at home. Therefore, it is considered good clinical practice

Table 17–3. SPIKES System for Ensuring Effective Patient-Clinician Communication

Guideline	Definition
Setting	Find a quiet place to sit down with the patient.
Permission	Ask the patient for permission to talk; give the patient the opportunity to choose a convenient time.
Information	Determine what information will define the purpose and form the outline of the discussion.
Knowledge	Determine the patient's level of knowledge about his or her cancer.
Emotions	Identify the patient's emotions; attach the emotion to an event in the past, present, or future; and acknowledge and normalize the emotion. Try to help the patient find a way to express this emotion in an individual way.
Support	Be aware of terminating communication (e.g., with false and early reassurances that affect the patient's willingness to talk openly about serious issues); overloading the patient with information; and focusing on physical issues while avoiding psychosocial, existential, and spiritual concerns.

Abbreviations: SPIKES, Setting, Permission, Information, Knowledge, Emotions, Support.

to routinely check the patient's prognosis and to ensure that her do-not-resuscitate orders are on file. It is also advisable to openly but respectfully discuss other legal issues early in the patient's disease course. This is another strategy used at M. D. Anderson to ensure that "bad news" is delivered in a sensitive and timely manner. This approach enables patients to finalize personal and business affairs, visit with loved ones, and attend to end-of-life issues. During this time, we encourage patients and family members to focus on the quality of the patient's final days.

When communicating with patients, physicians often encounter their own emotional issues, such as the perception that a patient's deteriorating condition is reflective of some failure on their part or that an open discussion of prognosis might decrease the patient's hope and cause feelings of abandonment. In addition, when counseling patients, clinicians are often compelled to face their own mortality. Members of the palliative care team also frequently need emotional support when planning the care of patients whose conditions are dismal or terminal, when attempting to normalize patients' illness experiences, and when assessing patients' symptom expression.

Palliative care team members might benefit from meeting regularly with other professionals in a support group to discuss potential problems and share their experiences (positive and negative). Crucial to the success of a support group for the palliative care team members is stressing the importance of confidentiality and, when necessary, obtaining the guidance of a trained psychological counselor.

KEY PRACTICE POINTS

- Disciplined, continual assessments of patients' palliative care needs should be routine clinical practice and should include early assessment and management of distressing symptoms, dissemination of essential information, and palliative cancer care that addresses psychosocial and end-of-life issues.

- Treatment of cancer pain should be decided on the basis of the following: risk factors for altered pain expression (incident pain vs neuropathic pain, psychosocial and existential distress, and cognitive impairment), the possible presence of 1 or more pain syndromes, misperceptions about and barriers to opiate treatment, and patient compliance or noncompliance with opiate treatment.

- Delirium often presents with mild cognitive deficits, perceptual disturbances such as tactile hallucinations, and emotional changes such as anxiety, sadness, irritability, or anger.

- Communication between patients with cancer and their family members and health care providers should be modeled after the SPIKES program (Table 17–3).

- Gastrointestinal dysfunction syndromes, especially constipation, are underdiagnosed syndromes that contribute substantially to morbidity in the cancer patient.

- Constipation is a syndrome rather than a symptom and requires careful daily assessment of the frequency, amount, and consistency of bowel movements as reported by the patient.

- Depression is an underrecognized condition in patients with advanced cancer. Patients with cancer exhibit many of the features of major depression (e.g., fatigue and anorexia). In addition, the depressed cancer patient might exhibit feelings of inappropriate guilt, pervasive hopelessness, worthlessness, and passive or active suicidal ideations. In patients with depressive symptoms, the differential diagnosis to delirium is crucial.

- Routine screening for involuntary weight loss and reduced oral intake in cancer patients is a worthwhile clinical practice. When paraneoplastic anorexia/cachexia syndrome is diagnosed in combination with secondary anorexia/cachexia, special treatment interventions are required.

Suggested Readings

Baile WF, Buckman R, Lenzi R, Glober G, Beale EA, Kudelka AP. SPIKES-A six-step protocol for delivering bad news: application to the patient with cancer. *Oncologist* 2000;5:302–311.

Bruera E, Schoeller T, Wenk R, et al. A prospective multicenter assessment of the Edmonton Staging System for cancer pain. *J Pain Symptom Manage* 1995;10:348–355.

Bruera E, Suarez-Almazor M, Velasco A, Bertolino M, MacDonald SM, Hanson J. The assessment of constipation in terminal cancer patients admitted to a palliative care unit: a retrospective review. *J Pain Symptom Manage* 1994;9:515–519.

Cherny N, Ripamonti C, Pereira J, et al. Expert Working Group of the European Association of Palliative Care Network. Strategies to manage the adverse effects of oral morphine: an evidence-based report. *J Clin Oncol* 2001;19:2542–2554.

Fainsinger RL, Nekolaichuk CL, Lawlor PG, Neumann CM, Hanson J, Vigano A. A multicenter study of the revised Edmonton Staging System for classifying cancer pain in advanced cancer patients. *J Pain Symptom Manage* 2005;29:224–237.

Hanks GW, Conno F, Cherny N, et al. Morphine and alternative opioids in cancer pain: the EAPC recommendations. *Br J Cancer* 2001;84:587–593.

Indelicato RA, Portenoy RK. Opioid rotation in the management of refractory cancer pain. *J Clin Oncol* 2002;20:348–352.

Lawlor PG, Bruera ED. Delirium in patients with advanced cancer. *Hematol Oncol Clin North Am* 2002;16:701–714.

Pereira J, Lawlor P, Vigano A, et al. Equianalgesic dose ratios for opioids. A critical review and proposals for long-term dosing. *J Pain Symptom Manage* 2001;22:672–687.

Ripamonti C, Fusco F. Respiratory problems in advanced cancer. *Support Care Cancer* 2002;10:204–216.

Ripamonti C, Twycross R, Baines M, et al. Working Group of the European Association for Palliative Care. Clinical-practice recommendations for the management of bowel obstruction in patients with end-stage cancer. *Support Care Cancer* 2001;9:223–233.

Stiefel R, Die Trill M, Berney A, Olarte JM, Razavi A. Depression in palliative care: a pragmatic report from the Expert Working Group of the European Association for Palliative Care. *Support Care Cancer* 2001;9:477–488.

Strasser F, Bruera ED. Update on anorexia and cachexia. *Hematol Oncol Clin North Am* 2002;16:589–617.

Strasser F, Walker P, Bruera E. Palliative pain management: when both pain and suffering hurt. *J Pall Care* 2005;21:68–79.

INDEX

Page numbers with t and f represent tables and figures, respectively.